ATLS

Advanced Trauma Life Support®

Program for Doctors

This Seventh Edition is dedicated to the families
and professional colleagues of the ATLS Instructors and Students

This program is dedicated to the care of all victims of trauma.

Advanced Trauma Life Support® and the acronym ATLS® are marks of the American College of Surgeons

Seventh Edition

Published 2004. Second Impression, 2005.

Printed in the United States of America.

Advanced Trauma Life Support® Program for Doctors   ISBN 1-880696-14-2

TABLE OF CONTENTS

Preface

■ THE ROLE OF THE AMERICAN COLLEGE OF SURGEONS COMMITTEE ON TRAUMA

The American College of Surgeons (ACS), founded to improve the care of the surgical patient, has long been a leader in establishing and maintaining the high quality of surgical practice in North America. In accordance with that role, and recognizing that trauma is a surgical disease, the ACS Committee on Trauma (COT) has worked to establish guidelines for the care of the trauma patient.

Accordingly, the COT sponsors and contributes to the continued development of the Advanced Trauma Life Support (ATLS) Program for Doctors. The ATLS Student Course does not present new concepts in the field of trauma care. Established treatment methods are taught in the course. A systematic, concise approach to the early care of the trauma patient is the hallmark of the ATLS Program.

This edition is prepared for the ACS by members of the Subcommittee on ATLS and the ACS COT, other individual Fellows of the College, members of the international ATLS community, and nonsurgical consultants to the Subcommittee who were selected for their special competence in trauma care and for their expertise in medical education. The COT believes that those having the responsibility for such patients will find the information valuable. The principles of patient care presented in this manual may also be beneficial for the care of patients with nontrauma-related diseases.

Injured patients present a wide range of complex problems. The ATLS Student Course presents a concise approach to assessing and managing the multiply injured patient. The course presents doctors with knowledge and techniques that are comprehensive and easily adapted to fit their needs. The skills presented in this manual recommend one, safe way to perform each technique. The ACS recognizes that there are other acceptable approaches. However, the knowledge and skills taught in the course are easily adapted to all venues for the care of these patients.

The ATLS Course is revised by the ATLS Subcommittee approximately every 4 years to respond to changes in available knowledge, and to incorporate newer and perhaps even safer skills. ATLS Committees in other countries, where the program has been introduced, have participated in the revision process and the ATLS Subcommittee appreciates their outstanding contributions. National and international educators review the educational materials to ensure that the course is conducted in a manner that facilitates learning. All of the course content is available in other resources, ie, textbooks and journals. However, the ATLS Course is a specific entity, and the manuals, slides, skills procedures, and other resources are all used for the entire course only and cannot be fragmented into separate freestanding lectures or practical sessions. Members of the ACS COT and the ACS Regional and State/Provincial Committees, as well as the ACS ATLS Program Office staff members, are responsible for maintaining the high quality of the program. By introducing this course and maintaining its high quality, the COT hopes to provide another instrument by which to reduce the mortality and morbidity related to trauma. The COT recommends that doctors participating in the ATLS Student Course reverify their status every 4 years to maintain both their current status in the program and their knowledge of current ATLS core content.

■ American College of Surgeons Committee on Trauma

David B. Hoyt, MD, FACS
Chair, 1998–2002

J. Wayne Meredith, MD, FACS
Chair, 2002–2006

■ Subcommittee on Advanced Trauma Life Support of the American College of Surgeons Committee on Trauma 1997–2001, 2002–2007

Steven N. Parks, MD, FACS
Chair, 1998–2002

Christoph Kaufmann, MD, FACS
Chair, 2003–2007

Jameel Ali, MD, FACS
Charles Aprahamian, MD, FACS*
Richard M. Bell, MD, FACS
Don E. Boyle, MD, FACS
Paul E. Collicott, MD, FACS*
Gerald Demarest, MD, FACS
Lawrence M. Gentilello, MD, FACS
Michael L. Hawkins, MD, FACS
Gregory J. Jurkovich, MD, FACS
James F. Kellam, MD, FACS
John B. Kortbeek, MD, FACS
Brent E. Krantz, MD, FACS
West Livaudais, Jr., MD, FACS
Fred Luchette, MD, FACS

Donald W. Marion, MD, FACS
Philip S. Metz, MD, FACS
Frank L. Mitchell, III, MD, FACS
Charles N. Mock, MD, FACS
Raj K. Narayan, MD, FACS
Steven N. Olson, MD, FACS
Galen V. Poole, MD, FACS
Max L. Ramenofsky, MD, FACS*
Charles F. Rinker, MD, FACS
R. Stephen Smith, MD, FACS
Thomas M. Scalea, MD, FACS
J. Octavio Ruiz Speare, MD, FACS
Gregory A. Timberlake, MD, FACS
John A. Weigelt, MD, FACS

*Consultant to the Subcommittee

■ Associate Members to the Subcommittee on Advanced Trauma Life Support of the American College of Surgeons Committee on Trauma

Frederick D. Brenneman, MD, FACS
Arthur Cooper, MD, FACS
Jésus R. Diaz-Portocarrero, MD, FACS
Francisco Holguin R., MD, FACS
Dennis G. Leland, MD, FACS
Lawrence Lottenberg, MD, FACS

Richard S. Miller, MD, FACS
Martin J. Odriozola, MD, FACS
Frank D. Sacco, MD, FACS
Marc J. Shapiro, MD, FACS
Richard K. Simons, MB BCh, FACS

■ American College of Emergency Physicians Liaisons to the Subcommittee on Advanced Trauma Life Support of the American College of Surgeons Committee on Trauma

Richard C. Hunt, MD, FACEP, and Jon R. Krohmer, MD, FACEP

As representatives of the American College of Emergency Physicians (ACEP), an organization that represents over 21,000 emergency doctors nationwide, we appreciate the opportunity to work closely with the ATLS Subcommittee to the ACS COT on this revision of the ATLS Course manual. We believe that sharing the emergency doctor's perspective in this important revision and participating in the productive trauma care debates benefits patients.

We are particularly pleased with the emphasis on making the ATLS Course as evidence based as possible. These revisions follow a deliberate and careful review process that provided an opportunity for appropriate and timely input. We also appreciate the opportunity to share drafts of the manual with ACEP's Trauma Care and Injury Control Committee, whose valuable feedback guided our comments and suggestions to the ATLS Subcommittee.

The ATLS Course is a critically important tool in guiding care for injured patients in emergency department trauma rooms. The course training provides a common framework of communication that can save lives in critical situations. We anticipate that this collaborative, collegial effort will serve as a model for providing the best possible emergency care to patients.

The American College of Surgeons COT and its ATLS Subcommittee take this opportunity to recognize the valuable contributions of the representatives of ACEP to the ATLS Subcommittee in preparation of this edition of the course materials and program. Richard C. Hunt, MD, FACEP and Jon R. Krohmer, MD, FACEP participated fully in the revision of this seventh edition of course materials and program. Their valuable contributions included feedback from the ACEP membership on proposed changes to the materials. The ACS COT and the ATLS Subcommittee appreciate the time, expertise, and commitment that these colleagues have given to the ATLS Program.

■ Editorial Notes

The ACS Committee on Trauma hereafter is referred to as the ACS COT or the Committee, and the State/Provincial Chair(s) is referred to as S/P Chair(s).

The international nature of this edition of the ATLS Program has necessitated some change in commonly used terms to facilitate understanding by all students and teachers of the program.

Advanced Trauma Life Support® and ATLS® are proprietary trademarks and service marks owned by the American College of Surgeons and cannot be used by individuals or entities outside the ACS Committee on Trauma organization for their goods and services without ACS approval. Accordingly, any reproduction of either or both marks in direct conjunction with the ACS ATLS Program within the ACS Committee on Trauma organization must be accompanied by the common law symbol of trademark ownership.

Contributing Authors

The Committee gratefully acknowledges these individuals for their medical expertise and support in the development of the ATLS Course materials.

Joe E. Acker, III, MS, MPH, EMTP
Executive Director, Birmingham Regional EMS, Birmingham, Alabama.

Jameel Ali, MD, MMed Ed, FRCS(C), FACS
Professor of Surgery, Department of Surgery, University of Toronto, Toronto, Ontario, Canada.

Charles Aprahamian, MD, FACS
Retired Professor of Surgery, Medical College of Wisconsin, Milwaukee, Wisconsin.

Richard M. Bell, MD, FACS
Professor and Chair of Surgery, University of South Carolina School of Medicine, Columbia, South Carolina.

Don E. Boyle, MD, FACS
Retired Clinical Assistant Professor of Surgery, University of Iowa College of Medicine, Iowa City, Iowa; Okoboji, Iowa.

Paul E. Collicott, MD, FACS
Director, Member Services, American College of Surgeons, Chicago, Illinois.

Arthur Cooper, MD, MS, FACS
Associate Professor and Chief, Division of Pediatric Surgery; Director of Trauma Center, Columbia University College of Physicians and Surgeons, Harlem Hospital Center, New York, New York.

Frank X. Doto, MS
Professor of Health Education, County College of Morris, Randolph, New Jersey.

John H. George, PhD
Vice-chair for Educational Affairs, Department of Family and Community Medicine; Senior Advisor to the Vice-dean for Educational Affairs, Pennsylvania State College of Medicine, Hershey, Pennsylvania.

Michael L. Hawkins, MD, FACS
Professor of Surgery and Anesthesia, Chief of Trauma/Surgical Critical Care, Medical College of Georgia, Augusta, Georgia.

Irvene K. Hughes, RN
Manager, ATLS Program, Division of Research and Optimal Patient Care, Trauma Section, American College of Surgeons, Chicago, Illinois.

Richard C. Hunt, MD, FACEP
Professor and Chair, Department of Emergency Medicine, State University of New York, Upstate Medical University, Syracuse, New York.

Gregory J. Jurkovich, MD, FACS
Professor of Surgery, Chief of Trauma Service, University of Washington; Harborview Medical Center, Seattle, Washington.

Christoph R. Kaufmann, MD, FACS
Associate, Trauma Director, Legacy Emanuel Hospital, Portland, Oregon.

John B. Kortbeek, MD, FACS
Clinical Associate Professor of Surgery, University of Calgary; Director of Trauma Services, Calgary Regional Health Authority, Calgary, Alberta, Canada.

Brent E. Krantz, MD, FACS
Professor of Surgery, University of South Carolina School of Medicine, Columbia, South Carolina.

Jon R. Krohmer, MD, FACEP
Associate Professor, Section of Emergency Medicine, College of Human Medicine, Michigan State University, Grand Rapids, Michigan.

Dennis G. Leland, MD, FACS
Director of Trauma, Queen of Peace Hospital, Mitchell, South Dakota.

Donald W. Marion, MD, FACS
Professor and Chair, Neurologic Surgery, Boston Medical Center, Boston, Massachusetts.

Philip S. Metz, MD, FACS
Clinical Assistant Professor, Department of Surgery, University of Nebraska Medical Center, Omaha, Nebraska; Private Practice, Lincoln, Nebraska.

Raj K. Narayan, MD, FACS
Professor and Chairman, Department of Neurosurgery, Temple University School of Medicine, Philadelphia, Pennsylvania.

James B. Nichols, DVM, MS
Director, Animal Care, University of Vermont, Burlington, Vermont.

Franklin C. Olson, EdD
Retired Professor of Education, Pacific Lutheran University, Tacoma, Washington; Ocean Park, Washington.

Steven N. Parks, MD, FACS
Clinical Professor of Surgery, University of California at San Francisco, Fresno, California.

Galen V. Poole, MD, FACS
Professor of Surgery, University of Mississippi Medical Center, Jackson, Mississippi.

Max L. Ramenofsky, MD, FACS
Professor of Surgery, Drexel University School of Medicine, St. Christopher's Hospital for Children, Philadelphia, Pennsylvania; Chief, Pediatric Surgery, St. Luke's Hospital and Health Network, Bethlehem, Pennsylvania.

Charles F. Rinker, MD, FACS
Director of Trauma, Bozeman Deaconess Hospital, Bozeman, Montana.

J. Octavio Ruiz Speare, MD, MS, FACS
Chief, Transplant Services, Department of Surgery, American British Cowdray Medical Center, Mexico City, Mexico.

Richard C. Simmonds, DVM, MS
Director of Laboratory Animal Medicine, University of Nevada System; Professor of Physiology, University of Nevada School of Medicine, Reno, Nevada.

Gregory A. Timberlake, MD, FACS
Professor of Surgery, Physiology, and Biophysics, University of Mississippi School of Medicine, Jackson, Mississippi.

John A. Weigelt, MD, FACS
Professor and Vice-Chair of Surgery, Medical College of Wisconsin, Milwaukee, Wisconsin.

■ Acknowledgments

The Committee also gratefully acknowledges members from these international committees and specific individuals who reviewed the core medical content for its validity and relevance to private and academic practice and/or contributed to media resources for the course materials.

INTERNATIONAL COMMITTEES

Argentina
Committee on Trauma, Argentina
Chapter—American College of Surgeons

Australia
EMST/ATLS Committee,
Royal Australasian College of Surgeons

Bolivia
Committee on Trauma,
Bolivian Surgeons Society

Brazil
Committee on Trauma, Brazil
Chapter—American College of Surgeons

Canada
Provincial Committees on Trauma, Canadian Chapters—American College of Surgeons: Alberta, British Columbia, Manitoba, Maritime Provinces, Newfoundland, Ontario, Quebec, and Saskatchewan

Chile
Committee on Trauma, Chile
Chapter—American College of Surgeons

Colombia
Committee on Trauma, Colombia
Chapter—American College of Surgeons

Denmark
ATLS Denmark

Ecuador
Committee on Trauma, Ecuador
Chapter—American College of Surgeons

Germany
German Society for Trauma Surgery and Task Force for Early Trauma Care

Greece
Committee on Trauma, Greece
Chapter—American College of Surgeons

Hong Kong
Committee on Trauma, Hong Kong
Chapter—American College of Surgeons

Hungary
Committee on Trauma,
Hungarian Trauma Society

Indonesia
Committee on Trauma,
Indonesian Surgeons Association

Ireland
Committee on Trauma,
Royal College of Surgeons in Ireland

Israel
Israel Association for the Advancement of Trauma Care, Israel Surgical Society

Italy
Committee on Trauma, Italy
Chapter—American College of Surgeons

Kingdom of Saudi Arabia
Committee on Trauma, Saudi Arabia
Chapter—American College of Surgeons

Mexico
Committee on Trauma, Mexico
Chapter—American College of Surgeons

Netherlands, The
ATLS® Foundation,
Dutch Trauma Society

New Zealand
EMST/ATLS® Committee,
Royal Australasian College of Surgeons

Panama
Committee on Trauma, Panama
Chapter—American College of Surgeons

Peru
Committee on Trauma, Peru
Chapter—American College of Surgeons

Portugal
Committee on Trauma,
Portuguese Society of Surgeons

Republic of China, Taiwan
Committee on Trauma,
Surgical Association of the Republic of China,
Taiwan

Republic of Singapore
Chapter of Surgeons, Academy of Medicine,
Singapore

Republic of South Africa
South African Trauma Society

Spain
Committee on Trauma,
Spanish Society of Surgeons

Sweden
Committee on Trauma,
Swedish Society of Surgeons

Switzerland
Committee on Trauma
Swiss Society of Surgeons

Thailand
Committee on Trauma,
Royal College of Surgeons of Thailand

Trinidad and Tobago, West Indies
Society of Surgeons of Trinidad and Tobago

United Arab Emirates
Committee on Trauma,
Surgical Advisory Committee

United Kingdom
ATLS Steering Committee,
Royal College of Surgeons of England

United States of America
State Committees on Trauma,
Chapters — American College of Surgeons

Uruguay
Committee on Trauma
Society of Surgery in Uruguay

Venezuela
Committee on Trauma, Venezuela
Chapter — American College of Surgeons

SPECIFIC INDIVIDUALS

Fareed Ali, MD, FRCS (C)
Toronto, Ontario, Canada

David G. Burris, MD, FACS
Bethesda, Maryland (U.S. Army)

Subrato J. Deb, MD
Herndon, Virginia (U.S. Navy)

John J. Fildes, MD, FACS
Las Vegas, Nevada

James A. Geiling, MD, FCCP
Kensington, Maryland (U.S. Army)

John E. Hutton, Jr, MD, FACS
Bethesda, Maryland (U.S. Army)

Edward B. Lucci, MD, FACEP
Columbia, Maryland (U.S. Army)

Michael R. Marohn, DO, FACS
Andrews AFB, Maryland (U.S. Air Force)

Barry D. Martin, MD
Silver Spring, MD (U.S. Army)

Philip W. Perdue, MD, FACS
Derwood, Maryland (U.S. Navy)

Paul Pudimat, MD
Potomac, Maryland (U.S. Navy)

Thomas E. Scott, MD, FACS
Bolling AFB, District of Columbia
(U.S. Air Force)

Course Overview:
The Purpose, History, and Concepts of the ATLS Program for Doctors

▊ PROGRAM GOALS:

The Advanced Trauma Life Support (ATLS) Course provides the participant with a safe, reliable method for immediate management of the injured patient and the basic knowledge necessary to:

1. Assess the patient's condition rapidly and accurately.
2. Resuscitate and stabilize the patient according to priority.
3. Determine if the patient's needs exceed a facility's resources and/or doctor's capabilities.
4. Arrange appropriately for the patient's interhospital transfer (what, who, when, and how)
5. Assure that optimum care is provided and that the level of care does not deteriorate at any point during the evaluation, resuscitation, or transfer process.

▊ COURSE OBJECTIVES:

The content and skills presented in this course are designed to assist doctors in providing emergency care for the trauma patient. The concept of the "golden hour" emphasizes the urgency necessary for successful management of the injured patient and is not intended to represent a "fixed" time period of 60 minutes. It is the window of opportunity for the doctor to have a positive impact on the morbidity and mortality associated with injury. The ATLS Course provides the essential information and skills that the doctor may apply to the identification and treatment of life-threatening or potentially life-threatening injuries under the extreme pressures associated with the care of these patients in the fast-paced environment and anxiety of the resuscitation room.

Upon completion of the ATLS Student Course, the participant will be able to:

A. Demonstrate concepts and principles of primary and secondary patient assessment.

B. Establish management priorities in a trauma situation.

C. Initiate primary and secondary management necessary within the "golden hour" for the emergency care of acute life-threatening conditions.

D. Demonstrate, in a given simulated clinical and surgical skills practicum, the following skills that are often required in the initial assessment and management of patients with multiple injuries:

1. Primary and secondary assessment of a patient with simulated, multiple injuries

2. Establishment of a patent airway and initiation of one- and two-person ventilation

3. Orotracheal and nasotracheal intubation on adult and infant manikins

4. Pulse oximetry and carbon dioxide detection in exhaled gas

5. Cricothyroidotomy

6. Assessment and management of the patient in shock, especially recognition of life-threatening hemorrhage

7. Venous and intraosseous access

8. Pleural decompression via needle thoracentesis and chest tube insertion

9. Recognition of cardiac tamponade and performance of pericardiocentesis

10. Clinical and radiographic identification of thoracic injuries

11. Peritoneal lavage, ultrasound, and computed tomography (CT) evaluation of the abdomen

12. Evaluation and management of the patient with brain injury, including the use of the Glasgow Coma Scale Score and CT of the brain

13. Assessment of head and facial trauma by physical examination

14. Protection of the spinal cord, and radiographic and clinical evaluation of spine injuries

15. Musculoskeletal trauma assessment and management

16. Estimation of the size and depth of burn injury and volume resuscitation

I. THE NEED

Trauma-related dollar costs exceed $400 billion annually in the United States (U.S.). These costs are accounted for by lost wages, medical expenses, insurance administration costs, property damage, fire loss, employer costs, and indirect loss from work-related injuries. Despite these staggering costs, less than 4 cents of each federal research dollar is expended on trauma research. As monumental as these data are, the true cost to society can be measured only when it is realized that trauma strikes down its youngest and potentially most productive members. As tragic as is any "accidental" death, the loss of life in the early years is the most tragic of all. Research dollars spent on communicable diseases, eg, polio and diphtheria, have nearly eliminated the incidence of these diseases in the U.S. Amazingly, the disease of trauma has not captured the public attention in the same way.

Unintentional injury accounted for over 3.2 million deaths and caused more than 312 million patients worldwide to seek medical attention in 1990. The number of deaths was expected to exceed 3.8 million by 2000, and by 2020 injury may advance to become the second or third leading cause of death in all age groups. Figure 2 demonstrates conclusively that the problem of injury is a significant world health issue. (See Figure 2, Death Rates from Injury per 100,000 Population, at conclusion of chapter.) Injury does not discriminate based on age, race, sex, or economic status. It is the leading cause of death in persons aged 1 through 44 years in most developed countries and is assuming a more prominent position in lower-income nations as infectious diseases are eradicated.

Motor vehicle crashes (MVC) account for the majority of injuries and deaths in 70% of the 39 countries for which data are available. MVCs are the second leading cause of injury and death in 10 additional countries and achieve their lowest ranking, third, in only 1 nation, Finland. The incidence of fatal mechanisms of injury varies from country to country. For example, the rate for vehicular mortality is highest in New Zealand, being nearly 2.5 times the rates in the Bahamas and the United Kingdom. Falls, drownings, and burns generally follow traffic crashes as leading injury mechanisms.

Deaths from firearms are a particular problem in the U.S., Norway, Israel, and France. The mortality rate in the U.S. from guns approaches the rate due to vehicular trauma for the age group of 15 to 24 years, 13.7 vs 16.2 per 100,000 population. The availability of weapons in the U.S., compared with other nations of the world, may be a contributing factor to this problem. The mortality rates from firearms are so low in 25 of the 39 countries that the rates are not reported.

Data reflecting the rates of disability from injury in the U.S. and Portugal show that permanent disability dwarfs the mortality rate by 3 to 1. In 1998, over 19.4 million disabling injuries occurred in the U.S., 1 every 2 seconds. For each vehicular fatality in Portugal in 1996, 31 people sustained some disability.

Over 60 million injuries occur in the U.S. each year, resulting in an average of 36.8 million visits to emergency centers. This figure represents 40% of all emergency department visits. Fifty-four percent of these visits were by children, ages 5 to 14 years. For every injury death there are 19 hospital admissions, 233 emergency department visits, and 450 office-based doctor visits for medical attention related to injury. These data indicate that care for the injured patient consumes a significant proportion of the health care resources of any nation.

Injury is a disease. It has a host (the patient), and it has a vector of transmission (motor vehicle, firearm, etc). Great strides have been made in the eradication of infectious diseases. Cancer and heart disease prevention and treatment have extended the life expectancy of the populations in developed countries. Compared with other diseases, only a small amount of money and effort has been expended to combat this disease, which affects the potentially most productive members of any society and its most valuable national resource, the children. Further, the economic impact is staggering. Lost wages, medical expenses, administration costs, property damage, and indirect costs contribute to the annual price tag of over $400 billion in the U.S., or $1522 for every citizen. Unfortunately, the problem of injury has not captured the attention of the public and the lawmakers in the same way that other health care issues have.

Many significant changes have improved the care of the injured patient since the first edition of the ATLS Program appeared in 1980. The need for the program, and for sustained aggressive efforts to prevent injuries, is as great now as it has ever been.

II. HISTORY

A. The Nebraska Conception and Inception

The delivery of trauma care by doctors in the U.S. was at best inconsistent before 1980. A tragedy occurred in February 1976 that changed trauma care in the "first hour" for the injured patient in the U.S. and in much of the rest of the world. An orthopaedic surgeon, piloting his plane, crashed in a rural Nebraska cornfield. The surgeon sustained serious injuries, 3 of his children sustained critical injuries, and 1 child sustained minor injuries. His wife was killed instantly. The care he and his family received was inadequate by the day's standards. The surgeon, recognizing how inadequate his treatment was, stated: "When I can provide better care in the field with limited resources than what my children and I received at the primary care facility, there is something wrong with the system and the system has to be changed."

A group of private-practice surgeons and doctors in Nebraska, the Lincoln Medical Education Foundation, and the Lincoln-area Mobile Heart Team Nurses, with the help of the University of Nebraska Medical Center, the Nebraska State Committee on Trauma (COT) of the American College of Surgeons (ACS), and the Southeast Nebraska Emergency Medical Services, identified the need for training in advanced trauma life support. A combined educational format of lectures, associated with lifesaving skill demonstrations and practical laboratory experiences, formed the first prototype ATLS Course for doctors.

A new approach to the provision of care for individuals suffering major, life-threatening injury premiered in 1978, the year of the first ATLS Course. This prototype ATLS Course was field-tested in conjunction with the Southeast Nebraska Emergency Medical Services. One year later, the ACS COT, recognizing trauma as a surgical disease, enthusiastically adopted the course under the imprimatur of the College and incorporated it as an educational program.

This course was based on the assumption that appropriate and timely care could significantly improve the outcome of the injured. The original intent of the ATLS Program was to train doctors who do not manage major trauma on a daily basis. The original audience for the course has not changed.

However, today the ATLS method is accepted as a standard for the "first hour" of trauma care by many who provide care for the injured, whether the patient is treated in an isolated rural area or a state-of-the-art trauma center.

B. Trimodal Death Distribution

Death due to injury occurs in 1 of 3 time periods or peaks. (See Figure 1, Trimodal Death Distribution.) The **first peak** occurs within seconds to minutes of injury. During this early period, deaths generally result from apnea due to severe brain or high spinal cord injury; or rupture of the heart, aorta, or other large blood vessels. Very few of these patients can be salvaged due to the severity of their injuries. Only prevention can significantly reduce this peak of trauma-related deaths.

The **second peak** occurs within minutes to several hours following injury. Deaths occurring during this period are usually due to subdural and epidural hematomas, hemopneumothorax, ruptured spleen, lacerations of the liver, pelvic fractures, and/or other multiple injuries associated with significant blood loss. The "golden hour" of care after injury is characterized by the need for rapid assessment and resuscitation, which are the fundamental principles of Advanced Trauma Life Support.

The **third peak**, which occurs several days to weeks after the initial injury, is most often due to sepsis and multiple organ system dysfunction. Care provided during each of the preceding periods impacts on patient outcome during this stage. The first and every subsequent person to care for the injured patient has a direct effect on long-term outcome.

III. THE CONCEPT

The concept behind this course was and is simple. The approach to the injured patient, as taught in medical schools, was the same as that for a patient with a previously undiagnosed medical condition, ie, an extensive history including past medical history, a physical examination starting at the top of the head and progressing down the body, the development of a differential diagnosis, and a list of adjuncts to confirm the diagnosis. This approach was quite adequate for a patient with diabetes mellitus or even many acute surgical illnesses, but it did not satisfy the needs of the patient suffering life-threatening injury. The approach required change.

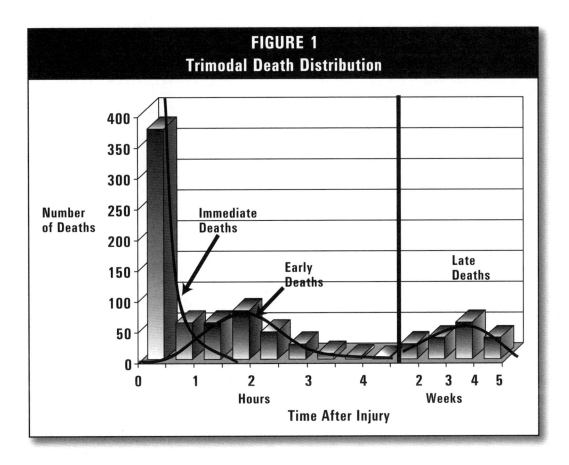

FIGURE 1
Trimodal Death Distribution

Three underlying concepts of the ATLS Program were initially difficult to accept. The most important of these premises was to treat the greatest threat to life first. Secondly, the lack of a definitive diagnosis should never impede the application of an indicated treatment. Finally, a detailed history was not essential to begin the evaluation of an acutely injured patient. The result was the development of the "ABCDE" approach to the evaluation and treatment of the injured. These concepts are also in keeping with the observation that the care of the injured patient in many circumstances is a team effort, allowing medical personnel with special skills and expertise to provide care simultaneously with surgical leadership of the process.

The ATLS Course emphasizes that injury kills in certain reproducible time frames. For example, the loss of an airway kills more quickly than does the loss of the ability to breathe. The latter kills more quickly than loss of circulating blood volume. The presence of an expanding intracranial mass lesion is the next most lethal problem. Thus, the mnemonic "ABCDE" defines the specific, ordered evaluations and interventions that should be followed in all injured patients:

A Airway with cervical spine protection

B Breathing

C Circulation, stop the bleeding

D Disability or neurologic status

E Exposure (undress) and Environment (temperature control)

IV. COURSE OVERVIEW

The ATLS Course emphasizes the rapid initial assessment and primary management of the injured patient, starting at the time of injury and continuing through initial assessment, lifesaving intervention, reevaluation, stabilization, and, when needed, transfer to a trauma center. The course consists of pre- and postcourse tests, core content lectures, interactive case presentations, discussions, development of lifesaving skills, practical laboratory experiences, and a final performance proficiency evaluation. Upon completion of the course, doctors should feel confident in implementing the skills taught in the ATLS Course.

Based on well-established principles and objectives of trauma management, the course is intended to provide doctors with 1 acceptable method for safe, immediate management and the basic knowledge necessary to:

1. Assess the patient's condition rapidly and accurately.
2. Resuscitate and stabilize the patient according to priority.
3. Determine if the patient's needs exceed a facility's capabilities.
4. Arrange appropriately for the patient's interhospital or intrahospital transfer.
5. Assure that optimum care is provided.

These appendices, designed to enhance the core content, are included as supplemental materials.

1. Triage Scenarios
2. Injury Prevention
3. Biomechanics of Injury
4. Tetanus Immunization
5. Trauma Scores: Revised and Pediatric
6. Sample Trauma Flow Sheet
7. Ocular Trauma (Optional Lecture)
8. Injury Care in Austere and Hostile Environments (Optional Lecture)

V. COURSE DEVELOPMENT AND DISSEMINATION

A. The 1980s and 1990s

The ATLS Course was given nationally for the first time under the auspices of the American College of Surgeons in January 1980. Canada became an active participant in the ATLS Program in 1981. Countries in Latin and South America joined the ACS COT in 1986 and implemented the ATLS Program. Under the auspices of the ACS Military Committee on Trauma, the program has been conducted for U.S. military doctors in other countries.

The program has grown both in the number of courses and participants each year. By 2004, the course had trained approximately 500,000 doctors in more than 25,000 courses around the world. Currently, an average of 24,000 doctors are trained each year in approximately 1700 courses. The greatest growth in recent years has been in the international community, and this group currently represents approximately 43% of all ATLS activity.

The text for the course is revised approximately every 4 years and incorporates new modalities of evaluation and treatment that have become accepted parts of the armamentarium of doctors who treat trauma patients. Course revisions incorporate suggestions from members of the Subcommittee on ATLS; members of the ACS COT; members of the international ATLS family; representatives from the American College of Emergency Physicians to the ATLS Subcommittee; and course instructors, coordinators, educators, and participants. Changes that are made to the program reflect accepted, verified practice patterns, not "cutting edge" technology nor experimental methods. The international nature of the program mandates that the course be adaptable to a variety of geographic, economic, social, and medical practice situations. To retain a current status in the ATLS Program, an individual must reverify with the latest edition of the materials.

A parallel course to the ATLS Course is the Prehospital Trauma Life Support (PHTLS) course sponsored by the National Association of Emergency Medical Technicians (NAEMT). The PHTLS Course, developed in cooperation with the ACS COT, is based on the concepts of the ACS ATLS Program for Doctors and is conducted for emergency medical technicians, paramedics, and nurses who are providers of prehospital trauma care. Other courses have been developed with similar concepts and philosophies. For example, the Society of Trauma Nurses offers the Advanced Trauma Course for Nurses (ATCN), which is also done in cooperation with the ACS COT. The ATCN and ATLS are conducted parallel to each other with the nurses auditing the ATLS lectures and then participating in skills stations separate from the ATLS skills stations conducted for doctors. The benefits of having both prehospital and inhospital trauma personnel speaking the same "language" are apparent.

B. International Dissemination

As a pilot project, the ATLS Program was exported outside of North America in 1986 to the Republic of Trinidad and Tobago. The ACS Board of Regents gave permission in 1987 for promulgation of the

ATLS Program in other countries. The ATLS Program may be requested by a recognized surgical organization or ACS Chapter in another country by corresponding with the ATLS Subcommittee Chairperson, care of the ACS ATLS Program Office, Chicago, IL, USA. At the time of publication, 41 countries were actively providing the ATLS Course to their doctors. These countries include:

1. Argentina (ACS Chapter and Committee on Trauma)
2. Australia (Royal Australasian College of Surgeons)
3. Bahrain (Kingdom of Saudi Arabia ACS Chapter and Committee on Trauma)
4. Bolivia (Bolivian Surgeons Society)
5. Brazil (ACS Chapter and Committee on Trauma)
6. Canada (ACS Chapters and Provincial Committees on Trauma)
7. Chile (ACS Chapter and Committee on Trauma)
8. Colombia (ACS Chapter and Committee on Trauma)
9. Cyprus (ACS Chapter and Committee on Trauma, Greece)
10. Denmark (ATLS Denmark)
11. Ecuador (ACS Chapter and Committee on Trauma)
12. Fiji (Royal Australasian College of Surgeons)
13. Germany (German Society for Trauma Surgery and Task Force for Early Trauma Care)
14. Greece (ACS Chapter and Committee on Trauma)
15. Hong Kong (ACS Chapter and Committee on Trauma)
16. Hungary (Hungarian Trauma Society)
17. Indonesia (Indonesian Surgeons Association)
18. Ireland (Royal College of Surgeons in Ireland)
19. Israel (Israel Surgical Society)
20. Italy (ACS Chapter and Committee on Trauma)
21. Jamaica (Society of Surgeons of Trinidad and Tobago)
22. Kingdom of Saudi Arabia (ACS Chapter and Committee on Trauma)
23. Lithuania (Lithuanian Society of Traumatology and Orthopaedics)
24. Mexico (ACS Chapter and Committee on Trauma)
25. Netherlands, The (Dutch Trauma Society)
26. New Zealand (Royal Australasian College of Surgeons)
27. Norway (Norwegian Surgical Society)
28. Pakistan (College of Physicians and Surgeons of Pakistan)
29. Panama (ACS Chapter and Committee on Trauma)
30. Papua New Guinea (Royal Australasian College of Surgeons)
31. Peru (ACS Chapter and Committee on Trauma)
32. Portugal (Portuguese Society of Surgeons)
33. Qatar (Kingdom of Saudi Arabia ACS Chapter and Committee on Trauma)
34. Republic of China, Taiwan (Surgical Association of the Republic of China, Taiwan)
35. Republic of Singapore (Chapter of Surgeons, Academy of Medicine)
36. Republic of South Africa (South African Trauma Society)
37. Spain (Spanish Society of Surgeons)
38. Sweden (Swedish Society of Surgeons)
39. Switzerland (Swiss Society of Surgeons)
40. Thailand (Royal College of Surgeons of Thailand)
41. Trinidad and Tobago (Society of Surgeons of Trinidad and Tobago)
42. United Arab Emirates (Surgical Advisory Committee)
43. United Kingdom (Royal College of Surgeons of England)
44. United States, U.S. territories (ACS Chapters and State Committees on Trauma)
45. Uruguay (Society of Surgery of Uruguay)
46. Venezuela (ACS Chapter and Committee on Trauma)

VI. THE IMPACT

Data exist (Class II and Class III) that document improvements in the care of injured patients following the implementation of the ATLS Program. ATLS training for doctors in a developing country has resulted in a decrease in injury mortality. Lower per capita injury death rates are observed in areas where doctors have ATLS training. In one study, a small trauma team led by a doctor with ATLS experience had equivalent patient survival when compared with a larger team with more doctors in an urban setting. Additionally, there were more unexpected survivors than fatalities. There is abundant evidence that ATLS training improves the knowledge base, the psychomotor skills and their use in resuscitation, and the confidence and performance of doctors who have been students in the program. The organization and procedural skills taught in the course are retained by course participants for at least 6 years. This may be the most significant impact of all.

VII. ACKNOWLEDGMENTS

The COT of the ACS and the ATLS Subcommittee gratefully acknowledge these organizations for their time and efforts in developing and field-testing the Advanced Trauma Life Support concept: The Lincoln Medical Education Foundation, Southeast Nebraska Emergency Medical Services, the University of Nebraska College of Medicine, and the Nebraska State Committee on Trauma of the ACS. The committee also is indebted to those Nebraska doctors who supported the development of this course and to the Lincoln Area Mobile Heart Team Nurses who shared their time and ideas to help build it. Appreciation is extended to those organizations identified previously in this chapter for their support of the worldwide promulgation of the course. Special recognition is given to the spouses, significant others, children, and practice partners of the ATLS Instructors and Students. The time spent away from their homes and practices and effort afforded to this voluntary program are essential components for the existence and success of the ATLS Program.

VIII. SUMMARY

The ATLS Course provides an easily remembered approach to the evaluation and treatment of the injured patient for any doctor, irrespective of practice specialty, even under the stress, anxiety, and intensity that accompanies the resuscitation process. In addition, the program provides a common language to all that care for the injured patient. The ATLS Course provides a foundation for evaluation, treatment, education, and quality assurance—in short, a system of trauma care that is measurable, reproducible, and comprehensive.

The ATLS Program has had a positive impact on the care provided to injured patients worldwide. This has resulted from the improved skills and knowledge of the doctors and other health care providers who have been course participants. The ATLS Course establishes an organized and systematic approach for the evaluation and treatment of patients, promotes minimum standards of care, and recognizes injury as a world health care issue. Morbidity and mortality have been reduced, but the need to eradicate injury remains. The ATLS Program has changed and will continue to change as advances occur in medicine and the needs/expectations of our societies change.

■ BIBLIOGRAPHY

1. Ali J, Adam R, Butler AK, et al: Trauma outcome improves following the Advanced Trauma Life Support program in a developing country. **Journal of Trauma** 1993; 34:890–899.

2. Ali J, Adam R, Josa D, et al: Comparison of interns completing the old (1993) and new interactive (1997) Advanced Trauma Life Support courses. **Journal of Trauma** 1999; 46:80–86.

3. Ali J, Adam R, Stedman M, et al: Advanced Trauma Life Support program increases emergency room application of trauma resuscitative procedures in a developing country. **Journal of Trauma** 1994; 36:391–394.

4. Ali J, Adam R, Stedman M, et al: Cognitive and attitudinal impact of the Advanced Trauma Life Support Course in a developing country. **Journal of Trauma** 1994; 36:695–702.

5. Ali J, Cohen R, Adams R, et al: Attrition of cognitive and trauma skills after the Advanced Trauma Life Support (ATLS) course. **Journal of Trauma** 1996; 40:860–866.

6. Ali J, Cohen R, Adam R, et al: Teaching effectiveness of the Advanced Trauma Life Support program as demonstrated by an objective structured clinical examination for practicing physicians. **World Journal of Surgery** 1996; 20: 1121–1125.

7. Ali J, Howard M: The Advanced Trauma Life Support Program in Manitoba: A 5–year review. **Canadian Journal of Surgery** 1993; 36:181–183.

8. Anderson ID, Anderson IW, Clifford P, et al: Advanced Trauma Life Support in the UK: 8 years on. **British Journal of Hospital Medicine** 1997; 57:272–273.

9. Aprahamian C, Nelson KT, Thompson BM, et al: The relationship of the level of training and area of medical specialization with registrant performance in the Advanced Trauma Life Support course. **Journal of Emergency Medicine** 1984; 2:137-140.

10. Ben Abraham R, Stein M, Kluger Y, et al: ATLS course in emergency medicine for physicians. **Harefuah** 1997; 132:695-697, 743.

11. Ben Abraham R, Stein M, Kluger Y, et al: The impact of Advanced Trauma Life Support Course on graduates with non-surgical medical background. **European Journal of Emergency Medicine** 1997; 4:11-14.

12. Berger LR, Mohan D: **Injury Control: A Global View.** Delhi, India, Oxford University Press, 1996.

13. Blumenfield A, Ben Abraham R, Stein M, et al: Cognitive knowledge decline after Advanced Trauma Life Support courses. **Journal of Trauma** 1998; 44:513-516.

14. Burt CW: Injury-related visits to hospital emergency departments: United States, 1992. **Advance Data from Vital Health Statistics**; no 261. Hyattsville, MD, National Center for Health Statistics, 1995.

15. Deo SD, Knottenbelt JD, Peden MM: Evaluation of a small trauma team for major resuscitation. **Injury** 1997; 28:633-637.

16. Direccao Geral de Vicao, Lisboa, Portugal, data provided by Pedro Ferreira Moniz Pereira, MD, FACS.

17. Fingerhut LA, Cox CS, Warner M, et al: International comparative analysis of injury mortality: Findings from the ICE on injury statistics. **Advance Data from Vital Health Statistics**; no 303. Hyattsville, MD, 1998 (www.cdc.gov/nchs/releases/98facts/98sheets/ineinj.htm).

18. Firdley FM, Cohen DJ, Bienbaum ML, et al: Advanced Trauma Life Support: Assessment of cognitive achievement. **Military Medicine** 1993; 158:623-627.

19. Gautam V, Heyworth J: A method to measure the value of formal training in trauma management: Comparison between ATLS and induction courses. **Injury** 1995; 26:253-255.

20. Greenslade GL, Taylor RH: Advanced Trauma Life Support aboard the RFA Argus. **Journal of the Royal Naval Medical Services** 1992; 78: 23-26.

21. Leibovici D, Fedman B, Gofrit ON, et al: Prehospital cricothyroidotomy by physicians. **American Journal of Emergency Medicine** 1997; 15: 91-93.

22. Mock CJ: International approaches to trauma care. **Trauma Quarterly** 1998; 14:191-348.

23. Murray CJ, Lopez A: The global burden of disease: I. A comprehensive assessment of mortality and disability from diseases, and injuries and risk factors in 1990 and projected to 2020. Cambridge, MA, USA, Harvard University Press, 1996.

24. National Center for Health Statistics: Injury visits to emergency departments. 1998 Fact Sheet.

25. National Safety Council: **Injury Facts (1999)**. Itasca, IL, USA.

26. Nourjah P: National hospital ambulatory medical care survey: 1997 Emergency department summary. **Advance Data from Vital Health Statistics**; no 304. Hyattsville, MD, National Center for Health Statistics, 1999.

27. Rutledge R, Fakhry SM, Baker CC, et al: A population-based study of the association of medical manpower with county trauma death rates in the United States. **Annals of Surgery** 1994; 219: 547-563.

28. Walsh DP, Lammert GR, Devoll J: The effectiveness of the advanced trauma life support system in a mass casualty situation by non-trauma experienced physicians: Grenada 1983. **Journal of Emergency Medicine** 1989; 7:175-180.

29. Williams MJ, Lockey AS, Culshaw MC: Improved trauma management with Advanced Trauma Life Support (ATLS) training. **Journal of Accident and Emergency Medicine** 1997; 14: 81-83.

30. World Health Organization: Detailed data files of WHO mortality data base, 1998 (http://www.who.int/shosis/mort/download.htm).

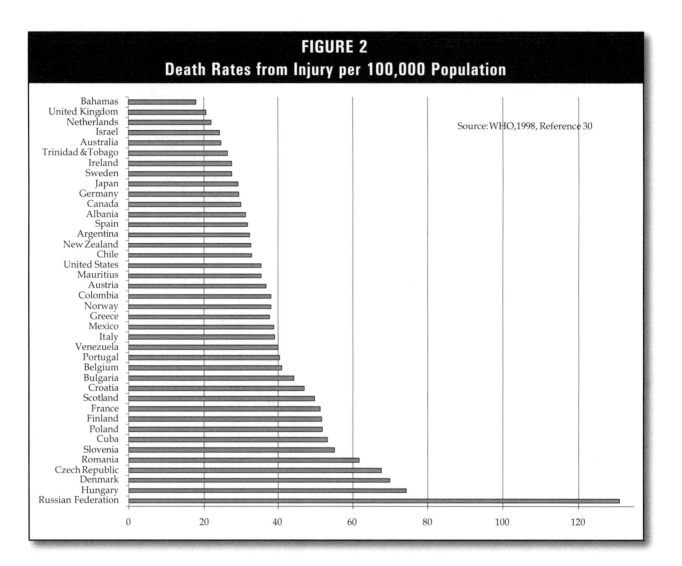

FIGURE 2
Death Rates from Injury per 100,000 Population

Source: WHO, 1998, Reference 30

CHAPTER 1

Initial Assessment and Management

■ OBJECTIVES:

Upon completion of this topic, the student will be able to demonstrate the ability to apply the principles of emergency medical care to the multiply injured patient.

Specifically, the doctor will be able to:

A. Identify the correct sequence of priorities in assessing the multiply injured patient.

B. Apply the principles outlined in the primary and secondary evaluation surveys to the assessment of the multiply injured patient.

C. Apply guidelines and techniques in the initial resuscitative and definitive-care phases of treatment of the multiply injured patient.

D. Identify how the patient's medical history and the mechanism of injury contribute to the identification of injuries.

E. Anticipate the pitfalls associated with the initial assessment and management of the injured patient and apply steps to minimize their impact.

F. Conduct an initial assessment survey on a simulated multiply injured patient, using the correct sequence of priorities and explaining management techniques for primary treatment and stabilization.

INITIAL ASSESSMENT AND MANAGEMENT

I. INTRODUCTION

The treatment of the seriously injured patient requires rapid assessment of the injuries and institution of life-preserving therapy. Because time is of the essence, a systematic approach that can be easily reviewed and practiced is desirable. This process is termed "initial assessment" and includes:

1. Preparation
2. Triage
3. Primary survey (ABCDEs)
4. Resuscitation
5. Adjuncts to primary survey and resuscitation
6. Secondary survey (head-to-toe evaluation and history)
7. Adjuncts to the secondary survey
8. Continued postresuscitation monitoring and reevaluation
9. Definitive care

The primary and secondary surveys should be repeated frequently to ascertain any deterioration in the patient's status and any necessary treatment to be instituted at the time an adverse change is identified.

This sequence is presented in this chapter as a longitudinal progression of events. **In the actual clinical situation, many of these activities occur in parallel or simultaneously.** The linear or longitudinal progression allows the doctor an opportunity to mentally review the progress of an actual trauma resuscitation.

ATLS® is intended to guide the assessment and resuscitation of injured patients. Judgment is required to determine what procedures are necessary, because not all patients require all of these procedures.

II. PREPARATION

Preparation for the trauma patient occurs in 2 different clinical settings. First, during the **prehospital phase**, all events must be coordinated with the doctors at the receiving hospital. Second, during the **hospital phase**, preparations must be made to rapidly facilitate the resuscitation of the trauma patient.

A. Prehospital Phase

Coordination with the prehospital agency and personnel can greatly expedite the treatment in the field. The prehospital system should be set up such that the receiving hospital is notified **before** the prehospital personnel transport the patient from the scene. This allows mobilization of the hospital's trauma team members so that all necessary personnel and resources are present in the emergency department at the time of the patient's arrival. Emphasis in the prehospital phase should be placed on airway maintenance, control of external bleeding and shock, immobilization of the patient, and immediate transport to the **closest appropriate facility**, preferably a verified trauma center. Every effort should be made to minimize scene time. (See Flowchart 1, Triage Decision Scheme.) The National Association of Emergency Medical Technicians' Prehospital Trauma Life Support Committee, in cooperation with the Committee on Trauma (COT) of the American College of Surgeons (ACS), has developed a course with a format similar to the ATLS Course that addresses the prehospital care issues for the injured patient. Emphasis also should be placed on obtaining and reporting information needed for triage at the hospital, eg, time of injury, events related to the injury, and patient history. The mechanisms of injury may suggest the degree of injury as well as specific injuries for which the patient must be evaluated.

B. Inhospital Phase

Advanced planning for the trauma patient's arrival is essential. Ideally, a resuscitation area should be available for trauma patients. Proper airway equipment (eg, laryngoscopes, tubes) should be organized, tested, and placed where it is immediately accessible. Warmed intravenous crystalloid solutions (eg, Ringer's lactate) should be available and ready to infuse when the patient arrives. Appropriate monitoring capabilities should be immediately available. A method to summon extra medical assistance should be in place. A means to assure prompt response by laboratory and radiology personnel is necessary. Transfer agreements with a verified trauma center should be established and operational. (Reference: ACS Committee on Trauma, *Resources for Optimal Care of the Injured Patient.*) Periodic review of patient care through the quality improvement process is an essential component of the hospital's trauma program.

All personnel who have contact with the patient must be protected from communicable diseases. Most prominent among these diseases are hepatitis and the acquired immune deficiency syndrome (AIDS). The Centers for Disease Control and Prevention (CDC) and other health agencies strongly recommend the use of standard precautions (eg, facemask, eye protection, water-impervious apron, leggings, and gloves) when coming in contact with body fluids. The ACS COT considers these to be **minimum** precautions and protection for all health care providers. This also is an Occupational Safety and Health Administration (OSHA) requirement in the United States.

III. TRIAGE

Triage is the sorting of patients based on the need for treatment and the available resources to provide that treatment. Treatment is rendered based on the ABC priorities (Airway with cervical spine protection, Breathing, and Circulation with hemorrhage control) as outlined later in this chapter.

Triage also pertains to the sorting of patients in the field and the medical facility to which they are to be transported. It is the responsibility of the prehospital personnel and their medical director to see that the appropriate patients arrive at the appropriate hospital. It is inappropriate for prehospital personnel to deliver a severely traumatized patient to a nontrauma center hospital if a trauma center is available. (See Flowchart 1, Triage Decision Scheme, adapted with permission from ACS Committee on Trauma, *Resources for Optimal Care of the Injured Patient.*) Prehospital trauma scoring is helpful in identifying those severely injured patients who should be transported to a trauma center. (See Appendix 1, Triage Scenarios and Appendix 5, Trauma Scores: Revised and Pediatric.) Two types of triage situations usually exist:

A. Multiple Casualties

The number of patients and the severity of their injuries do not exceed the ability of the facility to render care. In this situation, patients with life-threatening problems and those sustaining multiple-system injuries are treated first.

The use of prehospital care protocols and online medical direction can facilitate and improve care initiated in the field. Periodic multidisciplinary review

of the care provided through quality assurance/ improvement activities is essential.

B. Mass Casualties

The number of patients and the severity of their injuries exceed the capability of the facility and staff. In this situation, those patients with the greatest chance of survival and with the least expenditure of time, equipment, supplies, and personnel, are managed first.

IV. PRIMARY SURVEY

Patients are assessed and their treatment priorities established based on their injuries, their vital signs, and the injury mechanism. In the severely injured patient, logical sequential treatment priorities must be established based on overall patient assessment. The patient's vital functions must be assessed quickly and efficiently. Patient management must consist of a rapid primary evaluation, resuscitation of vital functions, a more detailed secondary assessment, and, finally, the initiation of definitive care. This process constitutes the ABCDEs of trauma care and identifies life-threatening conditions by adhering to this sequence:

A **A**irway maintenance with cervical spine protection

B **B**reathing and ventilation

C **C**irculation with hemorrhage control

D **D**isability: Neurologic status

E Exposure/Environmental control: Completely undress the patient, but prevent hypothermia

During the primary survey, life-threatening conditions are identified and management is instituted **simultaneously**. The prioritized assessment and management procedures reviewed in this chapter are identified as sequential steps in order of importance and for the purpose of clarity. However, these steps are frequently accomplished simultaneously.

Priorities for the care of the **pediatric patient** are the same as those for adults. Although the quantities of blood, fluids, and medications, the size of the child, degree and rapidity of heat loss, and injury patterns may differ, assessment and management priorities are identical. Specific problems of the pediatric trau-

INITIAL ASSESSMENT AND MANAGEMENT

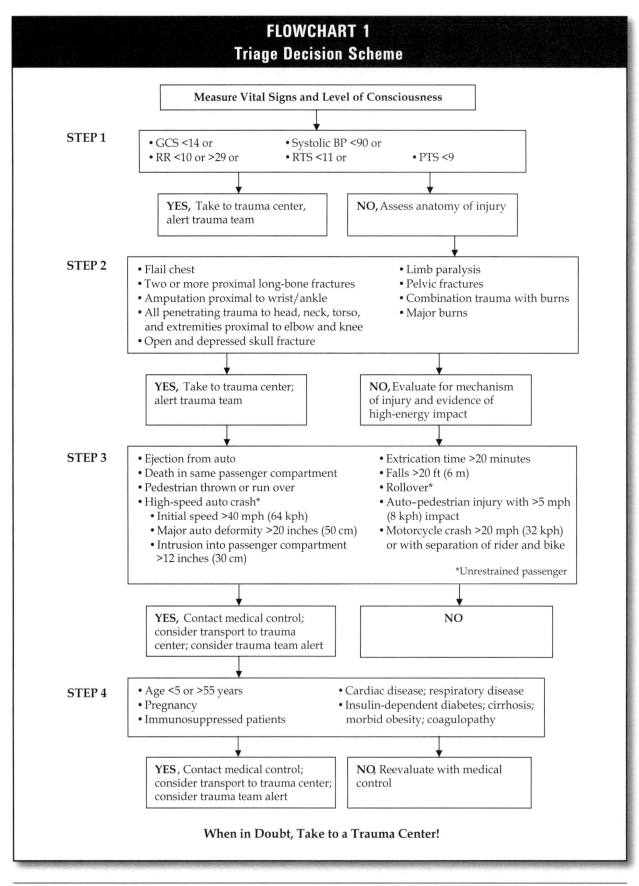

FLOWCHART 1
Triage Decision Scheme

Measure Vital Signs and Level of Consciousness

STEP 1
- GCS <14 or
- RR <10 or >29 or
- Systolic BP <90 or
- RTS <11 or
- PTS <9

YES, Take to trauma center, alert trauma team

NO, Assess anatomy of injury

STEP 2
- Flail chest
- Two or more proximal long-bone fractures
- Amputation proximal to wrist/ankle
- All penetrating trauma to head, neck, torso, and extremities proximal to elbow and knee
- Open and depressed skull fracture
- Limb paralysis
- Pelvic fractures
- Combination trauma with burns
- Major burns

YES, Take to trauma center; alert trauma team

NO, Evaluate for mechanism of injury and evidence of high-energy impact

STEP 3
- Ejection from auto
- Death in same passenger compartment
- Pedestrian thrown or run over
- High-speed auto crash*
  - Initial speed >40 mph (64 kph)
  - Major auto deformity >20 inches (50 cm)
  - Intrusion into passenger compartment >12 inches (30 cm)
- Extrication time >20 minutes
- Falls >20 ft (6 m)
- Rollover*
- Auto–pedestrian injury with >5 mph (8 kph) impact
- Motorcycle crash >20 mph (32 kph) or with separation of rider and bike

*Unrestrained passenger

YES, Contact medical control; consider transport to trauma center; consider trauma team alert

NO

STEP 4
- Age <5 or >55 years
- Pregnancy
- Immunosuppressed patients
- Cardiac disease; respiratory disease
- Insulin-dependent diabetes; cirrhosis; morbid obesity; coagulopathy

YES, Contact medical control; consider transport to trauma center; consider trauma team alert

NO, Reevaluate with medical control

When in Doubt, Take to a Trauma Center!

ma patient are addressed in Chapter 10, Extremes of Age: A. Pediatric Trauma.

Priorities for the care of the **pregnant woman** are similar to the nonpregnant patient, but the anatomic and physiologic changes of pregnancy may modify the patient's response to injury. Early recognition of pregnancy by palpation of the abdomen for a gravid uterus and laboratory testing (HCG), and early fetal assessment are important for maternal and fetal survival. Specific problems of the pregnant patient are addressed in Chapter 11, Trauma in Women.

Trauma is a common cause of death in the **elderly**. With increasing age, cardiovascular disease and cancer overtake the incidence of injury as the leading causes of death. Interestingly, the risk of death for any given injury at the lower and moderate Injury Severity Score (ISS) levels is greater for the elderly man than for the elderly woman. Resuscitation of the elderly patient necessitates special attention. The aging process diminishes the physiologic reserve of the elderly trauma patient. Chronic cardiac, respiratory, and metabolic diseases may reduce the ability of the patient to respond to injury in the same manner that younger patients are able to compensate for the physiologic stress imposed by injury. Comorbidities such as diabetes, congestive heart failure, coronary artery disease, restrictive and obstructive pulmonary disease, coagulopathy, liver disease, and peripheral vascular disease are more common in and adversely affect outcome following injury to the older patient. The chronic use of medications may alter the usual physiologic response to injury. The narrow therapeutic window frequently leads to over- or underresuscitation in this patient population, and early invasive monitoring is frequently a valuable adjunct to management. Despite these facts, most elderly trauma patients recover and return to their preinjury level of independent activity if appropriately managed. Prompt aggressive resuscitation and the early recognition of preexisting medical conditions and medication use can improve the survival of this group. (See Chapter 10, Extremes of Age: B. Trauma in the Elderly.)

A. Airway Maintenance with Cervical Spine Protection

Upon initial evaluation of the trauma patient, the airway should be assessed first to ascertain patency. This rapid assessment for signs of airway obstruction should include inspection for foreign bodies and facial, mandibular, or tracheal/laryngeal fractures that may result in airway obstruction. Measures to establish a patent airway should be instituted while protecting the cervical spine. Initially, the chin lift or jaw thrust maneuvers are recommended to achieve this task.

If the patient is able to communicate verbally, the airway is not likely to be in immediate jeopardy; however, repeated assessment of airway patency is prudent. Additionally, severe head-injury patients with an altered level of consciousness or a Glasgow Coma Scale (GCS) Score of 8 or less usually require the placement of a definitive airway. The finding of nonpurposeful motor responses strongly suggests the need for definitive airway management. Management of the pediatric airway requires knowledge of the unique anatomic features of the position and size of the larynx in children, as well as special equipment. (See Chapter 10, Extremes of Age: A. Pediatric Trauma.)

While assessing and managing the patient's airway, great care should be taken to prevent excessive movement of the cervical spine. The patient's head and neck should not be hyperextended, hyperflexed, or rotated to establish and maintain the airway. Based on the history of the trauma incident, the loss of stability of the cervical spine should be suspected. Neurologic examination alone does not exclude a cervical spine injury. Protection of the patient's spinal cord with appropriate immobilization devices should be accomplished and maintained. If immobilizing devices must be removed temporarily, 1 member of the trauma team should manually stabilize the patient's head and neck using inline immobilization techniques. Stabilization equipment used to protect the patient's spinal cord should be left in place until cervical spine injury is excluded. **Protection of the spine and spinal cord is the important management principle.** Cervical spine x-rays may be obtained to confirm or exclude injury once immediate or potentially life-threatening conditions have been addressed. **Remember: Assume a cervical spine injury in any patient with multisystem trauma, especially with an altered level of consciousness or a blunt injury above the clavicle.** (See Chapter 7, Spine and Spinal Cord Trauma.)

Every effort should be made to promptly identify airway compromise and secure a definitive airway. Equally important is the necessity to recognize the potential for progressive airway loss. Frequent re-

INITIAL ASSESSMENT AND MANAGEMENT

evaluation of airway security is essential to identify the patient who is losing the ability to maintain an adequate airway.

Pitfalls:

1. Despite the efforts of even the most prudent and attentive doctor, there are circumstances where airway management proves to be exceptionally difficult and occasionally impossible to achieve. Equipment failure often cannot be anticipated, eg, the light on the laryngoscope burns out or the cuff on the endotracheal tube that was placed with exceptional difficulty leaks because it was torn on the patient's teeth during the intubation struggle.

2. Another tragic pitfall is the patient who cannot be intubated after paralysis or the patient in whom a surgical airway cannot be performed expediently due to the patient's obesity.

3. Endotracheal intubation of a patient with an unknown laryngeal fracture or incomplete upper airway transection may precipitate total airway occlusion or complete airway transection. This can occur in the absence of clinical findings suggesting the potential for an airway problem or when the urgency of the situation dictates the immediate need for a secure airway or ventilation.

These pitfalls cannot always be prevented. However, they should be **anticipated** and preparations should be made to minimize their impact.

B. Breathing and Ventilation

Airway patency alone does not assure adequate ventilation. Adequate gas exchange is required to maximize oxygenation and carbon dioxide elimination. Ventilation requires adequate function of the lungs, chest wall, and diaphragm. Each component must be examined and evaluated rapidly.

The patient's chest should be exposed to adequately assess chest wall excursion. Auscultation should be performed to assure gas flow in the lungs. Percussion may demonstrate the presence of air or blood in the chest. Visual inspection and palpation may detect injuries to the chest wall that may compromise ventilation.

Injuries that may acutely impair ventilation are tension pneumothorax, flail chest with pulmonary contusion, massive hemothorax, and open pneumothorax. These injuries should be identified in the primary survey. Simple pneumo- or hemothorax, fractured ribs, and pulmonary contusion may compromise ventilation to a lesser degree and are usually identified in the secondary survey.

Pitfalls: Differentiation of ventilation problems from airway compromise may be difficult.

1. A patient may be profoundly dyspneic and tachypneic, giving the impression that the primary problem may be related to an inadequate airway. If the ventilation problem is produced by a pneumothorax or tension pneumothorax, intubation with vigorous bag-valve ventilation could lead to further deterioration of the patient.

2. When intubation and ventilation are necessary in the unconscious patient, the procedure itself may unmask or aggravate a pneumothorax, and the patient's chest must be reevaluated. Chest x-rays should be obtained as soon after intubation and initiation of ventilation as is practical.

C. Circulation with Hemorrhage Control

1. Blood volume and cardiac output

Hemorrhage is the predominant cause of preventable postinjury deaths. Hypotension following injury must be considered to be hypovolemic in origin until proved otherwise. Rapid and accurate assessment of the injured patient's hemodynamic status is therefore essential. The elements of clinical observation that yield important information within seconds are level of consciousness, skin color, and pulse.

a. Level of consciousness

When circulating blood volume is reduced, cerebral perfusion may be critically impaired, resulting in altered levels of consciousness. However, a conscious patient also may have lost a significant amount of blood.

b. Skin color

Skin color can be helpful in evaluating the injured patient who is hypovolemic. A patient with pink skin, especially in the face and extremities, is rarely critically hypovolemic after injury. Conversely, the ashen, gray skin of the face and the white skin of the exsanguinate extremities are ominous signs of hypovolemia.

c. Pulse

Pulses, usually an easily accessible central pulse (femoral or carotid artery), should be assessed bilaterally for quality, rate, and regularity. Full, slow, and regular peripheral pulses are **usually** signs of relative normovolemia in a patient who has not been taking beta-adrenergic-blocking medications. A rapid, thready pulse is usually a sign of hypovolemia, but may have other causes as well. A normal pulse rate does not ensure that the patient is normovolemic. An irregular pulse usually is a warning of potential cardiac dysfunction. Absent central pulses, not attributable to local factors, signify the need for immediate resuscitative action to restore depleted blood volume and effective cardiac output if death is to be avoided.

2. Bleeding

External hemorrhage is identified and controlled in the primary survey.

Rapid, external blood loss is managed by direct manual pressure on the wound. Pneumatic splinting devices also may help control hemorrhage. These devices should be transparent to allow monitoring of underlying bleeding. Tourniquets should **not** be used (except in unusual circumstances such as a traumatic amputation of an extremity) because they crush tissues and cause distal ischemia. The use of hemostats is time consuming, and surrounding structures, such as nerves and veins, can be injured. Hemorrhage into the thoracic or abdominal cavities, into soft tissue surrounding a major long-bone fracture, into the retroperitoneal space from a pelvic fracture, or as a result of a penetrating torso injury are the major sources of occult blood loss.

Pitfalls: Trauma respects no patient population barrier. The elderly, children, athletes, and others with chronic medical conditions do not respond to volume loss in a similar or even in a "normal" manner.

1. Healthy elderly patients have a limited ability to increase their heart rate in response to blood loss, obscuring one of the earliest signs of volume depletion, tachycardia. Blood pressure has little correlation with cardiac output in the older patient group.

2. Children, at the other extreme, usually have abundant physiologic reserve and often demonstrate few signs of hypovolemia even after severe volume depletion. When deterioration does occur, it is precipitous and catastrophic.

3. The well-trained athlete has similar compensatory mechanisms, is normally relatively bradycardic, and does not demonstrate the usual level of tachycardia with blood loss.

4. It also is common that the "AMPLE" history, described subsequently in this chapter, is not available, and the health care team is not aware of the patient's use of medications for chronic conditions.

Anticipation and an attitude of skepticism regarding the patient's "normal" hemodynamic status are appropriate.

D. Disability (Neurologic Evaluation)

A rapid neurologic evaluation is performed at the end of the primary survey. This neurologic evaluation establishes the patient's level of consciousness, pupillary size and reaction, lateralizing signs, and spinal cord injury level.

The GCS is a quick, simple method for determining the level of consciousness, and is predictive of patient outcome (particularly the best motor response). If not done in the primary survey, the GCS should be performed as part of the more detailed, quantitative neurologic examination in the secondary survey. (See Chapter 6, Head Trauma and Appendix 5, Trauma Scores: Revised and Pediatric.)

A decrease in the level of consciousness may indicate decreased cerebral oxygenation and/or perfusion or may be due to direct cerebral injury. An altered level of consciousness indicates the need for immediate reevaluation of the patient's oxygenation, ventilation, and perfusion status. Hypoglycemia, alcohol, narcotics, and/or other drugs also may alter the patient's level of consciousness. However, if these are excluded, changes in the level of consciousness should be considered to be of traumatic central nervous system origin until proven otherwise.

Pitfalls: Despite proper attention to all aspects of managing the patient with a closed head injury,

INITIAL ASSESSMENT AND MANAGEMENT

neurologic deterioration can occur, often rapidly. The lucid interval classically associated with acute epidural hematoma is an example of a situation where the patient will "talk and die." (See Chapter 6, Head Trauma.) Frequent neurologic **reevaluation** can minimize this problem by allowing early detection of changes. It may be necessary to return to the primary survey and to confirm that the patient has a secure airway, adequate ventilation and oxygenation, and adequate cerebral perfusion. Early consultation with the neurosurgeon also is necessary to guide additional management efforts.

E. Exposure/Environmental Control

The patient should be completely undressed, usually by cutting off the garments to facilitate thorough examination and assessment. After the patient's clothing is removed and assessment is completed, it is imperative to cover the patient with warm blankets or an external warming device to prevent hypothermia in the emergency department. Intravenous fluids should be warmed before infusion, and a warm environment (room temperature) should be maintained. **It is the patient's body temperature that is most important, not the comfort of the health care providers.**

Pitfalls: Injured patients may arrive in the emergency department hypothermic, and some of those who require massive transfusions and crystalloid resuscitation become hypothermic despite aggressive efforts to maintain body heat. The problem is best minimized by early control of hemorrhage. This may require operative intervention or the application of an external device to reduce the pelvic volume for certain types of pelvic fractures. Efforts to rewarm the patient and to prevent hypothermia should be considered as important as any other component of the primary survey or resuscitation phase.

V. RESUSCITATION

Aggressive resuscitation and the management of life-threatening injuries, as they are identified, are essential to maximize patient survival.

A. Airway

The airway should be protected in all patients and secured when the potential for airway compromise exists. The jaw thrust or chin lift maneuver may suffice. A nasopharyngeal airway may initially estab-lish and maintain airway patency in the conscious patient. If the patient is unconscious and has no gag reflex, an oropharyngeal airway may be helpful temporarily. **However, a definitive airway should be established if there is any doubt about the patient's ability to maintain airway integrity.**

B. Breathing/Ventilation/Oxygenation

Definitive control of the airway in patients who have compromised airways due to mechanical factors, have ventilatory problems, or are unconscious is achieved by endotracheal intubation, either nasally or orally. This procedure should be accomplished with continuous protection of the cervical spine. A surgical airway should be performed if oral or nasal intubation is contraindicated or cannot be accomplished. (See Chapter 2, Airway and Ventilatory Management.) A tension pneumothorax compromises ventilation and circulation dramatically and acutely, and, if suspected, chest decompression should be accomplished immediately. Every injured patient should receive supplemental oxygen. If not intubated, the patient should have oxygen delivered by a mask/reservoir device to achieve optimal oxygenation. The use of the pulse oximeter is valuable in ensuring adequate hemoglobin saturation. (See Chapter 2, Airway and Ventilatory Management.)

C. Circulation

Control bleeding by direct pressure or operative intervention.

A minimum of 2 large-caliber intravenous (IV) catheters should be established. The maximum rate of fluid administration is determined by the internal diameter of the catheter and inversely by its length, not by the size of the vein in which the catheter is placed. Establishment of upper extremity peripheral IV access is preferred. Other peripheral lines, cutdowns, and central venous lines should be utilized as necessary in accordance with the skill level of the doctor caring for the patient. (See Skills Station IV, Shock Assessment and Management, and Skills Station V, Venous Cutdown, in Chapter 3, Shock.)

At the time of IV insertion, draw blood for type and crossmatch and for baseline hematologic studies, including a pregnancy test for all females of childbearing age.

Aggressive and continued volume resuscitation is not a substitute for manual or operative control

of hemorrhage. Intravenous fluid therapy with a balanced salt solution should be initiated. Ringer's lactate solution is preferred as the initial crystalloid solution and should be administered rapidly. Such bolus IV therapy may require the administration of 2–3 liters of solution to achieve an appropriate patient response in the adult patient. All IV solutions should be warmed either by storage in a warm environment (37°C to 40°C or 98.6°F to 104°F) or by fluid-warming devices.

Shock associated with injury is most often hypovolemic in origin. If the patient remains unresponsive to bolus IV therapy, type-specific blood may be administered as necessary. If type-specific blood is not available, O-negative blood is considered as a substitute. For life-threatening blood loss, the use of unmatched, type-specific blood is preferred over type O blood unless multiple, unidentified casualties are being treated simultaneously. Hypovolemic shock should not be treated by vasopressors, steroids, sodium bicarbonate, or by continued crystalloid/blood infusion. If blood loss continues, it should be controlled by operative intervention. The process of operative resuscitation provides the surgeon the opportunity to stop the bleeding in addition to the maintenance and restoration of intravascular volume.

Hypothermia may be present when the patient arrives, or it may develop quickly in the emergency department in the uncovered patient and by rapid administration of room-temperature fluids or refrigerated blood. Hypothermia is a potentially lethal complication in the injured patient, and aggressive measures should be taken to prevent the loss of body heat and to restore body temperature to normal. The temperature of the resuscitation area should be increased to minimize the loss of body heat. The use of a high-flow fluid warmer or microwave oven to heat crystalloid fluids to 39°C (102.2°F) is recommended. Blood products should not be warmed in a microwave oven. (See Chapter 3, Shock.)

VI. ADJUNCTS TO PRIMARY SURVEY AND RESUSCITATION

A. Electrocardiographic Monitoring

Electrocardiographic (ECG) monitoring of all trauma patients is important. Dysrhythmias, including unexplained tachycardia, atrial fibrillation, premature ventricular contractions, and ST seg-

ment changes, may indicate blunt cardiac injury. Pulseless electrical activity (PEA, formerly termed electromechanical dissociation) may indicate cardiac tamponade, tension pneumothorax, and/or profound hypovolemia. When bradycardia, aberrant conduction, and premature beats are present, hypoxia and hypoperfusion should be suspected immediately. Extreme hypothermia also produces these dysrhythmias. (See Chapter 3, Shock.)

B. Urinary and Gastric Catheters

The placement of urinary and gastric catheters should be considered as part of the resuscitation phase. A urine specimen should be submitted for routine laboratory analysis.

1. Urinary catheters

Urinary output is a sensitive indicator of the volume status of the patient and reflects renal perfusion. Monitoring of urinary output is best accomplished by the insertion of an indwelling bladder catheter. Transurethral bladder catheterization is contraindicated in patients in whom urethral transection is suspected. Urethral injury should be suspected if there is (1) blood at the penile meatus, (2) perineal ecchymosis, (3) blood in the scrotum, (4) a high-riding or nonpalpable prostate, or (5) a pelvic fracture. Accordingly, the urinary catheter should not be inserted before an examination of the rectum and genitalia. If urethral injury is suspected, urethral integrity should be confirmed by a retrograde urethrogram before the catheter is inserted.

Pitfalls: The doctor may encounter situations in which anatomic abnormalities (eg, urethral stricture or prostatic hypertrophy) preclude placement of an indwelling bladder catheter despite meticulous technique. Excessive manipulation of the urethra or the use of specialized instrumentation by the nonspecialist must be avoided. Consult a urologist early.

2. Gastric catheters

A gastric tube is indicated to reduce stomach distention and decrease the risk of aspiration. Decompression of the stomach reduces the risk of aspiration, but **does not prevent it entirely.** Thick or semisolid gastric contents will not return through the tube, and actual passage of the tube may induce vomiting. For the tube to be effective,

INITIAL ASSESSMENT AND MANAGEMENT

it must be positioned properly, attached to appropriate suction, and be functioning. Blood in the gastric aspirate may represent oropharyngeal (swallowed) blood, traumatic insertion, or actual injury to the upper digestive tract. If the cribriform plate is fractured or a fracture is suspected, the gastric tube should be inserted orally to prevent intracranial passage. In this situation, any nasopharyngeal instrumentation is potentially dangerous.

Pitfalls: Placement of a gastric catheter may induce vomiting or gagging and produce the specific problem that its placement is intended to prevent: aspiration. Functional suction equipment should be immediately available.

C. Monitoring

Adequate resuscitation is best assessed by improvement in physiologic parameters, ie, pulse rate, blood pressure, pulse pressure, ventilatory rate, arterial blood gas analysis, body temperature, and urinary output, rather than the qualitative assessment done in the primary survey. **Actual values for these parameters should be obtained as soon as practical after completing the primary survey. Periodic reevaluation is prudent.**

1. **Ventilatory rate and arterial blood gases** should be used to monitor the adequacy of respirations. Endotracheal tubes can be dislodged whenever the patient is moved. A colorimetric carbon dioxide detector is a device capable of detecting carbon dioxide in exhaled gas. It is useful in confirming that the endotracheal tube is located somewhere in the airway of the ventilated patient and not in the esophagus. It does **not** confirm proper placement of the tube in the airway. A variety of quantitative devices are available for this purpose. (See Chapter 2, Airway and Ventilatory Management.)

Pitfalls: Combative trauma patients occasionally extubate themselves. They also may occlude their endotracheal tube or deflate the cuff by biting it. Frequent reevaluation of the airway is necessary.

2. **Pulse oximetry** is a valuable adjunct for monitoring oxygenation in injured patients. The pulse oximeter measures the oxygen saturation of hemoglobin colorimetrically, but does **not** measure the partial pressure of oxygen. It also does not measure the partial pressure of carbon dioxide, which reflects the adequacy of ventilation. A small sensor is placed on the finger, toe, earlobe, or some other convenient place. Most devices display pulse rate and oxygen saturation continuously.

Pitfalls: The pulse oximeter sensor should not be placed distal to the blood pressure cuff. Misleading information regarding hemoglobin saturation and pulse can be generated when the cuff is inflated and occludes blood flow.

Hemoglobin saturation from the pulse oximeter should be compared with the value obtained from the arterial blood gas analysis. Inconsistency indicates that at least 1 of the 2 determinations is in error.

3. The blood pressure should be measured, realizing that it may be a poor measure of actual tissue perfusion.

Pitfalls: Normalization of hemodynamics in injured patients requires more than simply being satisfied with a normal blood pressure. A return to normal peripheral perfusion must be established. This may be problematic in the elderly, as indicated previously, and consideration should be given to early invasive monitoring of cardiac function in these patients.

D. X-rays and Diagnostic Studies

X-rays should be used judiciously and should not delay patient resuscitation. The anteroposterior (AP) chest film and an AP pelvis may provide information that can guide resuscitation efforts of the patient with blunt trauma. Chest x-rays may detect potentially life-threatening injuries that require treatment, and pelvic films may demonstrate fractures of the pelvis that indicate the need for early blood transfusion. A lateral cervical spine x-ray that demonstrates an injury is an important finding, whereas a negative or inadequate film does not exclude cervical spine injury. These films can be taken in the resuscitation area, usually with a portable x-ray unit, but should not interrupt the resuscitation process. They may be deferred to the secondary survey when appropriate.

During the secondary survey, complete cervical and thoracolumbar spine films may be obtained with a portable x-ray unit if the patient's care is not compromised and if the mechanism of injury suggests the possibility of spinal injury. Spinal cord protection should have been performed in the primary survey and maintained. An AP chest film and films pertinent to the site(s) of suspected injury should be obtained. Essential diagnostic x-rays should not be avoided in the pregnant patient.

Diagnostic peritoneal lavage (DPL) and abdominal ultrasonography are useful tools for the quick detection of occult intraabdominal bleeding. Their use depends on the skill and experience level of the doctor. Early identification of the source of occult intraabdominal blood loss may indicate the need for operative control of hemorrhage.

Pitfalls: Technical problems can be encountered when performing any diagnostic procedure, including those necessary to identify intraabdominal hemorrhage. Obesity and intraluminal bowel gas may compromise the images obtained by abdominal ultrasonography. Obesity also can make DPL difficult. Even in the hands of an experienced surgeon, the effluent volume from the lavage may be minimal or zero. In these circumstances, an alternative diagnostic tool should be chosen. The surgeon should be involved in the evaluation process and guide further diagnostic or therapeutic procedures.

VII. CONSIDER NEED FOR PATIENT TRANSFER

During the primary survey and resuscitation phase, the evaluating doctor frequently has enough information to indicate the need for transfer of the patient to another facility. This transfer process may be initiated immediately by administrative personnel at the direction of the examining doctor while additional evaluation and resuscitative measures are being performed. Once the decision to transfer the patient has been made, referring doctor-to-receiving-doctor communication is essential. **Remember,** lifesaving measures are initiated when the problem is identified, rather than after the primary survey.

VIII. SECONDARY SURVEY

The secondary survey does not begin until the primary survey (ABCDEs) is completed, resuscitative efforts are well established, and the patient is demonstrating normalization of vital functions.

The secondary survey is a **head-to-toe evaluation** of the trauma patient, ie, a complete history and physical examination, including a **reassessment** of all vital signs. Each region of the body is completely examined. The potential for missing an injury or failure to appreciate the significance of an injury is great, especially in the unresponsive or unstable patient. (See Table 2, Secondary Survey, in Skills Station I, Initial Assessment and Management.)

In this survey a complete neurologic examination is performed, including a GCS Score determination, if not done during the primary survey. During this evaluation, examination-indicated x-rays are obtained. Such examinations can be interspersed into the secondary survey at appropriate times.

Special procedures, eg, specific radiographic evaluations and laboratory studies, also are obtained at this time. Complete evaluation of the patient requires repeated physical examinations.

A. History

Every complete medical assessment should include a history of the mechanism of injury. Many times such a history cannot be obtained from the patient. Prehospital personnel and family must be consulted to obtain information that may enhance an understanding of the patient's physiologic state. The AMPLE history is a useful mnemonic for this purpose.

> **A** Allergies
>
> **M** Medications currently used
>
> **P** Past illnesses/Pregnancy
>
> **L** Last meal
>
> **E** Events/Environment related to the injury

The patient's condition is greatly influenced by the mechanism of injury. Prehospital personnel can provide valuable information on such mechanisms and should report pertinent data to the examining doctor. Some injuries can be predicted based on the direction and amount of energy force. Injury usually is classified into 2 broad categories, blunt and penetrating. (See Appendix 3, Biomechanics of Injury.)

1. Blunt trauma

Blunt trauma results from automobile collisions, falls, and other transportation-, recreation-, and occupation-related injuries.

Important information to obtain about automobile collisions includes seat belt usage, steering

INITIAL ASSESSMENT AND MANAGEMENT

Table 1—Mechanisms of Injury and Related Suspected Injury Patterns

MECHANISM OF INJURY	SUSPECTED INJURY PATTERNS
Frontal Impact • Bent steering wheel • Knee imprint, dashboard • Bull's-eye fracture, windscreen	• Cervical spine fracture • Anterior flail chest • Myocardial contusion • Pneumothorax • Traumatic aortic disruption • Fractured spleen or liver • Posterior fracture/dislocation of hip, knee
Side Impact, automobile	• Contralateral neck sprain • Cervical spine fracture • Lateral flail chest • Pneumothorax • Traumatic aortic disruption • Diaphragmatic rupture • Fractured spleen/liver, kidney depending on side of impact • Fractured pelvis or acetabulum
Rear Impact, automobile collision	• Cervical spine injury • Soft-tissue injury to neck
Ejection, vehicle	• Ejection from the vehicle precludes meaningful prediction of injury patterns, but places patient at greater risk from virtually all injury mechanisms
Motor Vehicle Impact with Pedestrian	• Head injury • Traumatic aortic disruption • Abdominal visceral injuries • Fractured lower extremities/pelvis

wheel deformation, direction of impact, damage to the automobile in terms of major deformation or intrusion into the passenger compartment, and ejection of the passenger from the vehicle. Ejection from the vehicle greatly increases the chance of major injury.

Injury patterns may often be predicted by the mechanism of injury. Such injury patterns also are influenced by age groups and activities. (See Table 1, Mechanisms of Injury and Related Suspected Injury Patterns.)

2. Penetrating trauma

The incidence of penetrating trauma (injuries from firearms, stabbings, and impaling objects) is increasing rapidly. Factors determining the type and extent of injury and subsequent management include the region of the body injured, the organs in the proximity to the path of the penetrating object, and the velocity of the missile. Therefore, the velocity, caliber, presumed path of the bullet, and the distance from the weapon to the wound may provide important clues to the extent of injury. (See Appendix 3, Biomechanics of Injury, and related Table 1, Missile Kinetic Energy.)

3. Injuries due to burns and cold

Burns are another significant type of trauma that may occur alone or may be coupled with blunt and penetrating trauma resulting from a burning automobile, explosion, falling debris, the patient's attempt to escape a fire, or an assault with a firearm or knife. Inhalation injury and carbon monoxide poisoning often complicate burn injury. Therefore, it is important to know the circumstances of the burn injury. Specifically, knowledge of the environment in which the burn injury occurred (open or closed space), as well as of substances consumed by the flames (eg, plastics, chemicals) and possible associated injuries sustained, is critical in the treatment of the patient.

Acute or chronic hypothermia without adequate protection against heat loss produces either local or generalized cold injuries. Significant heat loss may occur at moderate temperatures (15°C to 20°C or 59°F to 68°F) if wet clothes, decreased activity, and/or vasodilatation caused by alcohol or drugs compromise the patient's ability to conserve heat. Such historical information can be obtained from prehospital personnel.

4. Hazardous environment

Histories of exposure to chemicals, toxins, and radiation are important to obtain for 2 reasons. First, these agents can produce a variety of pulmonary, cardiac, or internal organ dysfunction in the injured patient. Secondly, these same agents also present a hazard to health care providers. Frequently, the doctor's only means of preparation is to understand the general principles of management of such conditions and establish immediate contact with the Regional Poison Control Center.

B. Physical Examination

1. Head (See Chapter 6, Head Trauma)

The secondary survey begins with evaluating the head and identifying all related neurologic and significant injuries. The entire scalp and head should be examined for lacerations, contusions, and evidence of fractures. Because edema around the eyes may later preclude an in-depth examination, the eyes should be reevaluated for

   a. Visual acuity

   b. Pupillary size

   c. Hemorrhages of the conjunctiva and fundi

   d. Penetrating injury

   e. Contact lenses (remove before edema occurs)

   f. Dislocation of the lens

   g. Ocular entrapment

A quick visual acuity examination of both eyes can be performed by having the patient read

printed material, eg, a hand-held Snelling Chart, words on an IV container, or a 4 × 4 dressing package. Ocular mobility should be evaluated to exclude entrapment of extraocular muscles due to orbital fractures. These procedures frequently identify optic injuries not otherwise apparent. (See Appendix 7, Ocular Trauma.)

Pitfalls: Facial edema in patients with massive facial injury or patients in coma can preclude a complete eye examination. Such difficulties should not deter the doctor from performing those components of the ocular examination that are possible. (See Appendix 7, Ocular Trauma.)

2. Maxillofacial (See Chapter 6, Head Trauma, and Skills Station IX, Head and Neck Trauma Assessment and Management)

Maxillofacial trauma, not associated with airway obstruction or major bleeding, should be treated only after the patient is stabilized completely and life-threatening injuries have been managed. At the discretion of appropriate specialists, definitive management may be safely delayed without compromising care.

Patients with fractures of the midface may have a fracture of the cribriform plate. For these patients, gastric intubation should be performed via the oral route.

Pitfalls: Some maxillofacial fractures, eg, nasal fracture, nondisplaced zygomatic fractures, and orbital rim fractures, may be difficult to identify early in the evaluation process. Therefore, frequent reassessment is crucial.

3. Cervical spine and neck (See Chapter 7, Spine and Spinal Cord Trauma)

Patients with maxillofacial or head trauma should be presumed to have an unstable cervical spine injury (fracture and/or ligamentous injury), and the neck should be immobilized until all aspects of the cervical spine have been adequately studied and an injury has been excluded. The absence of neurologic deficit does not exclude injury to the cervical spine, and such injury should be presumed until a complete cervical spine radiographic series is reviewed by a doctor experienced in detecting cervical spine fractures radiographically.

INITIAL ASSESSMENT AND MANAGEMENT

Examination of the neck includes inspection, palpation, and auscultation. Cervical spine tenderness, subcutaneous emphysema, tracheal deviation, and laryngeal fracture may be discovered on a detailed examination. The carotid arteries should be palpated and auscultated for bruits. Evidence of blunt injury over these vessels should be noted and, if present, should arouse a high index of suspicion for carotid artery injury. Occlusion or dissection of the carotid artery may occur late in the injury process without antecedent signs or symptoms. Angiography or duplex ultrasonography may be required to exclude the possibility of major cervical vascular injury when the mechanism of injury suggests this possibility. Most major cervical vascular injuries are the result of penetrating injury. However, blunt force to the neck or a traction injury from a shoulder–harness restraint can result in intimal disruption, dissection, and thrombosis.

Protection of a potentially unstable cervical spine injury is imperative for patients wearing any type of protective helmet. Extreme care must be taken when removing the helmet. (See Chapter 2, Airway and Ventilatory Management.)

Penetrating injuries to the neck have the potential of injuring several organ systems. Wounds that extend through the platysma should not be explored manually or probed with instruments in the emergency department, or by individuals in the emergency department who are not trained to deal with such injuries. The emergency department usually is not equipped to deal with problems that may be encountered unexpectedly. These injuries require evaluation by a surgeon either operatively or with specialized diagnostic procedures under direct supervision by the surgeon. The finding of active arterial bleeding, an expanding hematoma, arterial bruit, or airway compromise usually requires surgical operative evaluation. Unexplained or isolated paralysis of an upper extremity should raise the suspicion signs of a cervical nerve root injury and be accurately documented.

Pitfalls:

1. Blunt injury to the neck may produce injuries in which clinical signs and symptoms develop late and may not be present during the initial examination. Injury to the intima of the carotid arteries is an example.

2. The identification of cervical nerve root or brachial plexus injury may not be possible in the comatose patient. Consideration of the mechanism of injury may be the only clue available to the doctor.

3. In some patients, a decubitus ulcer may develop quickly over the sacrum or other areas from immobilization on a rigid spine board or from the cervical collar. Efforts to exclude the possibility of spinal injury should be initiated as soon as practical and these devices removed. **However**, resuscitation and efforts to identify life-threatening or potentially life-threatening injuries should not be compromised.

4. Chest (See Chapter 4, Thoracic Trauma)

Visual evaluation of the chest, both anterior and posterior, identifies such conditions as open pneumothorax and large flail segments. A complete evaluation of the chest wall requires palpation of the entire chest cage, including the clavicle, ribs, and sternum. Sternal pressure may be painful if the sternum is fractured or costochondral separations exist. Contusions and hematomas of the chest wall should alert the doctor to the possibility of occult injury.

Significant chest injury may be manifested by pain, dyspnea, or hypoxia. Evaluation includes auscultation of the chest and a chest x-ray. Breath sounds are auscultated high on the anterior chest wall for pneumothorax and at the posterior bases for hemothorax. Auscultatory findings may be difficult to evaluate in a noisy environment, but may be extremely helpful. Distant heart sounds and narrow pulse pressure may indicate cardiac tamponade. Cardiac tamponade or tension pneumothorax may be suggested by the presence of distended neck veins, although associated hypovolemia may minimize this finding or eliminate it altogether. Decreased breath sounds, hyperresonance to percussion, and shock may be the only indications of tension pneumothorax and the need for immediate chest decompression.

The chest x-ray confirms the presence of a hemothorax or simple pneumothorax. Rib fractures may be present, but they may not be visible on the x-ray. A widened mediastinum or other radiographic signs may suggest an aortic rupture.

Pitfalls:

1. Elderly patients may not tolerate even relatively minor chest injuries. Progression to acute respiratory insufficiency must be anticipated and support instituted before collapse occurs.

2. Children often sustain significant injury to the intrathoracic structures without evidence of thoracic skeletal trauma. A high index of suspicion is essential.

5. Abdomen (See Chapter 5, Abdominal Trauma)

Abdominal injuries must be identified and treated aggressively. The specific diagnosis is not as important as recognizing that an injury exists and surgical intervention may be necessary. A normal initial examination of the abdomen does not exclude a significant intraabdominal injury. Close observation and frequent reevaluation of the abdomen, preferably by the same observer, is important in managing blunt abdominal trauma. Over time, the patient's abdominal findings may change. Early involvement by a surgeon is essential.

Patients with unexplained hypotension, neurologic injury, impaired sensorium secondary to alcohol and/or other drugs, and equivocal abdominal findings should be considered as candidates for peritoneal lavage, abdominal ultrasonography, or, if hemodynamically normal, computed tomography (CT) of the abdomen with IV and intragastric contrast. Fractures of the pelvis or the lower rib cage also may hinder accurate diagnostic examination of the abdomen, because pain from these areas may be elicited when palpating the abdomen.

Pitfalls:

1. Excessive manipulation of the pelvis should be avoided. The AP pelvic x-ray, performed as an adjunct to the primary survey and resuscitation, may provide valuable information as to the presence or absence of pelvic fractures, which have the potential of being associated with significant blood loss.

2. Injury to the retroperitoneal organs may be difficult to identify, even with the use of CT. Classic examples include hollow viscus and pancreatic injuries.

Knowledge of injury mechanism, associated injuries that can be identified, and a high index of suspicion are required. Despite the doctor's appropriate diligence, some of these injuries are not diagnosed initially.

6. Perineum/rectum/vagina (See Chapter 5, Abdominal Trauma)

The perineum should be examined for contusions, hematomas, lacerations, and urethral bleeding.

A rectal examination should be performed before placing a urinary catheter. Specifically, the doctor should assess for the presence of blood within the bowel lumen, a high-riding prostate, the presence of pelvic fractures, the integrity of the rectal wall, and the quality of the sphincter tone.

For the female patient, a vaginal examination also is an essential part of the secondary survey. The doctor should assess for the presence of blood in the vaginal vault and vaginal lacerations. Additionally, pregnancy tests should be performed on all females of childbearing age.

Pitfall: Female urethral injury, while uncommon, does occur in association with pelvic fractures and straddle injuries. When present, such injuries are difficult to detect.

7. Musculoskeletal (See Chapter 7, Spine and Spinal Cord Trauma, and Chapter 8, Musculoskeletal Trauma)

The extremities should be inspected for contusion or deformity. Palpation of the bones and examining for tenderness or abnormal movement aids in the identification of occult fractures.

Pelvic fractures can be suspected by the identification of ecchymosis over the iliac wings, pubis, labia, or scrotum. Pain on palpation of the pelvic ring is an important finding in the alert patient. Mobility of the pelvis in response to gentle anterior-to-posterior pressure with the heels of the hands on both anterior iliac spines and the symphysis pubis can suggest pelvic ring disruption in the unconscious patient. Since such manipulation can initiate unwanted bleeding, it should be done (if at all) only once, preferably by the orthopaedic surgeon responsible for the patient's care. Additionally, assessment of peripheral pulses can identify vascular injuries.

INITIAL ASSESSMENT AND MANAGEMENT

Significant extremity injuries may exist without fractures being evident on examination or x-rays. Ligament ruptures produce joint instability. Muscle-tendon unit injuries interfere with active motion of the affected structures. Impaired sensation and/or loss of voluntary muscle contraction strength may be due to nerve injury or to ischemia, including that due to compartment syndrome.

Thoracic and lumbar spinal fractures and/or neurologic injuries must be considered based on physical findings and mechanism of injury. Other injuries may mask the physical findings of spinal injuries, which may go unsuspected unless the doctor obtains the appropriate x-rays.

The doctor must remember that the musculo-skeletal examination is not complete without an examination of the patient's back. Unless the patient's back is examined, significant injuries may be missed.

Pitfalls:

1. Blood loss from pelvic fractures that increase pelvic volume can be difficult to control and fatal hemorrhage may result. A sense of urgency should accompany the management of these injuries.

2. Fractures involving the bones of the hands, wrists, and feet are often not diagnosed in the secondary survey performed in the emergency department. It may be only after the patient has regained consciousness or other major injuries are resolved that the patient indicates pain in the area of an occult injury.

3. Injuries to the soft tissues around joints are frequently diagnosed after the patient begins to recover. Therefore, frequent reevaluation is essential.

8. Neurologic (See Chapter 6, Head Trauma, and Chapter 7, Spine and Spinal Cord Trauma)

A comprehensive neurologic examination includes not only motor and sensory evaluation of the extremities, but also reevaluation of the patient's level of consciousness and pupillary size and response. The GCS Score facilitates detection of early changes and trends in the neurologic status. (See Appendix 5, Trauma Scores: Revised and Pediatric.)

Early consultation with a neurosurgeon is required for patients with neurologic injury. The patient should be frequently monitored for deterioration in the level of consciousness or changes in the neurologic examination, as these findings may reflect progression of the intracranial injury. If a patient with a head injury deteriorates neurologically, oxygenation and perfusion of the brain and the adequacy of ventilation (ABCDEs) must be reassessed. Intracranial surgical intervention may be necessary or measures instituted to reduce intracranial pressure. The neurosurgeon must make the decision whether such conditions as epidural and subdural hematomas require evacuation, or depressed skull fractures need operative intervention.

Pitfalls: Any increase in intracranial pressure (ICP) can reduce cerebral perfusion pressure and lead to secondary brain injury. Most of the diagnostic and therapeutic maneuvers necessary for the evaluation and care of the brain-injured patient increase ICP. Tracheal intubation is a classic example, and in the patient with brain injury, it should be performed expeditiously and as smoothly as possible. Rapid neurologic deterioration of the brain-injured patient can occur despite the application of all measures to control intracranial pressure and maintain appropriate support of the central nervous system.

Any evidence of loss of sensation, paralysis, or weakness suggests major injury to the spinal column or peripheral nervous system. Neurologic deficits should be documented when identified, even when transfer to another facility or doctor for specialty care is necessary. Immobilization of the **entire** patient, using a long spine board, a semirigid cervical collar, and/or other cervical immobilization devices, must be maintained until spinal injury can be excluded. The common mistake of immobilizing the head and freeing the torso allows the cervical spine to flex with the body as a fulcrum. **Protection of the spinal cord is required at all times until a spine injury is excluded. Early consultation with a neurosurgeon or orthopaedic surgeon is necessary.**

IX. ADJUNCTS TO THE SECONDARY SURVEY

Specialized diagnostic tests may be performed during the secondary survey to identify specific injuries.

These include additional x-rays of the spine and extremities; CT scans of the head, chest, abdomen, and spine; contrast urography and angiography; transesophageal ultrasound; bronchoscopy; esophagoscopy; and other diagnostic procedures. Often these procedures require transportation of the patient to other areas of the hospital where equipment and personnel to manage life-threatening contingencies are not immediately available. Therefore, these specialized tests should not be performed until the patient's hemodynamic status has been normalized and the patient has been carefully examined.

X. REEVALUATION

The trauma patient must be reevaluated constantly to assure that new findings are not overlooked, and to discover deterioration in previously noted findings. As initial life-threatening injuries are managed, other equally life-threatening problems and less severe injuries may become apparent. Underlying medical problems that may severely affect the ultimate prognosis of the patient may become evident. A high index of suspicion facilitates early diagnosis and management.

Continuous monitoring of vital signs and urinary output is essential. For the adult patient, maintenance of urinary output of 0.5 mL/kg/hour is desirable. In the pediatric patient more than 1 year old, an output of 1 mL/kg/hour should be adequate. Arterial blood gas analyses and cardiac monitoring devices should be used. Pulse oximetry on critically injured patients and end-tidal carbon dioxide monitoring on intubated patients should be considered.

The relief of severe pain is an important part of the management of the trauma patient. Many injuries, especially musculoskeletal injuries, produce pain and anxiety in the conscious patient. Effective analgesia usually requires the use of IV opiates or anxiolytics. Intramuscular injections should be avoided. These agents should be administered judiciously and in small doses to achieve the desired level of patient comfort and relief of anxiety while avoiding respiratory depression, the masking of subtle injuries, or changes in the patient's status.

XI. DEFINITIVE CARE

The interhospital triage criteria help determine the level, pace, and intensity of initial management of the multiple-injured patient. (Reference, American College of Surgeons Committee on Trauma, *Resources for Optimal Care of the Injured Patient*.) These criteria take into account the patient's physiologic status, obvious and anatomic injury, mechanisms of injury, concurrent diseases, and factors that may alter the patient's prognosis. Emergency department and surgical personnel should use these criteria to determine if the patient requires transfer to a trauma center or closest appropriate hospital capable of providing more specialized care. The closest appropriate local facility should be chosen based on its overall capabilities to care for the injured patient. (See Chapter 12, Transfer to Definitive Care and Flowchart 1, Triage Decision Scheme, in this chapter.)

XII. DISASTER

Disasters frequently overwhelm local and regional resources. Plans for management of such conditions must be developed, reevaluated, and rehearsed frequently to enhance the possibility of salvage of the maximum number of injured patients.

XIII. RECORDS AND LEGAL CONSIDERATIONS

A. Records

Meticulous record keeping with time documented for all events is very important. Often more than 1 doctor cares for the patient. Precise records are essential to evaluate the patient's needs and clinical status. Accurate records during the resuscitation can be facilitated by a member of the nursing staff whose sole job is to record and collate all patient care information.

Medicolegal problems arise frequently, and precise records are helpful for all concerned. Chronologic reporting with flowsheets helps both the attending doctor and consulting doctor to quickly assess changes in the patient's condition. (See Appendix 6, Sample Trauma Flowsheet, and Chapter 12, Transfer to Definitive Care, Table 2, Sample Transfer Form.)

B. Consent for Treatment

Consent is sought before treatment, if possible. In life-threatening emergencies it is often not possible to obtain such prospective consent. In such cases treatment should be given first and formal consent obtained later.

INITIAL ASSESSMENT AND MANAGEMENT

C. Forensic Evidence

If injury due to criminal activity is suspected, the personnel caring for the patient must preserve the evidence. All items, such as clothing and bullets, must be saved for law enforcement personnel. Laboratory determinations of blood alcohol concentrations and other drugs may be particularly pertinent and have substantial legal implications. (See Appendix 3, Biomechanics of Injury.)

XIV. SUMMARY

The injured patient must be evaluated rapidly and thoroughly. The doctor must develop treatment priorities for the overall management of the patient so that no steps in the process are omitted. An adequate patient history and accounting of the incident are important in evaluating and managing the trauma patient. Evaluation and care are divided into the following phases for the purposes of discussion and to provide clarity. In actual situations, assessment, resuscitation or treatment, reevaluation, and diagnosis may occur simultaneously, but priorities should not change.

A. Primary Survey Assessment of ABCDEs

1. Airway and cervical spine protection

2. Breathing

3. Circulation with control of external hemorrhage

4. Disability: Brief neurologic evaluation

5. Exposure/Environment: Completely undress the patient, but prevent hypothermia.

B. Resuscitation

1. Oxygenation and ventilation

2. Shock management, IV lines, warmed Ringer's lactate solution

3. Management of life-threatening problems identified in the primary survey is continued.

C. Adjuncts to Primary Survey and Resuscitation

1. **Monitoring**

   a. Arterial blood gas analysis and ventilatory rate

   b. End-tidal carbon dioxide

   c. Electrocardiograph

   d. Pulse oximetry

   e. Blood pressure

2. **Urinary and gastric catheters**

3. **X-rays and diagnostic studies**

   a. Chest

   b. Pelvis

   c. C-spine

   d. DPL or FAST

D. Secondary Survey, Total Patient Evaluation: Physical Examination and History

1. Head and skull

2. Maxillofacial and intraoral

3. Neck

4. Chest

5. Abdomen (including back)

6. Perineum/rectum/vagina

7. Musculoskeletal

8. Neurologic examination

E. Adjuncts to the Secondary Survey

Specialized diagnostic procedures that are utilized to confirm suspected injury should only be performed after the patient's life-threatening injuries have been identified and managed, and the patient's hemodynamic and ventilation status returned to normal.

1. Computed tomography

2. Contrast x-ray studies

3. Extremity x-rays

4. Endoscopy and ultrasonography

F. Definitive Care

After identifying the patient's injuries, managing life-threatening problems, and obtaining special studies, definitive care begins. Definitive care, associated with the major trauma entities, is described in later chapters.

G. Transfer

If the patient's injuries exceed the institution's immediate treatment capabilities, the process of transferring the patient is initiated as soon as the need is identified. Delay in transferring the patient to a facility with a higher level of care may significantly increase the patient's risk of mortality. (See Chapter 12, Transfer to Definitive Care.)

■ BIBLIOGRAPHY

1. American College of Surgeons Committee on Trauma: **Resources for Optimal Care of the Injured Patient.** Chicago, 1999 and In publication.

2. Battistella FD: Emergency department evaluation of the patient with multiple injuries. In: Wilmore DW, Cheung LY, Harken AH et al (eds): **Scientific American Surgery.** New York, Scientific American, 1988-2000.

3. Bell RM, Krantz BE: Initial assessment. In: Mattox KL, Feliciano DV, Moore EE (eds): **Trauma, 4th Edition.** New York, McGraw-Hill, 2000.

4. Blaisdell FW, Trunkey DD (eds): **Cervicothoracic Trauma, 2nd Edition.** New York, Thieme Medical Publishers, 1994.

5. Enderson BL, Reath DB, Meadors J, et al: The tertiary trauma survey: a prospective study of missed injury. **Journal of Trauma** 1990; 30: 666–670.

6. Esposito TJ, Kuby A, Unfred C, et al: General surgeons and the Advanced Trauma Life Support course: Is it time to refocus? **Journal of Trauma** 1995; 39:929–934.

7. Ivatury RR, Cayten CG (eds): **Textbook of Penetrating Trauma.** Baltimore, Williams and Wilkins, 1996.

8. Lucas CE, Ledgerwood AM: Initial evaluation and management of severely injured patients. In: Wilson RF, Walt AJ (eds): **Management of Trauma: Pitfalls and Practice, 2nd Edition.** Baltimore, Williams & Wilkins, 1996.

9. Mattox KL, Feliciano DV, Moore EE (eds): **Trauma, 4th Edition.** New York, McGraw-Hill, 2000.

10. McSwain NE Jr, Frame S, Salomone J, et al (eds): **Prehospital Trauma Life Support: Basic and Advanced, 4th Edition.** St. Louis, Mosby, 2003.

11. Morris JA, MacKinzie EJ, Daminso AM, et al: Mortality in trauma patients: Interaction between host factors and severity. **Journal of Trauma** 1990; 30:1476–1482.

12. Nahum AM, Melvin J (eds): **The Biomechanics of Trauma.** Norwalk, CT, Appleton-Century-Crofts, 1985.

13. Pepe PE: Prehospital management of trauma. In: Schwartz GR, et al (eds): **Principles and Practice of Emergency Medicine, 4th Edition.** Baltimore, Williams & Wilkins, 1999, pp 217–222.

14. Rhodes M, Brader A, Lucke J, et al: Direct transport to the operating room for resuscitation of trauma patients. **Journal of Trauma** 1989; 29: 907–915.

15. Wilson RF, Walt AJ (eds): **Management of Trauma. Pitfalls and Practice, 2nd Edition.** Baltimore, Williams & Wilkins, 1996.

Initial Assessment and Management

◼ OBJECTIVES:

Performance at this station will allow the participant to practice and demonstrate the following activities in a simulated clinical situation:

1. Communicate and demonstrate to the instructor the systematic initial assessment and management of each patient.

2. Using the primary survey assessment techniques, determine and demonstrate:
   a. Airway patency and cervical spine control
   b. Breathing efficacy
   c. Circulatory status with hemorrhage control
   d. Disability: Neurologic status
   e. Exposure/Environment: Undress the patient, but prevent hypothermia.

3. Establish resuscitation (management) priorities in the multiply injured patient based on findings from the primary survey.

4. Integrate appropriate history taking as an invaluable aid in the assessment of the patient situation.

5. Identify the injury-producing mechanism and discuss the injuries that may exist and/or may be anticipated as a result of the mechanism of injury.

6. Using secondary survey techniques, assess the patient from head to toe.

7. Using the primary and secondary survey techniques, reevaluate the patient's status and response to therapy instituted.

8. Given a series of x-rays:
   a. Diagnose fractures.
   b. Differentiate associated injuries.

9. Outline the definitive care necessary to stabilize each patient in preparation for possible transport to a trauma center or closest appropriate facility.

10. As referring doctor, communicate with the receiving doctor (instructor) in a logical, sequential manner:

---

a. Patient's history, including mechanism of injury

b. Physical findings

c. Management instituted

d. Patient's response to therapy

e. Diagnostic tests performed and results

f. Need for transport

g. Method of transportation

h. Anticipated time of arrival

INTERACTIVE SKILLS PROCEDURES

Initial Assessment and Management

I. PRIMARY SURVEY AND RESUSCITATION

The student should: (1) outline preparations that must be made to facilitate the rapid progression of assessing and resuscitating the patient; (2) indicate the need to wear appropriate clothing for self- and patient protection from communicable diseases; and (3) indicate that the patient is to be completely undressed, but that hypothermia should be prevented. **Note: Standard precautions are required whenever caring for the trauma patient.**

A. Airway with Cervical Spine Protection

1. **Assessment**

   a. Ascertain patency.

   b. Rapidly assess for airway obstruction.

2. **Management—Establish a patent airway**

   a. Perform a chin lift or jaw thrust maneuver.

   b. Clear the airway of foreign bodies.

   c. Insert an oropharyngeal or nasopharyngeal airway.

   d. Establish a definitive airway.

   1) Orotracheal or nasotracheal intubation

   2) Surgical cricothyroidotomy

   e. Describe jet insufflation of the airway, noting that it is only a temporary procedure.

3. Maintain the cervical spine in a neutral position with manual immobilization as necessary when establishing an airway.

4. Reinstate immobilization of the c-spine with appropriate devices after establishing an airway.

B. Breathing: Ventilation and Oxygenation

1. **Assessment**

   a. Expose the neck and chest: Assure immobilization of the head and neck.

   b. Determine the rate and depth of respirations.

   c. Inspect and palpate the neck and chest for tracheal deviation, unilateral and bilateral chest movement, use of accessory muscles, and any signs of injury.

   d. Percuss the chest for presence of dullness or hyperresonance.

   e. Auscultate the chest bilaterally.

INITIAL ASSESSMENT AND MANAGEMENT   *Initial Assessment and Management*

2. Management

   a. Administer high concentrations of oxygen.

   b. Ventilate with a bag-valve-mask device.

   c. Alleviate tension pneumothorax.

   d. Seal open pneumothorax.

   e. Attach a CO_2 monitoring device to the endotracheal tube.

   f. Attach the patient to a pulse oximeter.

C. Circulation with Hemorrhage Control

1. Assessment

   a. Identify source of external, exsanguinating hemorrhage.

   b. Identify potential source(s) of internal hemorrhage.

   c. Pulse: Quality, rate, regularity, and paradox

   d. Skin color

   e. Blood pressure, time permitting

2. Management

   a. Apply direct pressure to external bleeding site.

   b. Consider presence of internal hemorrhage and potential need for operative intervention, and obtain surgical consult.

   c. Insert 2 large-caliber IV catheters.

   d. Simultaneously obtain blood for hematologic and chemical analyses, pregnancy test, type and cross-match, and arterial blood gases.

   e. Initiate IV fluid therapy with warmed Ringer's lactate solution and blood replacement.

   f. Apply the pneumatic antishock garment or pneumatic splints as indicated to control hemorrhage.

   g. Prevent hypothermia.

D. Disability: Brief Neurologic Examination

   1. Determine the level of consciousness using the GCS Score.

   2. Assess the pupils for size, equality, and reaction.

E. Exposure/Environment: Completely undress the patient, but prevent hypothermia.

F. Adjuncts to Primary Survey and Resuscitation

   1. Obtain arterial blood gas analysis and ventilatory rate.

   2. Monitor the patient's exhaled CO_2 with an appropriate monitoring device.

   3. Attach the patient to an ECG monitor.

   4. Insert urinary and gastric catheters unless contraindicated and monitor the patient's hourly urinary output.

   5. Consider the need for and obtain (1) an AP chest x-ray, (2) an AP pelvis x-ray, and (3) a lateral, cross-table cervical spine x-ray.

   6. Consider the need for and perform DPL or abdominal ultrasonography.

G. Reassess the Patient's ABCDEs and Consider Need for Patient Transfer

II. SECONDARY SURVEY AND MANAGEMENT (See Table 2, Secondary Survey, in this skills station)

A. AMPLE History and Mechanism of Injury

1. Obtain AMPLE history from patient, family, or prehospital personnel.

2. Obtain history of injury-producing event and identify injury mechanisms.

B. Head and Maxillofacial

1. **Assessment**

   a. Inspect and palpate entire head and face for lacerations, contusions, fractures, and thermal injury.

   b. Reevaluate pupils.

   c. Reevaluate level of consciousness and GCS Score.

   d. Assess eyes for hemorrhage, penetrating injury, visual acuity, dislocation of the lens, and presence of contact lenses.

   e. Evaluate cranial nerve function.

   f. Inspect ears and nose for cerebrospinal fluid leakage.

   g. Inspect mouth for evidence of bleeding and cerebrospinal fluid, soft-tissue lacerations, and loose teeth.

2. **Management**

   a. Maintain airway; continue ventilation and oxygenation as indicated.

   b. Control hemorrhage.

   c. Prevent secondary brain injury.

   d. Remove contact lenses.

C. Cervical Spine and Neck

1. **Assessment**

   a. Inspect for signs of blunt and penetrating injury, tracheal deviation, and use of accessory respiratory muscles.

   b. Palpate for tenderness, deformity, swelling, subcutaneous emphysema, tracheal deviation, and symmetry of pulses.

   c. Auscultate the carotid arteries for bruits.

   d. Obtain a lateral, crosstable cervical spine x-ray.

2. **Management:** Maintain adequate in-line immobilization and protection of the cervical spine.

D. Chest

1. **Assessment**

   a. Inspect the anterior, lateral, and posterior chest wall for signs of blunt and penetrating injury, use of accessory breathing muscles, and bilateral respiratory excursions.

   b. Auscultate the anterior chest wall and posterior bases for bilateral breath sounds and heart sounds.

   c. Palpate the entire chest wall for evidence of blunt and penetrating injury, subcutaneous emphysema, tenderness, and crepitation.

d. Percuss for evidence of hyperresonance or dullness.

2. Management

a. Perform needle decompression of pleural space or tube thoracostomy, as indicated.

b. Attach the chest tube to an underwater seal drainage device.

c. Correctly dress an open chest wound.

d. Pericardiocentesis, as indicated.

e. Perform transfer the patient to the operating room, if indicated.

E. Abdomen

1. Assessment

a. Inspect the anterior and posterior abdomen for signs of blunt and penetrating injury and internal bleeding.

b. Auscultate for presence/absence of bowel sounds.

c. Percuss the abdomen to elicit subtle rebound tenderness.

d. Palpate the abdomen for tenderness, involuntary muscle guarding, unequivocal rebound tenderness, or a gravid uterus.

e. Obtain a pelvic x-ray.

f. Perform DPL/abdominal ultrasound, if warranted.

g. Obtain CT of the abdomen if the patient is hemodynamically normal.

2. Management

a. Transfer the patient to the operating room, if indicated.

b. Apply the pneumatic antishock garment or wrap a sheet around the pelvis as indicated to reduce pelvic volume and control hemorrhage from a pelvic fracture.

F. Perineum/Rectum/Vagina

1. Perineal assessment

a. Contusions and hematomas

b. Lacerations

c. Urethral bleeding

2. Rectal assessment

a. Rectal blood

b. Anal sphincter tone

c. Bowel wall integrity

d. Bony fragments

e. Prostate position

3. Vaginal assessment

a. Presence of blood in the vaginal vault

b. Vaginal lacerations

INITIAL ASSESSMENT AND MANAGEMENT

G. Musculoskeletal

1. Assessment

a. Inspect the upper and lower extremities for evidence of blunt and penetrating injury, including contusions, lacerations, and deformity.

b. Palpate the upper and lower extremities for tenderness, crepitation, abnormal movement, and sensation.

c. Palpate all peripheral pulses for presence, absence, and equality.

d. Assess the pelvis for evidence of fracture and associated hemorrhage.

e. Inspect and palpate the thoracic and lumbar spine for evidence of blunt and penetrating injury, including contusions, lacerations, tenderness, deformity, and sensation.

f. Evaluate the pelvic x-ray for evidence of a fracture.

g. Obtain x-rays of suspected fracture sites as indicated.

2. Management

a. Apply and/or readjust appropriate splinting devices for extremity fractures as indicated.

b. Maintain immobilization of the patient's thoracic and lumbar spine.

c. Apply the pneumatic antishock garment or wrap a sheet around the pelvis as indicated to reduce pelvic volume and control hemorrhage associated with a pelvic fracture.

d. Apply a splint to immobilize an extremity injury.

e. Administer tetanus immunization.

f. Administer medications as indicated or as directed by specialist.

g. Consider the possibility of compartment syndrome.

h. Perform a complete neurovascular examination of the extremities.

H. Neurologic

1. Assessment

a. Reevaluate the pupils and level of consciousness.

b. Determine the GCS Score.

c. Evaluate the upper and lower extremities for motor and sensory functions.

d. Observe for lateralizing signs.

2. Management

a. Continue ventilation and oxygenation.

b. Maintain adequate immobilization of the entire patient.

I. Adjuncts to the Secondary Survey

Consider the need for and obtain these diagnostic tests as the patient's condition permits and warrants:

1. Additional spinal x-rays

2. CT of the head, chest, abdomen, and/or spine

3. Contrast urography

4. Angiography

5. Extremity x-rays

6. Transesophageal ultrasound

INITIAL ASSESSMENT AND MANAGEMENT *Initial Assessment and Management*

7. Bronchoscopy

8. Esophagoscopy

III. PATIENT REEVALUATION

Reevaluate the patient, noting, reporting, and documenting any changes in the patient's condition and responses to resuscitative efforts. Judicious use of analgesics may be employed. Continuous monitoring of vital signs, urinary output, and the patient's response to treatment is essential.

IV. TRANSFER TO DEFINITIVE CARE

Outline rationale for patient transfer, transfer procedures, patient's needs during transfer, and indicate need for direct doctor-to-doctor communication.

Table 2—Secondary Survey

ITEM TO ASSESS	ESTABLISHES/ IDENTIFIES	ASSESS	FINDING	CONFIRM BY
Level of Consciousness	• Severity of head injury	• GCS Score	• ≤8, Severe head injury • 9–12, Moderate head injury • 13–15, Minor head injury	• CT scan • Repeat without paralyzing agents
Pupils	• Type of head injury • Presence of eye injury	• Size • Shape • Reactivity	• Mass effect • Diffuse brain injury • Ophthalmic injury	• CT scan
Head	• Scalp injury • Skull injury	• Inspect for lacerations and skull fractures • Palpable defects	• Scalp laceration • Depressed skull fracture • Basilar skull fracture	• CT scan
Maxillofacial	• Soft-tissue injury • Bone injury • Nerve injury • Teeth/mouth injury	• Visual deformity • Malocclusion • Palpation for crepitus	• Facial fracture • Soft-tissue injury	• Facial-bone x-ray • CT scan of facial bones
Neck	• Laryngeal injury • C-spine injury • Vascular injury • Esophageal injury • Neurologic deficit	• Visual inspection • Palpation • Auscultation	• Laryngeal deformity • Subcutaneous emphysema • Hematoma • Bruit • Platysmal penetration • Pain, tenderness of c-spine	• C-spine x-ray • Angiography/ duplex exam • Esophagoscopy • Laryngoscopy
Thorax	• Thoracic wall injury • Subcutaneous emphysema • Pneumo/ hemothorax • Bronchial injury • Pulmonary contusion • Thoracic aortic disruption	• Visual inspection • Palpation • Auscultation	• Bruising, deformity, or paradoxical motion • Chest-wall tenderness, crepitus • Diminished breath sounds • Muffled heart tones • Mediastinal crepitus • Severe back pain	• Chest x-ray • CT scan • Angiography • Bronchioscopy • Tube thoracostomy • Pericardiocentesis • TE ultrasound

INITIAL ASSESSMENT AND MANAGEMENT *Initial Assessment and Management*

Table 2—Secondary Survey (continued)

ITEM TO ASSESS	ESTABLISHES/ IDENTIFIES	ASSESS	FINDING	CONFIRM BY

Abdomen/ Flank	• Abdominal wall injury
	 • Intraperitoneal injury
	 • Retroperitoneal injury
		• Visual inspection
		 • Palpation
		 • Auscultation
		 • Determine path of penetration
			• Abdominal wall pain/tenderness
			 • Peritoneal irritation
			   • Visceral injury
			   • Retroperitoneal organ injury
				• DPL/ultrasound
				 • CT scan
				 • Celiotomy
				 • Contrast GI x-ray studies
				 • Angiography

Pelvis	• GU tract injuries
	 • Pelvic fracture(s)
		• Palpate symphysis pubis for widening
		 • Palpate bony pelvis for tenderness
		 • Determine pelvic stability only once
		 • Inspect perineum
		 • Rectal/vaginal exam
			• GU tract injury (hematuria)
			 • Pelvic fracture
			 • Rectal, vaginal, and/or perineal injury
				• Pelvic x-ray
				 • GU contrast studies
				   • Urethrogram
				   • Cystogram
				   • IVP
				 • Contrast-enhanced CT

Spinal Cord	• Cranial injury • Cord injury • Peripheral nerve(s) injury	• Motor response • Pain response	• Unilateral cranial mass effect • Quadriplegia • Paraplegia • Nerve root injury	• Plain spine x-rays • MRI
Vertebral Column	• Column injury • Vertebral instability • Nerve injury	• Verbal response to pain, lateralizing signs • Palpate for tenderness • Deformity	• Fracture vs dislocation	• Plain x-rays • CT scan
Extremities	• Soft-tissue injury • Bony deformities • Joint abnormalities • Neurovascular defects	• Visual inspection • Palpation	• Swelling, bruising, pallor • Malalignment • Pain, tenderness, crepitus • Absent/ diminished pulses • Tense muscular compartments • Neurologic deficits	• Specific x-rays • Doppler examination • Compartment pressures • Angiography

CHAPTER 2

Airway and Ventilatory Management

■ OBJECTIVES:

Upon completion of this chapter, the student will be able to identify actual or impending airway obstruction, explain the techniques of establishing and maintaining a patent airway, and confirm the adequacy of ventilation. Specifically, the doctor will be able to:

A. Identify the clinical settings in which airway compromise is likely to occur.

B. Recognize the signs and symptoms of acute airway obstruction.

C. Describe the techniques to establish and maintain a patent airway and confirm the adequacy of ventilation and oxygenation, including pulse oximetry and carbon dioxide (CO_2) colorimetric monitoring.

D. Define the term "definitive airway" and outline the steps needed to maintain oxygenation before, during, and after establishing a definitive airway.

AIRWAY AND VENTILATORY MANAGEMENT

I. INTRODUCTION

Inadequate delivery of oxygenated blood to the brain and other vital structures is the quickest killer of the injured. Prevention of hypoxemia requires a protected, unobstructed airway and adequate ventilation that must take priority over all other conditions. An airway must be secured, oxygen delivered and ventilatory support provided. **Supplemental oxygen must be administered to all trauma patients.**

Early preventable deaths from airway problems after trauma often result from:

1. Failure to recognize the need for an airway.
2. Inability to establish an airway.
3. Failure to recognize an incorrectly placed airway.
4. Displacement of a previously established airway.
5. Failure to recognize the need for ventilation.
6. Aspiration of gastric contents.

Remember: Airway and ventilation are the first priorities.

II. AIRWAY

A. Problem Recognition

Airway compromise may be sudden and complete, insidious and partial, and progressive and/or recurrent. Although often related to pain and/or anxiety, tachypnea may be a subtle but early sign of airway or ventilatory compromise. Therefore, assessment and frequent reassessment of airway patency and adequacy of ventilation are important. The patient with an altered level of consciousness is at particular risk for airway compromise and often requires provision of a definitive airway. The unconscious head-injured patient, the patient obtunded from alcohol and/or other drugs, and the patient with thoracic injuries may have compromised ventilatory effort. In these patients, endotracheal intubation is intended to (1) provide an airway, (2) deliver supplementary oxygen, (3) support ventilation, and (4) prevent aspiration. **Maintaining oxygenation and preventing hypercarbia are critical in managing the trauma patient, especially if the patient has sustained a head injury.**

The doctor should anticipate vomiting in all injured patients and be prepared. The presence of gastric contents in the oropharynx confirms a significant risk of aspiration with the patient's very next breath. Immediate suctioning and rotation of the **entire patient** to the lateral position are indicated.

1. Maxillofacial trauma

Trauma to the face demands aggressive airway management. The mechanism for this injury is exemplified by the unbelted passenger/driver who is thrown into the windshield and dashboard. Trauma to the midface may produce fractures/dislocations with compromise to the nasopharynx and oropharynx. Facial fractures may be associated with hemorrhage, increased secretions, and dislodged teeth, causing additional problems in maintaining a patent airway. Fractures of the mandible, especially bilateral body fractures, may cause loss of normal support. Airway obstruction results if the patient is in a supine position. Patients who refuse to lie down may be indicating difficulty in maintaining their airway or handling secretions.

2. Neck trauma

Penetrating injury to the neck may result in vascular injury with significant hemorrhage. This may result in displacement and obstruction of the airway. An urgent surgical airway may be necessary if this displacement and obstruction make endotracheal intubation impossible. Hemorrhage from adjacent vascular injury may be massive and operative control may be required.

Blunt or penetrating injury to the neck may cause disruption of the larynx or trachea, resulting in airway obstruction or severe bleeding into the tracheobronchial tree. A definitive airway is urgently required.

Neck injuries may cause partial airway obstruction by disruption of the larynx and trachea or by compression of the airway from hemorrhage into the soft tissues of the neck. Initially, a patient with this type of serious airway injury may be able to maintain airway patency and ventilation. However, if airway compromise is suspected, a definitive airway must be established. To prevent extending an existing airway injury, an endotracheal tube must be inserted cautiously. When the patient loses airway patency, it may be

AIRWAY AND VENTILATORY MANAGEMENT

precipitous, and an early surgical airway usually is indicated.

3. Laryngeal trauma

Although fracture of the larynx is a rare injury, it can present with acute airway obstruction. It is indicated by the following triad:

a. Hoarseness

b. Subcutaneous emphysema

c. Palpable fracture

If the patient's airway is totally obstructed or the patient is in severe respiratory distress, an attempt at intubation is warranted. Flexible endoscopic-guided intubation may be helpful in this situation, but only if it can be performed promptly. If intubation is unsuccessful, an emergency tracheostomy is indicated, followed by operative repair. However, a tracheostomy, when done under emergency conditions, is difficult to perform, may be associated with profuse bleeding, and may be time-consuming. Surgical cricothyroidotomy, although not preferred for this situation, may be a lifesaving option.

Penetrating trauma to the larynx or trachea is overt and requires immediate attention. Complete tracheal transection or occlusion of the airway with blood or soft tissue can cause acute airway compromise that requires immediate correction. These injuries are often associated with esophageal, carotid artery, or jugular vein trauma, as well as extensive tissue destruction surrounding the area due to blast effect.

Noisy breathing indicates partial airway obstruction that suddenly may become complete. Absence of breathing suggests that complete obstruction already exists. When the level of consciousness is depressed, detection of significant airway obstruction is more subtle. Labored respiratory effort may be the only clue to airway obstruction and tracheobronchial injury.

If a fracture of the larynx is suspected, based on the mechanism of injury and subtle physical findings, computed tomography (CT) may help to identify this injury.

During initial assessment of the airway, the "talking patient" provides reassurance (at least for the moment) that the airway is patent and not com-

promised. Therefore, the most important early measure is to talk to the patient and stimulate a verbal response. A positive, appropriate verbal response indicates that the airway is patent, ventilation is intact, and brain perfusion is adequate. Failure to respond or an inappropriate response suggests an altered level of consciousness or airway/ventilatory compromise.

B. Objective Signs—Airway Obstruction

1. Look to see if the patient is agitated or obtunded. Agitation suggests hypoxia, and obtundation suggests hypercarbia. Cyanosis indicates hypoxemia due to inadequate oxygenation and should be sought by inspection of the nail beds and circumoral skin. Look for retractions and the use of accessory muscles of ventilation that, when present, provide additional evidence of airway compromise.

2. Listen for abnormal sounds. Noisy breathing is obstructed breathing. Snoring, gurgling, and crowing sounds (stridor) may be associated with partial occlusion of the pharynx or larynx. Hoarseness (dysphonia) implies functional, laryngeal obstruction. The abusive or belligerent patient may be hypoxic and should not be presumed to be intoxicated.

3. Feel for location of the trachea and quickly determine if the trachea is midline.

III. VENTILATION

A. Problem Recognition

Assuring a patent airway is an important first step in providing oxygen to the patient but it is only a first step. An unobstructed airway is not likely to benefit the patient unless the patient also is ventilating adequately. Ventilation may be compromised by airway obstruction but also by altered ventilatory mechanics or central nervous system (CNS) depression. If breathing is not improved by clearing the airway, other etiologies must be sought. Direct trauma to the chest, especially with rib fractures, causes pain with breathing and leads to rapid, shallow ventilation and hypoxemia. Elderly patients and those with preexisting pulmonary dysfunction are at significant risk for ventilatory failure under these circumstances. Intracranial injury may cause abnormal patterns of breathing and compromise

AIRWAY AND VENTILATORY MANAGEMENT

adequacy of ventilation. Cervical spinal cord injury may result in diaphragmatic breathing and interfere with the ability to meet increased oxygen demands. Complete cervical cord transection, which spares the phrenic nerves (C-3, 4), results in abdominal breathing and paralysis of the intercostal muscles. Assisted ventilation may be required.

B. Objective Signs—Inadequate Ventilation

1. Look for symmetrical rise and fall of the chest and adequate chest wall excursion. Asymmetry suggests splinting or a flail chest and any labored breathing should be regarded as an imminent threat to the patient's oxygenation.

2. Listen for movement of air on both sides of the chest. Decreased or absent breath sounds over one or both hemithoraces should alert the examiner to the presence of thoracic injury. (See Chapter 4, Thoracic Trauma.) Beware of a rapid respiratory rate—tachypnea may indicate air hunger.

3. Use a pulse oximeter. This device gives information regarding the patient's oxygen saturation and peripheral perfusion, but does not assure adequate ventilation.

IV. MANAGEMENT

The assessment of airway patency and adequacy of ventilation must be done quickly and accurately. Pulse oximetry is essential. If problems are identified or **suspected**, measures should be instituted immediately to improve oxygenation and reduce the risk of further ventilatory compromise. These include airway maintenance techniques, definitive airway measures (including surgical airway), and methods to provide supplemental ventilation. Because all of these may require some neck motion, protection of the cervical spine must be provided in all patients, especially if the patient has a known, unstable cervical spine injury or is incompletely evaluated and at risk. The spinal cord must be protected until the possibility of a spinal injury has been excluded by clinical assessment and appropriate x-ray studies.

Patients wearing a helmet and requiring airway management should have the head and neck held in a neutral position while the helmet is removed. This is a 2-person procedure. One person provides in-line manual immobilization from below while the second person expands the helmet laterally and removes it from above. In-line manual immobilization is reestablished from above and the patient's head and neck are secured during airway management. Removal of the helmet using a cast cutter while stabilizing the head and neck minimizes cervical spine motion in the patient with a known cervical spine injury.

Supplemental oxygen should be provided before and immediately after airway management measures are instituted. A rigid suction device is essential and should be readily available. Patients with facial injuries may have associated cribriform plate fractures and the use of soft suction catheters (or nasogastric tube) inserted through the nose may result in passage of the tube into the cranial vault.

A. Airway Maintenance Techniques

The tongue may fall backward and obstruct the hypopharynx if the patient has a decreased level of consciousness. This form of obstruction can be corrected readily by the chin-lift or jaw-thrust maneuver. The airway can then be maintained with an oropharyngeal or nasopharyngeal airway. Maneuvers employed to establish an airway might produce or aggravate cervical spine injury. Therefore, in-line immobilization of the cervical spine is essential during these procedures.

1. Chin lift

The fingers of 1 hand are placed under the mandible, which is gently lifted upward to bring the chin anterior. The thumb of the same hand lightly depresses the lower lip to open the mouth. The thumb also may be placed behind the lower incisors and, simultaneously, the chin gently lifted. The chin-lift maneuver should not hyperextend the neck. This maneuver is useful for the trauma victim because it does not risk compromising a possible cervical spine fracture or converting a fracture without cord injury into one with cord injury.

2. Jaw thrust

The jaw-thrust maneuver is performed by grasping the angles of the lower jaw, one hand on each side, and displacing the mandible forward. When this method is used with the face mask of a bag-valve device, a good seal and adequate ventilation are achieved.

AIRWAY AND VENTILATORY MANAGEMENT

3. Oropharyngeal airway

The oral airway is inserted into the mouth behind the tongue. The preferred technique is to use a tongue blade to depress the tongue and then insert the airway posteriorly. The airway must not push the tongue backward and block, rather than clear, the airway. This device must not be used in the conscious patient because it may induce gagging, vomiting, and aspiration.

An alternative technique is to insert the oral airway upside down, so its concavity is directed upward, until the soft palate is encountered. At this point, with the device rotated 180°, the concavity is directed caudad and the device is slipped into place over the tongue. This method should not be used for children, because the rotation of the device may damage the mouth and pharynx.

4. Nasopharyngeal airway

The nasopharyngeal airway is inserted in 1 nostril and passed gently into the posterior oropharynx. The nasopharyngeal airway is preferred to the oropharyngeal airway in the responsive patient because it is better tolerated and less likely to induce vomiting. It should be well lubricated, then inserted into the nostril that appears to be unobstructed. If obstruction is encountered during introduction of the airway, stop and try the other nostril. If the tip of the nasopharyngeal tube is visible in the posterior oropharynx, it may provide safe passage of a nasogastric tube in the patient with facial fractures.

5. Multilumen esophageal airway device

The multilumen esophageal airway device is used by some prehospital personnel to achieve an airway when a definitive airway is not feasible. One of the ports communicates with the esophagus and one with the airway. The personnel who use these tubes are trained to observe which one is occluding the esophagus and which will provide air to the trachea. The esophageal port is occluded by a balloon and the other port ventilated. A CO_2 detector improves the accuracy with this apparatus. The multilumen esophageal airway device must be removed and/or a definitive airway provided by the doctor after appropriate assessment of the needs of the patient.

6. Laryngeal mask airway (LMA)

The LMA does not provide a definitive airway. Proper placement of this device is difficult without appropriate training. Its role in the resuscitation of the injured patient has not been defined. When a patient has an LMA in place on arrival in the emergency department, the doctor must decide after immediate assessment whether removal or replacement with an endotracheal tube is necessary.

B. Definitive Airway

A definitive airway requires a tube present in the trachea with the cuff inflated, the tube connected to some form of oxygen-enriched assisted ventilation, and the airway secured in place with tape. Definitive airways are of 3 varieties: orotracheal tube, nasotracheal tube, and surgical airway (cricothyroidotomy or tracheostomy). The decision to provide a definitive airway is based on clinical findings and includes (1) presence of apnea; (2) inability to maintain a patent airway by other means; (3) need to protect the lower airway from aspiration of blood or vomitus; (4) impending or potential compromise of the airway, eg, following inhalation injury, facial fractures, retropharyngeal hematoma, or sustained seizure activity; (5) presence of a closed head injury requiring assisted ventilation (GCS Score <8); and (6) inability to maintain adequate oxygenation by face-mask oxygen supplementation. (See Table 1, Indication for Definitive Airway, page 46.)

The urgency of the situation and circumstances determining the need for airway intervention dictate the specific route and method to be used. Continued assisted ventilation is aided by supplemental sedation, analgesics, or muscle relaxants, as indicated. The use of a pulse oximeter may be helpful in determining the need for a definitive airway, the urgency of the need, and, by inference, the effectiveness of airway placement. Orotracheal and nasotracheal intubations are the methods used most frequently. The potential for concomitant c-spine injury is of major concern in the patient requiring an airway. Figure 1, Airway Algorithm, page 47, provides a scheme by which decisions for the appropriate route of airway management can be made.

C. Definitive Airway—Endotracheal Intubation

It is important to establish the presence or absence of a cervical spine fracture. However, obtaining c-spine

AIRWAY AND VENTILATORY MANAGEMENT

Table 1—Indications for Definitive Airway

NEED FOR AIRWAY PROTECTION	NEED FOR VENTILATION
Unconscious	Apnea • Neuromuscular paralysis • Unconscious
Severe maxillofacial fractures	Inadequate respiratory efforts • Tachypnea • Hypoxia • Hypercarbia • Cyanosis
Risk for aspiration • Bleeding • Vomiting	Severe, closed head injury with need for brief hyperventilation if acute neurologic deterioration occurs
Risk for obstruction • Neck hematoma • Laryngeal, tracheal injury • Stridor	

x-rays should **not** impede or delay establishing a definitive airway when one is clearly indicated. The patient who has a GCS Score of 8 or less requires prompt intubation. If there is no immediate need for intubation, x-ray of the cervical spine may be obtained. **However, a normal lateral cervical spine film does not exclude a c-spine injury.**

Note: **The most important determinant of whether to proceed with orotracheal or nasotracheal intubation is the experience of the doctor. Both techniques are safe and effective when performed properly.** Esophageal occlusion by cricoid pressure is useful in preventing aspiration and providing better visualization of the airway.

If the decision is made that orotracheal intubation is indicated, the 2-person technique with in-line cervical spine immobilization should be used. If the patient is **apneic**, orotracheal intubation is indicated.

Following insertion of the orotracheal tube, the cuff should be inflated and assisted ventilation should be instituted. Proper placement of the tube is suggested but not confirmed by hearing equal breath sounds bilaterally and detecting no borborygmi in the epigastrium. The presence of gurgling noises in the epigastrium with inspiration suggests esophageal intubation and warrants repositioning of the tube. A carbon dioxide (CO_2) detector (colorimetric

CO_2 monitoring device) is indicated to help confirm proper intubation of the airway. The presence of CO_2 in exhaled air is an indication that the airway has been successfully intubated, but does not assure the correct position of the endotracheal tube. If CO_2 is not detected, esophageal intubation has occurred. Proper position of the tube is best confirmed by chest x-ray, once the possibility of esophageal intubation is excluded. Colorimetric CO_2 indicators are not useful for physiologic monitoring or assessing the adequacy of ventilation. When the proper position of the tube is determined, it should be secured in place. If the patient is moved, tube placement should be reassessed by auscultation of both lateral lung fields for equality of breath sounds and by reassessing for exhaled CO_2.

Nasotracheal intubation is a useful technique when urgency of airway management precludes a cervical spine x-ray. Blind nasotracheal intubation requires spontaneous breathing. It is **contraindicated in the apneic patient.** The deeper the patient breathes, the easier it is to follow the airflow through the larynx. Facial, frontal sinus, basilar skull, and cribriform plate fractures are relative contraindications to nasotracheal intubation. Evidence of nasal fracture, raccoon eyes, Battle sign, and possible cerebrospinal fluid leaks (rhinorrhea or otorrhea) identify patients with these injuries. Precautions regarding cervical spine immobilization should be followed as with orotracheal intubation.

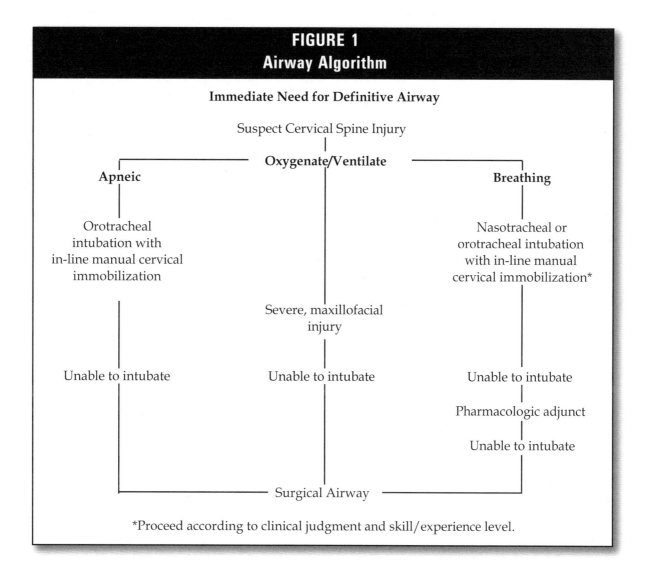

FIGURE 1
Airway Algorithm

Immediate Need for Definitive Airway

Suspect Cervical Spine Injury

Oxygenate/Ventilate

Apneic

Orotracheal intubation with in-line manual cervical immobilization

Breathing

Nasotracheal or orotracheal intubation with in-line manual cervical immobilization*

Severe, maxillofacial injury

Unable to intubate   Unable to intubate   Unable to intubate

Pharmacologic adjunct

Unable to intubate

Surgical Airway

*Proceed according to clinical judgment and skill/experience level.

Patients who arrive at the hospital with an endotracheal tube in place must have the proper position of the tube confirmed. This is important because the tube may have been inserted into the esophagus, a mainstem bronchus, or dislodged during patient transport from the field or another hospital. A chest x-ray, CO_2 monitoring, and physical examination are essential to assess the position of the tube. Carbon dioxide in the exhaled air will confirm that the tube is in the airway.

Patients with a cervical spine injury, severe arthritis of the cervical spine, a short muscular neck, or maxillofacial/mandibular injury may be technically difficult to intubate. The use of a flexible fiberoptic endoscope may facilitate these difficult intubations.

The use of anesthetic, sedative, and neuromuscular-blocking drugs for endotracheal intubation in the trauma patient is risky. In certain cases the need for an airway justifies the risk of these drugs. The doctor who uses these drugs must understand their pharmacology, be skilled in the techniques of endotracheal intubation, and be able to obtain a surgical airway if necessary. In many cases where an airway is acutely needed during the primary survey, the use of paralyzing or sedating drugs is not necessary.

The technique for rapid-sequence intubation is as follows:

1. Be prepared to perform a surgical airway in the event that airway control is lost

AIRWAY AND VENTILATORY MANAGEMENT

2. Preoxygenate the patient with 100% oxygen.

3. Apply pressure over the cricoid cartilage.

4. Administer a sedative (eg, etomidate, 0.3 mg/kg or 30 mg, or midazolam 2 to 5 mg intravenously)

5. Administer 1 to 2 mg/kg succinylcholine intravenously (usual dose, 100 mg).

6. After the patient relaxes, intubate the patient orotracheally.

7. Inflate the cuff and confirm tube placement (auscultate the patient's chest and determine presence of CO_2 in exhaled air).

8. Release cricoid pressure.

9. Ventilate the patient.

Etomidate does not have a significant effect on the blood or intracranial pressure. This drug does provide adequate sedation, which is advantageous in these patients. Etomidate or other sedatives must be used with great care to avoid loss of the airway as the patient becomes sedated. Then, succinylcholine, which is a short-acting drug, should be administered. It has a rapid onset of paralysis of less than 1 minute and duration of about 5 minutes or less. The most dangerous complication of using sedation and neuromuscular blocking agents is the inability to establish an airway. If endotracheal intubation is unsuccessful, the patient must be ventilated with a bag-valve-mask device until the paralysis resolves. Long-acting drugs are not used for this reason. Succinylcholine should not be used because of the potential for severe hyperkalemia in the patient with preexisting chronic renal failure, chronic paralysis, or chronic neuromuscular disease.

Induction agents, such as thiopental and sedatives, are dangerous to use in the hypovolemic trauma patient. Small doses of diazepam or midazolam are appropriate to reduce anxiety in the paralyzed patient. Flumazenil must be available to reverse the sedative effects after benzodiazepines have been administered. Practice patterns, drug preferences, and specific procedures for airway management vary between institutions. The principle that the individual utilizing these techniques be skilled in their use, knowledgeable of the inherent pitfalls associated with rapid sequence intubation, and capable of managing the potential complications cannot be overstated.

D. Definitive Airway—Surgical Airway

Inability to intubate the trachea is a clear indication for creating a surgical airway. A surgical airway is performed when edema of the glottis, fracture of the larynx, or severe oropharyngeal hemorrhage obstructs the airway and an endotracheal tube cannot be placed through the cords. A surgical cricothyroidotomy is preferable to a tracheostomy for most patients requiring an emergency surgical airway. A surgical cricothyroidotomy is easier to perform, is associated with less bleeding, and requires less time to perform than an emergency tracheostomy.

1. Jet insufflation of the airway (See Skills Station III, Cricothyroidotomy)

Insertion of a needle through the cricothyroid membrane or into the trachea is a useful technique in emergency situations that provides oxygen on a short-term basis until a definitive airway can be placed. Jet insufflation can provide temporary, supplemental oxygenation so that intubation can be accomplished on an urgent rather than an emergent basis. The jet insufflation technique is performed by placing a large-caliber plastic cannula, #12- to #14-gauge (#16- to #18-gauge in children), through the cricothyroid membrane into the trachea below the level of the obstruction. The cannula is then connected to wall oxygen at 15 L/minute (40 to 50 psi) with either a Y-connector or a side hole cut in the tubing attached between the oxygen source and the plastic cannula. Intermittent insufflation, 1 second on and 4 seconds off, can then be achieved by placing the thumb over the open end of the Y-connector or the side hole. The patient can be adequately oxygenated for only 30 to 45 minutes using this technique. However, only patients with normal pulmonary function who do not have a significant chest injury can be ventilated in this manner. During the 4 seconds that the oxygen is not being delivered under pressure, some exhalation occurs. Because of the inadequate exhalation, CO_2 slowly accumulates and limits the use of this technique, especially in head-injured patients.

Jet insufflation must be used with caution when complete foreign body obstruction of the glottic area is suspected. Although high pressure may expel the impacted material into the hypopharynx where it can be readily removed, significant barotrauma may occur, including pulmonary rupture with tension pneumothorax. Low flow rates (5 to 7 L/minute) should be used when persistent glottic obstruction is present.

2. Surgical cricothyroidotomy (See Skills Station III, Cricothyroidotomy)

Surgical cricothyroidotomy is performed by making a skin incision that extends through the cricothyroid membrane. A curved hemostat may be inserted to dilate the opening, and a small endotracheal tube or tracheostomy tube (preferably 5 to 7 mm OD) can be inserted. When the endotracheal tube is used, the cervical collar can be reapplied. One must be alert to the possibility that the endotracheal tube can become malpositioned and is easily advanced into a bronchus. Care must be taken, especially with children, to avoid damage to the cricoid cartilage, which is the only circumferential support to the upper trachea. Therefore, surgical cricothyroidotomy is not recommended for children under 12 years of age. (See Chapter 10, Extremes of Age: A. Pediatric Trauma.)

In recent years percutaneous tracheostomy has been reported as an alternative to open tracheostomy. This is not a safe procedure in the acute trauma situation, because the patient's neck must be hyperextended to properly position the head to perform the procedure safely. Percutaneous tracheostomy requires the use of a heavy guidewire and sharp dilator, or a guidewire and multiple dilators. This may be dangerous and/or time-consuming, depending on the type of equipment used.

E. Airway Decision Scheme

The airway decision scheme (Figure 1, Airway Algorithm, page 47) applies only to the patient who is in acute respiratory distress (or apneic) and in need of an immediate airway, **and** in whom a cervical spine injury is suspected by mechanism of injury or physical examination. The first priority is to assure continued oxygenation with maintenance of cervical spine immobilization. This is accomplished initially by position (ie, chin lift or jaw thrust) and preliminary airway techniques (ie, oropharyngeal airway or nasopharyngeal airway) already discussed.

In the patient who is still showing some respiratory effort, a nasotracheal tube may be passed if the doctor is skilled in this technique. Otherwise, an orotracheal tube should be passed while a second person provides in-line immobilization. If neither a nasotracheal nor an orotracheal tube can be inserted and the patient's respiratory status is in jeopardy, a cricothyroidotomy should be performed.

In the apneic patient, in-line immobilization should be maintained by 1 person and orotracheal intubation should be performed by another. If severe maxillofacial injury precludes nasotracheal intubation and orotracheal intubation cannot be achieved for any reason, a cricothyroidotomy is indicated.

Oxygenation and ventilation must be maintained before, during, and immediately upon completion of insertion of the definitive airway. Prolonged periods of inadequate or absent ventilation and oxygenation should be avoided.

F. Oxygenation

Oxygenated inspired air is best provided via a tight-fitting oxygen reservoir face mask with a flow rate of 11 L/minute. Other methods (eg, nasal catheter, nasal cannula, nonrebreather mask) can improve inspired oxygen concentration.

Because changes in oxygenation occur rapidly and are impossible to detect clinically, pulse oximetry should be used when difficulties are anticipated in intubation or ventilation. This includes the transport of the critically injured patient. Pulse oximetry is a noninvasive method to **continuously** measure oxygen saturation (O_2 sat) of arterial blood. It does **not** measure the partial pressure of oxygen (Pao_2) and, depending on the position of the oxyhemoglobin dissociation curve, the Pao_2 may vary widely. (See Table 2, Approximate Pao_2 Versus O_2 Hemoglobin Saturation Levels, page 50.) However, a measured saturation of 95% or greater by pulse oximetry is strong corroborating evidence of adequate, peripheral arterial oxygenation (Pao_2 >70 mm Hg or 9.3 kPa). Pulse oximetry requires intact peripheral perfusion and cannot distinguish oxyhemoglobin from carboxyhemoglobin or methemoglobin, which limits its usefulness in the severely vasoconstricted patient and in the patient with carbon monoxide poisoning. Profound anemia (hemoglobin <5 g/dL) and hypothermia (<30°C or 86°F) decrease the reliability of the technique. However, in most trauma patients pulse oximetry is not only useful, but also continuous monitoring of oxygen saturation provides an immediate assessment of therapeutic interventions.

AIRWAY AND VENTILATORY MANAGEMENT

(See Skills Station II, Airway and Ventilatory Management: VII., Pulse, Oximetry Monitoring, at the conclusion of this chapter.)

G. Ventilation

Effective ventilation can be achieved by bag-valve-face mask techniques. However, 1-person ventilation techniques, using a bag-valve mask, are less effective than 2-person techniques in which both hands can be used to assure a good seal. Bag-valve-mask ventilation should be performed by 2 people whenever possible.

Intubation of the hypoventilated and/or apneic patient may not be successful initially and may require multiple attempts. The patient **must be ventilated periodically** during prolonged efforts to intubate. The doctor should practice taking a deep breath when intubation is first attempted. When the doctor must breathe, the attempted intubation should be aborted and the patient ventilated.

With intubation of the trachea accomplished, assisted ventilation should follow using positive-pressure breathing techniques. A volume- or pressure-regulated respirator can be used, depending on availability of the equipment. The doctor should be alert to the complications secondary to changes in intrathoracic pressure, which can convert a simple pneumothorax to a tension pneumothorax, or even create a pneumothorax secondary to barotrauma.

H. Pitfalls

1. The inability to intubate the patient expediently or to provide a surgical airway results in hypoxia and patient deterioration. Remember that performing a needle cricothyroidotomy with jet insufflation may provide the time necessary to establish a definitive airway.

2. Trauma patients may vomit and aspirate. Functional suction equipment must be immediately available, and the doctor should ensure a secure, patent airway in all trauma patients.

3. Gastric distention may occur when ventilating the patient with a bag-valve-mask device, which may result in the patient vomiting and aspirating. It also may cause distention of the stomach against the vena cava, resulting in hypotension and bradycardia.

4. Equipment failure may occur at the most inopportune time and cannot always be anticipated, eg, the light on the laryngoscope burns out, the laryngoscope batteries are weak, the endotracheal tube cuff leaks, or the pulse oximeter does not function properly.

V. SUMMARY

A. Actual or impending airway obstruction should be suspected in all injured patients.

B. With all airway maneuvers, the cervical spine must be protected by in-line immobilization.

C. Clinical signs suggesting airway compromise should be managed by securing a patent airway and providing adequate oxygen-enriched ventilation.

Table 2–Approximate Pao_2 Versus O_2 Hemoglobin Saturation Levels

Pao_2 LEVELS	O_2 HEMOGLOBIN SATURATION LEVELS
90 mm Hg	100%
60 mm Hg	90%
30 mm Hg	60%
27 mm Hg	50%

D. A definitive airway should be inserted if there is any doubt on the part of the doctor as to the integrity of the patient's airway.

E. A definitive airway should be placed early after the patient has been ventilated with oxygen-enriched air, and prolonged periods of apnea must be avoided.

F. Airway management requires assessment and reassessment of airway patency, tube position, and ventilatory effectiveness.

G. The selection of orotracheal or nasotracheal routes for intubation is based on the experience and skill level of the doctor.

H. Surgical airway is indicated whenever an airway is needed and intubation is unsuccessful.

■ BIBLIOGRAPHY

1. Aprahamian C, Thompson BM, Finger WA, et al: Experimental cervical spine injury model: evaluation of airway management and splinting techniques. **Annals of Emergency Medicine** 1984; 13(8):584–587.

2. Bergen JM, Smith DC: A review of etomidate for rapid sequence intubation in the emergency department. **Journal of Emergency Medicine** 1997; 15(2): 221–230.

3. Brantigan CO, Grow JB Sr: Cricothyroidotomy: Elective use in respiratory problems requiring tracheotomy. **Journal of Thoracic and Cardiovascular Surgery** 1976; 71:72–81.

4. Danzl DF, Thomas DM: Nasotracheal intubation in the emergency department. **Critical Care Medicine** 1980; 8(11):667–682.

5. Frame SB, Simon JM, Kerstein MD, et al: Percutaneous transtracheal catheter ventilation (PTCV) in complete airway obstructions canine model. **Journal of Trauma** 1989; 29(6):774–781.

6. Fremstad JD, Martin SH: Lethal complication from insertion of nasogastric tube after severe basilar skull fracture. **Journal of Trauma** 1978; 18:820–822.

7. Guildner CV: Resuscitation—opening the airway. A comparative study of techniques for opening an airway obstructed by the tongue. **Journal of American College of Emergency Physicians** 1976; 5:588–590.

8. Iserson KV: Blind nasotracheal intubation. **Annals of Emergency Medicine** 1981; 10:468.

9. Jorden RC, Moore EE, Marx JA, et al: A comparison of PTV and endotracheal ventilation in an acute trauma model. **Journal of Trauma** 1985; 25(10):978–983.

10. Kress TD, et al: Cricothyroidotomy. **Annals of Emergency Medicine** 1982; 11:197.

11. Levinson MM, Scuderi PE, Gibson RL, et al: Emergency percutaneous and transtracheal ventilation. **Journal of American College of Emergency Physicians** 1979; 8(10):396–400.

12. Majernick TG, Bieniek R, Houston JB, et al: Cervical spine movement during orotracheal intubation. **Annals of Emergency Medicine** 1986; 15(4):417–420.

13. Seshul MB Sr, Sinn DP, Gerlock AJ Jr: The Andy Gump fracture of the mandible: a cause of respiratory obstruction or distress. **Journal of Trauma** 1978; 18:611–612.

14. Walter J, Doris PE, Shaffer MA: Clinical presentation of patients with acute cervical spine injury. **Annals of Emergency Medicine** 1984; 13(7):512–515.

15. Yeston NS: Noninvasive measurement of blood gases. **Infections in Surgery** 1990; 90:18–24.

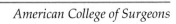

SKILLS STATION

Airway and Ventilatory Management

■ OBJECTIVES:

Performance at this station will allow the participant to evaluate a series of clinical situations and to acquire the cognitive skills related to decision making in airway and ventilatory management. The student will practice and demonstrate the following skills on adult and infant intubation manikins.

1. Insert oral and nasal pharyngeal airways.

2. Using both oral and nasal routes, intubate the trachea of an adult intubation manikin (within the guidelines listed), provide effective ventilation, and utilize the CO_2 colorimetric device to aid in determining proper placement of the endotracheal tube.

3. Intubate the trachea of an infant intubation manikin with an endotracheal tube within the guidelines listed, and provide effective ventilation.

4. Relate the indications of trauma to airway management when performing oral endotracheal intubation and nasotracheal intubation.

5. Using a pulse oximeter:
  a. Discuss the purpose of pulse oximetry monitoring.
  b. Demonstrate the proper use of the device.
  c. Discuss the indications for its use, its functional limits of accuracy, and reasons for malfunction or inaccuracy.
  d. Interpret accurately the pulse oximeter monitor readings and relate their significance to the care of the trauma patient.

■ PROCEDURES:

Eight procedures for acute airway management are outlined in Skills Station II:

  1. Oropharyngeal airway insertion

  2. Nasopharyngeal airway insertion

  3. Ventilation without intubation

  4. Orotracheal intubation

  5. Nasotracheal intubation

6. Infant endotracheal intubation

7. Pulse oximetry

8. Carbon dioxide detection

INTERACTIVE SKILLS PROCEDURES

Airway and Ventilatory Management

Note: Standard precautions are required whenever caring for the trauma patient.

Note: Scenarios are incorporated into the performance of some of these skills. The scenarios to be presented are included at the conclusion of the procedures. (See IX, Skills Scenarios.)

I. OROPHARYNGEAL AIRWAY INSERTION

A. This procedure is for temporary ventilation of the unconscious patient while preparing to intubate the patient.

B. Select the proper-sized airway. The correctly sized airway will extend from the corner of the patient's mouth to the external auditory canal.

C. Open the patient's mouth with either the chin-lift maneuver or the crossed-finger technique (scissors technique).

D. Insert a tongue blade on top of the patient's tongue far enough back to depress the tongue adequately, being careful not to gag the patient.

E. Insert the airway posteriorly, gently sliding the airway over the curvature of the tongue until the device's flange rests on top of the patient's lips. The airway must not push the tongue backward and block the airway.

F. Remove the tongue blade.

G. Ventilate the patient with a bag-valve-mask device.

II. NASOPHARYNGEAL AIRWAY INSERTION

A. This procedure is used when the patient would gag on an oropharyngeal airway.

B. Assess the nasal passages for any apparent obstruction (eg, polyps, fractures, hemorrhage).

C. Select the appropriately sized airway.

D. Lubricate the nasal pharyngeal airway with a water-soluble lubricant or tap water.

E. Insert the tip of the airway into the nostril and direct it posteriorly and toward the ear.

F. Gently insert the nasal pharyngeal airway through the nostril into the hypopharynx with a slight rotating motion, until the flange rests against the nostril.

G. Ventilate the patient with a bag-valve-mask device.

III. BAG-VALVE-MASK VENTILATION—2-PERSON TECHNIQUE

A. Select the appropriately sized mask to fit the patient's face.

B. Connect the oxygen tubing to the bag-valve device, and adjust the flow of oxygen to 12 L/minute.

AIRWAY AND VENTILATORY MANAGEMENT   *Airway and Ventilatory Management*

C. Assure that the patient's airway is patent and secured by previously described techniques.

D. The **first person** applies the mask to the patient's face, ascertaining a tight seal with both hands.

E. The **second person** ventilates the patient by squeezing the bag with both hands.

F. The adequacy of ventilation is assessed by observing the patient's chest movement.

G. The patient should be ventilated in this manner every 5 seconds.

IV. ADULT OROTRACHEAL INTUBATION

A. Assure that adequate ventilation and oxygenation are in progress, and that suctioning equipment is immediately available in the event that the patient vomits.

B. Inflate the cuff of the endotracheal tube to ascertain that the balloon does not leak, then deflate the cuff.

C. Connect the laryngoscope blade to the handle, and check the bulb for brightness.

D. Have an assistant manually immobilize the head and neck. The patient's neck must not be hyperextended or hyperflexed during this procedure.

E. Hold the laryngoscope in the left hand.

F. Insert the laryngoscope into the right side of the patient's mouth, displacing the tongue to the left.

G. Visually identify the epiglottis and then the vocal cords.

H. Gently insert the endotracheal tube into the trachea without applying pressure on the teeth or oral tissues.

I. Inflate the cuff with enough air to provide an adequate seal. **Do not overinflate the cuff.**

J. Check the placement of the endotracheal tube by bag-valve-to-tube ventilation.

K. Visually observe chest excursions with ventilation.

L. Auscultate the chest and abdomen with a stethoscope to ascertain tube position.

M. Secure the tube. If the patient is moved, the tube placement should be reassessed.

N. If endotracheal intubation is not accomplished within seconds or in the same time required to hold your breath before exhaling, discontinue attempts, ventilate the patient with a bag-valve-mask device, and try again.

O. Placement of the tube must be checked carefully. A chest x-ray is helpful to assess the position of the tube, but it cannot exclude esophageal intubation.

P. Attach a CO_2 colorimetric device to the endotracheal tube between the adapter and the ventilating device. Use of the colorimetric device provides a reliable means of confirming the position of the endotracheal tube in the airway.

Q. Attach a pulse oximeter device to one of the patient's fingers (intact peripheral perfusion must exist) to measure and monitor the patient's oxygen saturation levels. Pulse oximetry is useful to monitor oxygen saturation levels continuously and provides an immediate assessment of therapeutic interventions.

V. ADULT NASOTRACHEAL INTUBATION

Remember: Blind nasotracheal intubation is contraindicated in the apneic patient and whenever severe mid-face fractures or suspicion of basilar skull fracture exist.

A. If a cervical spine fracture is suspected, leave the cervical collar in place to assist in maintaining immobilization of the neck.

B. Assure that adequate ventilation and oxygenation are in progress.

C. Inflate the cuff of the endotracheal tube to ascertain that the balloon does not leak, then deflate the cuff.

D. If the patient is conscious, spray the nasal passage with an anesthetic and vasoconstrictor to anesthetize and constrict the mucosa. If the patient is **unconscious**, it is adequate to spray the nasal passage only with a vasoconstrictor.

E. Have an assistant maintain manual immobilization of the head and neck.

F. Lubricate the nasotracheal tube with a local anesthetic jelly and insert the tube into the nostril.

G. Guide the tube slowly but firmly into the nasal passage, going up from the nostril (to avoid the large inferior turbinate) and then backward and down into the nasopharynx. The curve of the tube should be aligned to facilitate passage along this curved course.

H. As the tube passes through the nose and into the nasopharynx, it must turn downward to pass through the pharynx.

I. Once the tube has entered the pharynx, listen to the airflow emanating from the endotracheal tube. Advance the tube until the sound of the moving air is maximal, suggesting location of the tip at the opening of the trachea. While listening to air movement, determine the point of inhalation and advance the tube quickly. If tube placement is unsuccessful, repeat the procedure by applying gentle pressure on the thyroid cartilage. **Remember, intermittently ventilate and oxygenate the patient.**

J. Inflate the cuff with enough air to provide an adequate seal. Avoid overinflation.

K. Check the placement of the endotracheal tube by bag-valve-to-tube ventilation.

L. Visually observe chest excursion with ventilation.

M. Auscultate the chest and abdomen with a stethoscope to ascertain tube position.

N. Secure the tube. If the patient is moved, the tube placement should be reassessed.

O. If endotracheal intubation is not accomplished within 30 seconds or in the same time required to hold your breath before exhaling, discontinue attempts, ventilate the patient with a bag-valve-mask device, and try again.

P. Placement of the tube must be checked carefully. A chest x-ray may be helpful to assess the position of the tube, but it cannot exclude esophageal intubation.

Q. Attach a CO_2 colorimetric device to the endotracheal tube, between the adapter and the ventilating device. The use of this device provides a reliable means of confirming the position of the endotracheal tube in the trachea.

R. Attach a pulse oximeter device to one of the patient's fingers (intact peripheral perfusion must exist) to measure and monitor the patient's oxygen saturation levels. Pulse oximetry is useful to monitor oxygen saturation levels continuously, and provides an immediate assessment of therapeutic interventions.

AIRWAY AND VENTILATORY MANAGEMENT *Airway and Ventilatory Management*

Complications of Orotracheal and Nasotracheal Intubation

1. *Esophageal intubation, leading to hypoxia and death*
2. *Right mainstem bronchus intubation, resulting in ventilation of the right lung only, collapse of the left lung*
3. *Inability to intubate, leading to hypoxia and death*
4. *Induction of vomiting, leading to aspiration, hypoxia, and death*
5. *Trauma to the airway, resulting in hemorrhage and potential aspiration*
6. *Chipping or loosening of the teeth (caused by levering of the laryngoscope blade against the teeth)*
7. *Rupture leak of the endotracheal tube cuff, resulting in loss of seal during ventilation, and necessitating reintubation*
8. *Conversion of a cervical vertebral injury without neurologic deficit to a cervical cord*
9. *Injury with neurologic deficit*

VI. INFANT OROTRACHEAL INTUBATION

A. Ensure that adequate ventilation and oxygenation are in progress.

B. Select the proper-sized uncuffed tube, which should be the same size as the infant's nostril or little finger.

C. Connect the laryngoscope blade and handle; check the light bulb for brilliance.

D. Hold the laryngoscope in the left hand.

E. Insert the laryngoscope blade in the right side of the mouth, moving the tongue to the left.

F. Observe the epiglottis, then the vocal cords.

G. Insert the endotracheal tube not more than 2 cm past the cords.

H. Check the placement of the tube by bag-valve-to-tube ventilation.

I. Check the placement of the endotracheal tube by observing lung inflations and auscultating the chest and abdomen with a stethoscope.

J. Secure the tube. If the patient is moved, the tube placement should be reassessed.

K. If endotracheal intubation is not accomplished within 30 seconds or in the same time required to hold your breath before exhaling, discontinue attempts, ventilate the patient with a bag-valve-mask device, and try again.

L. Placement of the tube must be checked carefully. A chest x-ray may be helpful to assess the position of the tube, but it cannot exclude esophageal intubation.

M. Attach a CO_2 colorimetric device to the endotracheal tube, between the adapter and the ventilating device. The use of this device provides a reliable means of confirming the position of the endotracheal tube in the trachea.

N. Attach a pulse oximeter device to one of the patient's fingers (intact peripheral perfusion must exist) to measure and monitor the patient's oxygen saturation levels. Pulse oximetry is useful to monitor oxygen saturation levels continuously, and provides an immediate assessment of therapeutic interventions.

Airway and Ventilatory Management **AIRWAY AND VENTILATORY MANAGEMENT**

VII. PULSE OXIMETRY MONITORING

The pulse oximeter is designed to measure oxygen saturation and pulse rate in peripheral circulation. This device is a microprocessor that calculates the percentage saturation of oxygen in each pulse of arterial blood that flows past a sensor. It also calculates the heart rate at the same time.

The pulse oximeter works by a low-intensity light beamed from a light-emitting diode (LED) to a photodiode that is a light receiver. Two thin beams of light, one red and the other infrared, are transmitted through blood and body tissue, a portion of which is absorbed by the blood and body tissue. The photodiode measures that portion of the light that passes through the blood and body tissue. The relative amount of light absorbed by oxygenated hemoglobin differs from that absorbed by nonoxygenated hemoglobin. The microprocessor evaluates these differences in the arterial pulse and reports the values as calculated oxyhemoglobin saturation (%SaO_2). Measurements are reliable and correlate well when compared with a cooximeter that directly measures hemoglobin saturation (SaO_2).

The accuracy of the pulse oximeter is **unreliable** when there is poor peripheral perfusion. This may be due to vasoconstriction, hypotension, a blood pressure cuff that is inflated above the sensor, hypothermia, and other

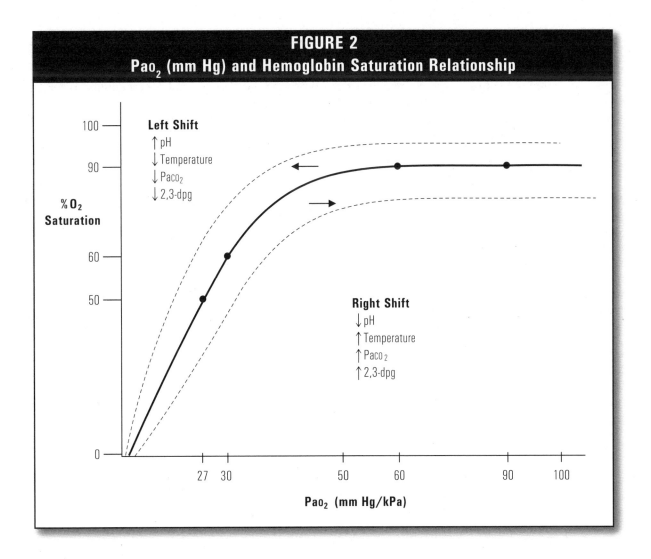

FIGURE 2
Pao₂ (mm Hg) and Hemoglobin Saturation Relationship

AIRWAY AND VENTILATORY MANAGEMENT *Airway and Ventilatory Management*

causes for poor blood flow. Severe anemia may likewise influence the reading. Significantly high levels of carboxyhemoglobin or methemoglobin may cause abnormalities, and circulating dye (eg, indocyanine green and methylene blue) may interfere with the measurement. Excessive patient movement, other electrical devices, or intense ambient light may cause malfunction of this device.

Using a pulse oximeter requires knowledge of the particular device being used. Various sensors are appropriate for different patients. The fingertip and earlobe are common sites where sensors are applied; however, both of these areas may be subject to vasoconstriction. The fingertip (or toe tip) of an injured extremity or below a blood pressure cuff should not be used.

When analyzing results of a pulse oximeter, evaluate the initial readings. Does the pulse rate correspond to the electrocardiogram monitor? Is the oxygen saturation appropriate? If the pulse oximeter is giving low readings or if they are very poor readings, look for a physiologic cause, not a mechanical one.

The relationship between partial pressure of oxygen in arterial blood (Pao_2) and $\%Sao_2$ is shown in Figure 2, page 59. The sigmoid shape of this curve indicates that the relationship between $\%Sao_2$ and Pao_2 is nonlinear. This is particularly important in the middle range of this curve, where small changes in Pao_2 will effect large changes in saturation. **Remember,** the pulse oximeter measures arterial oxygen saturation, not arterial oxygen partial pressure. (See Table 2, Approximate Pao_2 Versus O_2 Hemoglobin Saturation Levels in Chapter 2, Airway and Ventilatory Management, page 50.)

Standard blood gas measurements report both arterial oxygen pressure (Pao_2) and calculated hemoglobin saturation ($\%Sao_2$). When oxygen saturation is calculated from blood gas Pao_2, the calculated value may differ from the oxygen saturation measured by the pulse oximeter. This difference may occur because an oxygen saturation value that has been calculated from the blood gas Pao_2 has not necessarily been correctly adjusted for the effects of variables that shift the relationship between Pao_2 and saturation. These variables include temperature, pH, $Paco_2$ (partial pressure of carbon dioxide), 2,3-dpg (diphosphoglycerates), and the concentration of fetal hemoglobin.

VIII. END-TIDAL CO_2 DETECTORS

When a patient is intubated, it is essential to check the position of the endotracheal tube. If carbon dioxide is detected in the exhaled air, the tube is in the airway. Colorimetric end-tidal CO_2 detectors should be readily available in each emergency department. They can rapidly detect the presence of CO_2 in the exhaled air.

Colorimetric devices use a chemically treated indicator strip that generally reflects the CO_2 level. At very low levels of CO_2, eg, atmospheric air, the indicator turns purple. At higher CO_2 levels, eg, 2% to 5%, the indicator turns yellow. A tan color indicates detection of CO_2 levels that are generally lower than those found in the exhaled tracheal gases.

It is important to note that, on a rare occasion, patients with gastric distention may have elevated CO_2 levels in their esophagus. These elevated levels clear rapidly after several breaths, and the results of this colorimetric test should not be used until after at least 6 breaths. If the colorimetric device still shows an intermediate range, 6 additional breaths should be taken or given. If the patient sustains a cardiac arrest and has no cardiac output, CO_2 is not delivered to the lungs. In fact, with cardiac asystole, this may be a way of determining if cardiopulmonary resuscitation is adequate.

The colorimetric device is not used for the detection of elevated CO_2 levels. Similarly, it is not used to detect a main stem bronchial intubation. Physical examination and a chest x-ray are still required to determine that the endotracheal tube is properly positioned in the airway. In a noisy emergency department or when the patient is transported several times, this device is extremely reliable in differentiating between tracheal and esophageal intubation.

IX. SKILLS SCENARIOS

A. Scenario #1

A 22-year-old man is an unrestrained passenger in a motor vehicle that collides head-on into a retaining wall. He has a strong odor of alcohol on his breath. At the time of the collision, he hits the windshield and sustains a scalp laceration. At the injury scene he is combative and his GCS Score is 11. His blood pressure is 120/70 mm Hg, heart rate is 100 beats/minute, and respirations are 20 breaths/minute. A semirigid cervical collar is applied and he is immobilized on a long backboard. He is receiving oxygen via a high-flow oxygen mask. Shortly after his arrival in the emergency department, he begins to vomit.

B. Scenario #2

The patient described in the first scenario is now unresponsive and is endotracheally intubated. He is being ventilated with 100% oxygen. Part of his evaluation includes a CT scan of his brain. After he is transported to radiology for the scan, the pulse oximeter reveals 82% Sao_2.

C. Scenario #3

A 3-year-old unrestrained, front-seat passenger is injured when the car crashes into a stone wall. The child is unconscious at the injury scene. In the emergency department, bruises to the forehead, face, and chest wall are noted. There is blood around the mouth. Blood pressure is 105/70 mm Hg, heart rate is 120 beats/minute, and respirations are rapid and shallow. The child's GCS Score is 8.

D. Scenario #4

A 35-year-old man sustains blunt chest trauma during a single motor-vehicle collision. In the emergency department, he is alert and has evidence of a right chest wall contusion. He has point tenderness and fracture crepitus of several right ribs. His GCS Score is 14. He is immobilized with a semirigid cervical spine collar and is on a long backboard. High-flow oxygen is being administered via a face mask.

SKILLS STATION

Cricothyroidotomy

■ OBJECTIVES:

Performance at this station will allow the student to practice and demonstrate the techniques of needle crico-thyroidotomy and surgical cricothyroidotomy on a live, anesthetized animal; a fresh human cadaver; or an anatomic human body manikin. Specifically, the student will be able to:

1. Identify the surface markings and structures to be noted when performing needle and surgical crico-thyroidotomies.

2. Discuss the indications and complications of needle and surgical cricothyroidotomies.

3. Perform needle and surgical cricothyroidotomies on a live, anesthetized animal; a fresh human ca-daver; or an anatomic human body manikin as outlined in this skills station.

■ PROCEDURES:

1. Needle cricothyroidotomy

2. Surgical cricothyroidotomy

INTERACTIVE SKILLS PROCEDURES
Cricothyroidotomy

Note: **Standard precautions are required whenever caring for the trauma patient.**

I. NEEDLE CRICOTHYROIDOTOMY

A. Assemble and prepare oxygen tubing by cutting a hole toward one end of the tubing. Connect the other end of the oxygen tubing to an oxygen source, capable of delivering 50 psi or greater at the nipple, and assure free flow of oxygen through the tubing.

B. Place the patient in a supine position.

C. Assemble a #12- or #14-gauge, 8.5-cm, over-the-needle catheter to a 6- to 12-mL syringe.

D. Surgically prepare the neck, using antiseptic swabs.

E. Palpate the cricothyroid membrane, anteriorly, between the thyroid cartilage and cricoid cartilage. Stabilize the trachea with the thumb and forefinger of 1 hand to prevent lateral movement of the trachea during the procedure.

F. Puncture the skin in the midline with a #12- or #14-gauge needle attached to a syringe, directly over the cricothyroid membrane (ie, midsagittal). A small incision with a #11 blade facilitates passage of the needle through the skin.

G. Direct the needle at a 45° angle caudally, while applying negative pressure to the syringe.

H. Carefully insert the needle through the lower half of the cricothyroid membrane, aspirating as the needle is advanced.

I. Aspiration of air signifies entry into the tracheal lumen.

J. Remove the syringe and withdraw the stylet while gently advancing the catheter downward into position, being careful not to perforate the posterior wall of the trachea.

K. Attach the oxygen tubing over the catheter needle hub, and secure the catheter to the patient's neck.

L. Intermittent ventilation can be achieved by occluding the open hole cut into the oxygen tubing with your thumb for 1 second and releasing it for 4 seconds. After releasing your thumb from the hole in the tubing, passive exhalation occurs. **Note:** Adequate Pao_2 can be maintained for only 30 to 45 minutes, and CO_2 accumulation may occur more rapidly.

M. Continue to observe lung inflations and auscultate the chest for adequate ventilation.

Complications of Needle Cricothyroidotomy

1. *Inadequate ventilations leading to hypoxia and death*
2. *Aspiration (blood)*
3. *Esophageal laceration*
4. *Hematoma*
5. *Posterior tracheal wall perforation*

6. Subcutaneous and/or mediastinal emphysema

7. Thyroid perforation

II. SURGICAL CRICOTHYROIDOTOMY (See Figure 3, Surgical Cricothyroidotomy, page 67)

A. Place the patient in a supine position with the neck in a neutral position. Palpate the thyroid notch, cricothyroid interval, and the sternal notch for orientation. Assemble the necessary equipment.

B. Surgically prepare and anesthetize the area locally, if the patient is conscious.

C. Stabilize the thyroid cartilage with the left hand and maintain stabilization until the trachea is intubated.

D. Make a transverse skin incision over the cricothyroid membrane, and carefully incise through the membrane transversely.

E. Insert the scalpel handle into the incision and rotate it 90° to open the airway. (A hemostat or tracheal spreader also may be used instead of the scalpel handle.)

F. Insert an appropriately sized, cuffed endotracheal tube or tracheostomy tube (usually a #5 or #6) into the cricothyroid membrane incision, directing the tube distally into the trachea.

G. Inflate the cuff and ventilate the patient.

H. Observe lung inflations and auscultate the chest for adequate ventilation.

I. Secure the endotracheal or tracheostomy tube to the patient to prevent dislodging.

J. Caution: Do not cut or remove the cricoid and/or thyroid cartilages.

Complications of Surgical Cricothyroidotomy

1. Aspiration (eg, blood)

2. Creation of a false passage into the tissues

3. Subglottic stenosis/edema

4. Laryngeal stenosis

5. Hemorrhage or hematoma formation

6. Laceration of the esophagus

7. Laceration of the trachea

8. Mediastinal emphysema

9. Vocal cord paralysis, hoarseness

Cricothyroidotomy　　　**AIRWAY AND VENTILATORY MANAGEMENT**

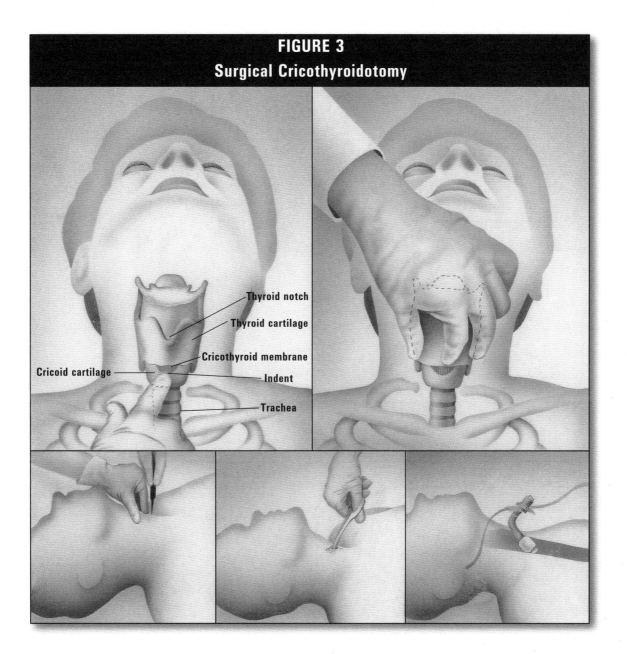

FIGURE 3
Surgical Cricothyroidotomy

Thyroid notch

Thyroid cartilage

Cricothyroid membrane

Cricoid cartilage

Indent

Trachea

THREE

CHAPTER

Shock

■ OBJECTIVES:

Upon completion of this topic, the participant will be able to identify and apply principles of management related to the initial diagnosis and treatment of shock in the injured patient. Specifically, the participant will be able to:

A. Define shock and apply this definition to clinical practice.

B. Recognize the clinical shock syndrome and correlate the patient's acute clinical signs with the degree of volume deficit.

C. Recognize the importance of early identification and control of the source of hemorrhage in the trauma patient.

D. Identify the similarities and differences in the clinical presentation of patients with the various etiologies of the shock state.

SHOCK

I. INTRODUCTION

The initial step in managing shock in the injured patient is to **recognize its presence**. No laboratory test diagnoses shock. The initial diagnosis is based on clinical appreciation of the presence of **inadequate tissue perfusion and oxygenation**. The definition of shock as an abnormality of the circulatory system that results in inadequate organ perfusion and tissue oxygenation also becomes an operative tool for diagnosis and treatment.

The second step in the initial management of shock is to **identify the probable cause** of the shock state. This process for the trauma patient is directly related to the mechanism of injury. Most injured patients in shock are hypovolemic, but they may suffer from cardiogenic, neurogenic, and even septic shock on occasion. Additionally, tension pneumothorax can reduce venous return and produce shock. This diagnosis should be considered in patients who may have injuries above the diaphragm. Neurogenic shock results from extensive injury to the central nervous system (CNS) or the spinal cord. For all practical purposes, **shock does not result from isolated brain injuries.** Patients with spinal cord injury may initially present in shock from both vasodilatation and relative hypovolemia. Septic shock is unusual but must be considered for patients whose arrival at the emergency facility has been delayed by many hours.

The doctor's management responsibilities begin with recognizing the presence of the shock state. Treatment should be initiated simultaneously with the identification of a probable cause of the shock state. The response to initial treatment, coupled with the findings during the primary and secondary patient surveys, usually provides sufficient information to determine the cause of the shock state. **Hemorrhage is the most common cause of shock in the injured patient.**

A. Basic Cardiac Physiology

Cardiac output is defined as the volume of blood pumped by the heart per minute and is determined by the product of heart rate and stroke volume. Stroke volume, the amount of blood pumped with each cardiac contraction, is classically determined by (1) preload, (2) myocardial contractility, and (3) afterload.

Preload denotes the volume of venous return to the heart and is determined by venous capacitance, volume status, and the difference between mean venous systemic pressure and right atrial pressure. This pressure differential determines venous flow. The venous system can be considered a reservoir or capacitance system in which the volume of blood can be divided into 2 components. One component does not contribute to the mean systemic venous pressure and represents the volume of blood that would remain in this capacitance circuit if the pressure in the system were zero.

The second, more important component represents the venous volume that contributes to the mean systemic venous pressure. Nearly 70% of the total blood volume is estimated to be located in the venous circuit. The relationship between venous volume and venous pressure describes the compliance of the system. Remember, it is this pressure gradient that drives venous flow and therefore the volume of venous return to the heart. Blood loss depletes this second component of venous volume, reduces the pressure gradient, and as a consequence, reduces venous return.

The volume of venous blood returned to the heart determines myocardial muscle fiber length after ventricular filling at end-diastole. Muscle fiber length is related to the contractile properties of myocardial muscle according to Starling's law. Myocardial contractility is the pump that drives the system. Afterload is systemic (peripheral) vascular resistance or, simply stated, the resistance to the forward flow of blood.

B. Blood Loss Pathophysiology

Early circulatory responses to blood loss are compensatory, ie, **progressive vasoconstriction** of cutaneous, muscle, and visceral circulation to preserve blood flow to the kidneys, heart, and brain. In association with injury, the response to acute circulating volume depletion is an increase in heart rate in an attempt to preserve cardiac output. In most cases, **tachycardia** is the earliest measurable circulatory sign of shock. The release of endogenous catecholamines increases peripheral vascular resistance. This increases diastolic blood pressure and reduces pulse pressure, but does little to increase organ perfusion. Other hormones with vasoactive properties are released into the circulation during shock, including histamine, bradykinin, beta-endorphins, and a cascade of prostanoids and other cytokines. These substances have profound effects on the microcirculation and vascular permeability.

Compensatory mechanisms preserve venous return to some degree in early hemorrhagic shock by contraction of the volume of blood in the venous system, which does not contribute to mean systemic venous pressure. This compensatory mechanism is limited. The most effective method to restore an adequate cardiac output and end-organ perfusion is to restore venous return to normal by volume repletion.

At the cellular level, inadequately perfused and oxygenated cells are deprived of essential substrates for normal aerobic metabolism and energy production. Initially, compensation occurs by shifting to anaerobic metabolism, which results in the formation of lactic acid and the development of metabolic acidosis. If shock is prolonged and substrate delivery for the generation of adenosine triphosphate (ATP) is inadequate, the cellular membrane loses the ability to maintain its integrity and the normal electrical gradient is lost.

Swelling of the endoplasmic reticulum is the first ultrastructural evidence of cellular hypoxia. Mitochondrial damage soon follows. Lysosomes rupture and release enzymes that digest other intracellular structural elements. Sodium and water enter the cell, and cellular swelling occurs. Intracellular calcium deposition also occurs. If the process is not reversed, progressive cellular damage, additional tissue swelling, and cellular death occur. This process compounds the impact of blood loss and hypoperfusion.

The administration of isotonic electrolyte solutions in sufficient quantities helps combat this process. Management is directed toward reversing this phenomenon by providing adequate oxygenation, ventilation, and appropriate fluid resuscitation. Resuscitation may be accompanied by a marked increase in interstitial edema, which is caused by the "reperfusion injury" to the capillary-interstitial membrane. As a result, larger volumes of fluid may be required for resuscitation than initially anticipated.

The initial treatment of shock is directed toward restoring cellular and organ perfusion with adequately oxygenated blood. Control of hemorrhage and restoration of adequate circulating volume are the goals of treatment of hemorrhagic shock.

With the possible exception of penetrating torso trauma without head injury, euvolemia should be maintained. **Vasopressors are contraindicated** for the treatment of hemorrhagic shock because they worsen tissue perfusion. Frequent monitoring of the patient's indices of perfusion is necessary to evaluate the response to therapy and detect deterioration in the patient's condition as early as possible.

Most injured patients who are in hypovolemic shock require early surgical intervention to reverse the shock state. **Therefore, the presence of shock in an injured patient demands the immediate involvement of a surgeon.**

II. INITIAL PATIENT ASSESSMENT

A. Recognition of Shock

Profound circulatory shock, evidenced by hemodynamic collapse with inadequate perfusion of the skin, kidneys, and central nervous system, is easy to recognize. However, after the airway and adequate ventilation have been ensured, careful evaluation of the patient's circulatory status is important to identify early manifestations of shock that include **tachycardia and cutaneous vasoconstriction.**

Sole reliance on systolic blood pressure as an indicator of shock results in delayed recognition of the shock state. Compensatory mechanisms may preclude a measurable fall in systolic pressure until up to 30% of the patient's blood volume is lost. Specific attention should be directed to pulse rate, respiratory rate, skin circulation, and pulse pressure (the difference between systolic and diastolic pressure). Tachycardia and cutaneous vasoconstriction are the usual and early physiologic responses to volume loss in most adults. **Accordingly, any injured patient who is cool and tachycardic is in shock until proven otherwise.** Occasionally, a normal heart rate, or even bradycardia, can be associated with the acute reduction of blood volume. Other indices of perfusion must be monitored in these situations.

The normal heart rate varies with age. Tachycardia is present when the heart rate is greater than 160 in an infant, 140 in a preschool-age child, 120 from school age to puberty, and 100 in an adult. The elderly patient may not exhibit tachycardia because of the limited cardiac response to catecholamine stimulation or the concurrent use of medications such as beta-adrenergic blocking agents. The ability

SHOCK

to increase the heart rate also may be limited by the presence of a pacemaker. **A narrowed pulse pressure** suggests significant blood loss and involvement of compensatory mechanisms.

Use of the hematocrit or hemoglobin concentration is unreliable for estimating acute blood loss and is inappropriate for diagnosing shock. Massive blood loss may produce only a minimal acute decrease in the hematocrit or hemoglobin concentration. Thus, a very low hematocrit obtained shortly after injury suggests massive blood loss or a preexisting anemia, while a normal hematocrit does not exclude significant blood loss.

B. Clinical Differentiation of Etiology of Shock

Shock in a trauma patient may be classified as hemorrhagic or nonhemorrhagic. A patient with injuries above the diaphragm may demonstrate evidence of inadequate organ perfusion due to poor cardiac performance from blunt myocardial injury, cardiac tamponade, or a tension pneumothorax that produces inadequate venous return (preload). A high index of suspicion and careful observation of the patient's response to initial treatment should enable the doctor to recognize and manage all forms of shock.

Initial determination of the etiology of shock depends on an appropriate history and careful physical examination. Selected additional tests, eg, central venous pressure (CVP), data from a pulmonary artery catheter, chest or pelvic x-rays, and ultrasonography, may provide confirmatory evidence for the etiology of the shock state, but should not delay aggressive volume restoration.

1. Hemorrhagic shock

Hemorrhage is the most common cause of shock after injury, and virtually all patients with multiple injuries have an element of hypovolemia. Additionally, most nonhemorrhagic shock states respond partially or briefly to volume resuscitation. Therefore, if the signs of shock are present, treatment usually is instituted as if the patient is hypovolemic. However, as treatment is instituted, it is important to identify the small number of patients whose shock has another etiology (eg, patients may have a secondary condition such as cardiac tamponade, tension pneumothorax, spinal cord injury, or blunt cardiac injury, which

complicates their hypovolemic/hemorrhagic shock). Specifics of the treatment of hemorrhagic shock are covered in greater detail in the next section of this chapter. The primary focus is to identify and stop hemorrhage promptly in the trauma patient in hemorrhagic shock.

2. Nonhemorrhagic shock

a. Cardiogenic shock

Myocardial dysfunction may occur from blunt cardiac injury, cardiac tamponade, air embolus, or rarely a myocardial infarction associated with the patient's injury. Blunt cardiac injury should be suspected when the mechanism of injury to the thorax is rapid deceleration. All patients with blunt thoracic trauma need constant ECG monitoring to detect injury patterns and dysrhythmias. Blood CPK isoenzymes and specific isotope studies of the myocardium rarely have any value in diagnosing or managing the patient in the emergency department. Echocardiography can be useful in the diagnosis of tamponade or valvular rupture, but it is often not practical or immediately available in the emergency department. "FAST" (Focused Assessment Sonography in Trauma) in the emergency department may identify pericardial fluid and the likelihood of cardiac tamponade as the cause of shock. Blunt cardiac injury may be an indication for early CVP monitoring to guide fluid resuscitation in this situation.

Cardiac tamponade is most commonly identified in penetrating thoracic trauma, but can occur as the result of blunt injuries to the thorax. Tachycardia, muffled heart sounds, and dilated, engorged neck veins with hypotension resistant to fluid therapy suggest cardiac tamponade. The absence of these classic findings does not exclude the presence of this condition. Tension pneumothorax may mimic cardiac tamponade, but is differentiated from the latter condition by the finding of absent breath sounds and a hyperresonant percussion note over the affected hemithorax. Appropriate placement of a needle into the pleural space in the case of tension pneumothorax or into the pericardial sac for tamponade temporarily relieves these 2 life-threatening conditions.

b. Tension pneumothorax

Tension pneumothorax is a true surgical emergency that requires immediate diagnosis and treatment. Tension pneumothorax develops when air enters the pleural space but a flap-valve mechanism prevents its escape. Intrapleural pressure rises, causing total lung collapse and a shift of the mediastinum to the opposite side with subsequent impairment of venous return and fall in cardiac output. The presence of acute respiratory distress, subcutaneous emphysema, absent breath sounds, hyperresonance to percussion, and tracheal shift supports the diagnosis and warrants immediate thoracic decompression without waiting for x-ray confirmation of the diagnosis.

c. Neurogenic shock

Isolated intracranial injuries do not cause shock. The presence of shock in a patient with a head injury necessitates a search for another cause of shock. Spinal cord injury may produce hypotension due to loss of sympathetic tone. **Remember,** loss of sympathetic tone compounds the physiologic effects of hypovolemia, and hypovolemia compounds the physiologic effects of sympathetic denervation. The classic picture of neurogenic shock is hypotension without tachycardia or cutaneous vasoconstriction. A narrowed pulse pressure is not seen in neurogenic shock. Patients sustaining a spinal injury often have concurrent torso trauma. Therefore, patients with known or suspected neurogenic shock should be treated initially for hypovolemia. Failure to restore organ perfusion with fluid resuscitation suggests either continuing hemorrhage or neurogenic shock. CVP monitoring may be helpful in managing this sometimes complex problem. (See Chapter 7, Spine and Spinal Cord Trauma.)

d. Septic shock

Shock due to infection immediately after injury is uncommon. However, if the patient's arrival at the emergency facility is delayed for several hours, this problem may occur. Septic shock may occur in patients with penetrating abdominal injuries and contamination of the peritoneal cavity with intestinal contents.

Septic patients who are hypotensive and afebrile are clinically difficult to distinguish from those in hypovolemic shock, as both groups may manifest tachycardia, cutaneous vasoconstriction, impaired urinary output, decreased systolic pressure, and narrow pulse pressure. Patients with early septic shock may have a normal circulating volume, a modest tachycardia, warm pink skin, a systolic pressure near normal, and a wide pulse pressure.

III. HEMORRHAGIC SHOCK IN THE INJURED PATIENT

Hemorrhage is the most common cause of shock in the trauma patient. The trauma patient's response to blood loss is made more complex by shifts of fluids among the fluid compartments in the body (particularly in the extracellular fluid compartment). The classic response to blood loss must be considered in the context of these fluid shifts associated with soft-tissue injury. Additionally, the changes associated with severe, prolonged shock and the pathophysiologic results of resuscitation and reperfusion must also be considered, as previously discussed.

A. Definition of Hemorrhage

Hemorrhage is defined as an **acute loss of circulating blood volume.** Although there is considerable variability, the normal adult blood volume is approximately 7% of body weight. For example, a 70-kilogram man has a circulating blood volume of approximately 5 liters. The blood volume of obese adults is estimated based on their ideal body weight. Calculation based on actual weight may result in significant overestimation. The blood volume for a child is calculated as 8% to 9% of the body weight (80 to 90 mL/kg). (See Chapter 10, Extremes of Age: A. Pediatric Trauma.)

B. Direct Effects of Hemorrhage

Classes of hemorrhage, based on percentage of acute blood volume loss, are outlined individually in this chapter for the purpose of understanding the physiologic and Class I to Class IV clinical manifestations of hemorrhagic shock. The distinction between classes of hemorrhagic shock may not be apparent in an individual patient, and **volume replacement should be directed by the response to initial therapy rather than by relying solely on the initial**

SHOCK

classification. This classification system is useful in emphasizing the early signs and pathophysiology of the shock state. **Class I** hemorrhage is exemplified by the condition of an individual who has donated a unit of blood. **Class II** is uncomplicated hemorrhage, but crystalloid fluid resuscitation is required. **Class III** is a complicated hemorrhagic state in which at least crystalloid infusion and perhaps blood replacement are required. **Class IV** hemorrhage should be considered a preterminal event, and unless very aggressive measures are taken, the patient will die within minutes. (See Table 1, Estimated Fluid and Blood Losses.)

Several confounding factors profoundly alter the classic hemodynamic response to an acute loss of circulating blood volume, and these must be promptly recognized by all individuals involved in the initial assessment and resuscitation of the injured patient who has the potential for hemorrhagic shock. These factors include (1) the patient's age; (2) severity of injury, with special attention to type and anatomic location of injury; (3) time lapse between injury and initiation of treatment; (4) prehospital fluid therapy and application of the pneumatic antishock garment (PASG); and (5) medications used for chronic conditions.

It is dangerous to wait until the trauma patient fits a precise physiologic classification of shock before initiating aggressive volume restoration. Fluid resuscitation must be initiated when early signs and symptoms of blood loss are apparent or suspected, not when the blood pressure is falling or absent.

Table 1—Estimated Fluid and Blood Losses[1]
Based on Patient's Initial Presentation

	CLASS I	CLASS II	CLASS III	CLASS IV
Blood loss (mL)	Up to 750	750–1500	1500–2000	>2000
Blood loss (% blood volume)	Up to 15%	15%–30%	30%–40%	>40%
Pulse rate	<100	>100	>120	>140
Blood pressure	Normal	Normal	Decreased	Decreased
Pulse pressure (mm Hg)	Normal or increased	Decreased	Decreased	Decreased
Respiratory rate	14–20	20–30	30–40	>35
Urine output (mL/hr)	>30	20–30	5–15	Negligible
CNS/Mental status	Slightly anxious	Mildly anxious	Anxious, confused	Confused, lethargic
Fluid replacement (3:1 rule)	Crystalloid	Crystalloid	Crystalloid and blood	Crystalloid and blood

[1]For a 70-kg man.

The guidelines in Table 1 are based on the 3-for-1 rule. This rule derives from the empiric observation that most patients in hemorrhagic shock require as much as 300 mL of electrolyte solution for each 100 mL of blood loss. Applied blindly, these guidelines can result in excessive or inadequate fluid administration. For example, a patient with a crush injury to the extremity may have hypotension out of proportion to his or her blood loss and require fluids in excess of the 3:1 guidelines. In contrast, a patient whose ongoing blood loss is being replaced by blood transfusion requires less than 3:1. The use of bolus therapy with careful monitoring of the patient's response can moderate these extremes.

1. Class I hemorrhage—Up to 15% blood volume loss

The clinical symptoms of this volume loss are minimal. In uncomplicated situations, minimal tachycardia occurs. No measurable changes occur in blood pressure, pulse pressure, or respiratory rate. For otherwise healthy patients, this amount of blood loss does not require replacement. Transcapillary refill and other compensatory mechanisms restore blood volume within 24 hours. However, in the presence of other fluid changes, this amount of blood loss can produce clinical symptoms. Replacement of the primary fluid losses corrects the circulatory state, usually without the need for blood transfusion.

2. Class II hemorrhage—15% to 30% blood volume loss

In a 70-kilogram male, this volume loss represents 750 to 1500 mL of blood. Clinical symptoms include tachycardia (heart rate above 100 in an adult), tachypnea, and a decrease in pulse pressure. This decrease in pulse pressure is primarily related to a rise in the diastolic component due to an increase in circulating catecholamines. These agents produce an increase in peripheral vascular tone and resistance. Systolic pressure changes minimally in early hemorrhagic shock; therefore, it is important to evaluate pulse pressure rather than systolic pressure. Other pertinent clinical findings with this degree of blood loss include subtle central nervous system changes such as anxiety, fright, or hostility. Despite the significant blood loss and cardiovascular changes, urinary output is only mildly affected. The measured urine flow is usually 20 to 30 mL/hour in an adult.

Accompanying fluid losses can exaggerate the clinical manifestations of this amount of blood loss. Some of these patients may eventually require blood transfusion, but can be stabilized initially with crystalloid solutions.

3. Class III hemorrhage—30% to 40% blood volume loss

This amount of blood loss (approximately 2000 mL in an adult) can be devastating. Patients almost always present with the classic signs of inadequate perfusion, including marked tachycardia and tachypnea, significant changes in mental status, and a measurable fall in systolic pressure. In an uncomplicated case, this is the least amount of blood loss that consistently causes a drop in systolic pressure. Patients with this degree of blood loss almost always require transfusion. However, priority should be to stop the hemorrhage, by emergency operation if necessary, in order to decrease the transfusion requirement. The decision to transfuse blood is based on the patient's response to initial fluid resuscitation and the adequacy of end-organ perfusion and oxygenation, as described later in this chapter.

4. Class IV hemorrhage—More than 40% blood volume loss

This degree of exsanguination is immediately life-threatening. Symptoms include marked tachycardia, a significant depression in systolic blood pressure, and a very narrow pulse pressure (or an unobtainable diastolic pressure). Urinary output is negligible, and mental status is markedly depressed. The skin is cold and pale. These patients frequently require rapid transfusion and immediate surgical intervention. These decisions are based on the patient's response to the initial management techniques described in this chapter. Loss of more than 50% of the patient's blood volume results in loss of consciousness, pulse, and blood pressure.

Clinical usefulness of this classification scheme can be illustrated by this example. Because Class III hemorrhage represents the smallest volume of blood loss that is consistently associated with a drop in systolic pressure, a 70-kilogram patient who arrives hypotensive has lost an estimated 1470 mL of blood (70 kg × 7% × 30% = 1.47 L, or 1470 mL). Using the 3-for-1 rule (discussed later in this chapter), this patient requires 4.4 liters of crystalloid fluid for resuscitation (1470 mL × 3 = 4410 mL). Nonresponse to fluid administration indicates (1) persistent blood loss, (2) unrecognized fluid losses, or (3) nonhemorrhagic shock.

C. Fluid Changes Secondary to Soft-Tissue Injury

Major soft-tissue injuries and fractures compromise the hemodynamic status of the injured patient in 2 ways. First, blood is lost into the site of injury, particularly in cases of major fractures. A fractured tibia or humerus may be associated with the loss of as much as 1.5 units (750 mL) of blood loss. Twice

SHOCK

that amount (up to 1500 mL) is commonly associated with femur fractures, and **several liters of blood may accumulate in a retroperitoneal hematoma associated with a pelvic fracture.**

The second factor to be considered is the obligatory edema that occurs in injured soft tissues. The degree of this additional volume loss is related to the magnitude of the soft-tissue injury. Tissue injury results in the activation of a systemic inflammatory response and the production and release of multiple cytokines. Many of these locally active hormones have profound effects on vascular endothelium, which increases permeability. The development of tissue edema is the result of shifts in fluid primarily from the plasma into the extravascular, extracellular space. Such shifts produce an additional depletion in intravascular volume.

IV. INITIAL MANAGEMENT OF HEMORRHAGIC SHOCK

The diagnosis and treatment of shock must occur almost simultaneously. For most trauma patients, treatment is instituted as if the patient has hypovolemic shock, unless there is clear evidence that the shock state is caused by an etiology other than hypovolemia. **The basic management principle to follow is to stop the bleeding and replace the volume loss.**

A. Physical Examination

The physical examination is directed at the immediate diagnosis of life-threatening injuries and includes assessment of the ABCDEs. Baseline recordings are important to monitor the patient's response to therapy. Vital signs, urinary output, and level of consciousness are essential. A more detailed examination of the patient follows as the situation permits.

1. Airway and breathing

Establishing a patent airway with adequate ventilation and oxygenation is the first priority. Supplementary oxygen is supplied to maintain oxygen saturation at greater than 95%.

2. Circulation—Hemorrhage control

Priorities include controlling obvious hemorrhage, obtaining adequate intravenous access, and assessing tissue perfusion. Bleeding from external wounds usually can be controlled by direct pressure to the bleeding site. The PASG may be used to control bleeding from pelvic or lower extremity fractures, but its use should **not** interfere with rapid reestablishment of intravascular volume by intravenous fluid infusion. The adequacy of tissue perfusion dictates the amount of fluid resuscitation required. Operative control of internal hemorrhage may be required.

3. Disability—Neurologic examination

A brief neurologic examination that determines the level of consciousness, eye motion and pupillary response, best motor function, and degree of sensation is performed. This information is useful in assessing cerebral perfusion, following the evolution of neurologic disability, and prognosticating future recovery. Alterations in CNS function in the patient who is hypotensive from hypovolemic shock do not necessarily imply direct intracranial injury and may reflect inadequate brain perfusion. Restoration of cerebral perfusion and oxygenation must be achieved before these findings can be ascribed to intracranial injury. (See Chapter 6, Head Trauma.)

4. Exposure—Complete examination

After lifesaving priorities are addressed, the patient must be completely undressed and carefully examined from "head to toe" as part of the search for associated injuries. **When undressing the patient, preventing hypothermia is essential.** The use of fluid warmers as well as external passive and active warming techniques are essential to prevent hypothermia.

5. Gastric dilatation—Decompression

Gastric dilatation often occurs in the trauma patient, **especially in children,** and may cause unexplained hypotension or cardiac dysrhythmia, usually bradycardia from excessive vagal stimulation. **In the unconscious patient, gastric distention increases the risk of aspiration of gastric contents, a potentially fatal complication.** Gastric decompression is accomplished by intubating the stomach with a tube passed nasally or orally and attaching it to suction to evacuate gastric contents. However, proper positioning of the tube does not completely obviate the risk of aspiration.

6. Urinary catheter insertion

Bladder catheterization allows for the assessment of urine for hematuria and continuous evaluation of renal perfusion by monitoring urinary output. Blood at the urethral meatus or a high-riding, mobile, or nonpalpable prostate in the male is an absolute contraindication to the insertion of a transurethral catheter prior to radiographic confirmation of an intact urethra. (See Chapter 5, Abdominal Trauma.)

B. Vascular Access Lines

Access to the vascular system must be obtained promptly. This is best done by the insertion of 2 large-caliber (minimum of #16-gauge) peripheral intravenous catheters before any consideration is given to a central venous line. The rate of flow is proportional to the fourth power of the radius of the cannula, and is inversely related to its length (Poiseuille's law). Hence, short, large-caliber peripheral IVs are preferred for the rapid infusion of large volumes of fluid. Use fluid warmers and rapid infusion pumps in the presence of massive hemorrhage and severe hypotension.

The most desirable sites for peripheral, percutaneous intravenous lines in the adult are the forearm or antecubital veins. If circumstances prevent the use of peripheral veins, large-caliber, central venous (femoral, jugular, or subclavian vein) access using the Seldinger technique or saphenous vein cutdown is indicated, depending on the skill and experience level of the doctor. Frequently, central venous access in an emergency situation is not accomplished under tightly controlled or totally sterile conditions. These lines should be changed in a more controlled environment as soon as the patient's condition permits. Consideration also must be given to the potential for serious complications related to attempted central venous catheter placement, ie, pneumo- or hemothorax, in a patient who may already be unstable. In children younger than 6 years, the placement of an intraosseous needle should be attempted before central line insertion. The important determinant for selecting a procedure or route for establishing vascular access is the experience and skill level of the doctor. Intraosseous access with specially designed equipment also is possible in adults.

As intravenous lines are started, blood samples are drawn for type and crossmatch, appropriate labora-tory analyses, toxicology studies, and testing of all females of childbearing age for pregnancy. Arterial blood gas analysis should be obtained at this time. A chest x-ray must be obtained after attempts at inserting a subclavian or internal jugular CVP monitoring line to document its position and evaluate for a pneumo- or hemothorax.

C. Initial Fluid Therapy

Warmed isotonic electrolyte solutions are used for initial resuscitation. This type of fluid provides transient intravascular expansion and further stabilizes the vascular volume by replacing accompanying fluid losses into the interstitial and intracellular spaces. Ringer's lactate solution is the initial fluid of choice. Normal saline is the second choice. Although normal saline is a satisfactory replacement fluid, it has the potential to cause hyperchloremic acidosis. This potential is enhanced if renal function is impaired.

An initial, warmed fluid bolus is given as rapidly as possible. The usual dose is 1 to 2 liters for an adult and 20 mL/kg for a pediatric patient. This often requires application of pumping devices (mechanical or manual) to the fluid administration sets. The patient's response is observed during this initial fluid administration, and further therapeutic and diagnostic decisions are based on this response.

The amount of fluid and blood required for resuscitation is difficult to predict on initial evaluation of the patient. Table 1, Estimated Fluid and Blood Losses, provides general guidelines for establishing the amount of fluid and blood the patient probably requires. A rough guideline for the total amount of crystalloid volume acutely required is to replace each milliliter of blood loss with 3 mL of crystalloid fluid, thus allowing for restitution of plasma volume lost into the interstitial and intracellular spaces. This is known as the 3-for-1 rule mentioned previously in this chapter. **However, it is more important to assess the patient's response to fluid resuscitation and evidence of adequate end-organ perfusion and oxygenation, eg, urinary output, level of consciousness, and peripheral perfusion.** If, during resuscitation, the amount of fluid required to restore or maintain adequate organ perfusion greatly exceeds these estimates, a careful reassessment of the situation and a search for unrecognized injuries or other causes of shock are necessary.

SHOCK

V. EVALUATION OF FLUID RESUSCITATION AND ORGAN PERFUSION

A. General

The same signs and symptoms of inadequate perfusion that are used to diagnose shock are useful determinants of patient response. The return of normal blood pressure, pulse pressure, and pulse rate are positive signs that suggest perfusion is returning to normal. However, these observations give no information regarding organ perfusion. Improvements in the CVP status and skin circulation are important evidence of enhanced perfusion, but are difficult to quantitate. The volume of urinary output is a reasonably sensitive indicator of renal perfusion. Normal urine volumes generally imply adequate renal blood flow, if not modified by the administration of diuretic agents. For this reason, urinary output is one of the prime monitors of resuscitation and patient response. Changes in central venous pressure can provide useful information, and the risks incurred in the placement of a CVP line are justified for complex cases. Measurement of CVP is adequate for most cases.

B. Urinary Output

Within certain limits, urinary output is used as a monitor of renal blood flow. Adequate resuscitation volume replacement should produce a urinary output of approximately 0.5 mL/kg/hour in the adult. One mL/kg/hour is an adequate urinary output for the **pediatric patient.** For children **under 1 year of age, 2 mL/kg/hour** should be maintained. Inability to obtain urinary output at these levels or a decreasing urinary output with an increasing specific gravity suggests inadequate resuscitation. This situation should stimulate further volume replacement and diagnostic endeavors.

C. Acid/base Balance

Patients in early hypovolemic shock have respiratory alkalosis due to tachypnea. Respiratory alkalosis is frequently followed by mild metabolic acidosis in the early phases of shock and does not require treatment. Severe metabolic acidosis may develop from long-standing or severe shock. Metabolic acidosis is due to anaerobic metabolism resulting from inadequate tissue perfusion and the production of lactic acid. Persistent acidosis is usually due to inadequate resuscitation or ongoing blood loss and, in the normothermic patient in shock, should be treated with fluids, blood, and consideration of **operative intervention for control of hemorrhage.** The base deficit obtained from the arterial blood gas analysis may be useful in estimating the severity of the acute perfusion deficit. Sodium bicarbonate should **not** be used routinely to treat metabolic acidosis secondary to hypovolemic shock.

VI. THERAPEUTIC DECISIONS BASED ON RESPONSE TO INITIAL FLUID RESUSCITATION

The patient's response to initial fluid resuscitation is the key to determining subsequent therapy. (See Table 2, Responses to Initial Fluid Resuscitation.) Having established a preliminary diagnosis and plan based on the initial evaluation of the patient, the doctor can now modify management based on the patient's response to the initial fluid resuscitation. Observing the response to the initial resuscitation identifies those patients whose blood loss was greater than estimated and those with ongoing bleeding who require operative control of internal hemorrhage. Resuscitation in the operating room can accomplish simultaneously the direct control of bleeding by the surgeon and the restoration of intravascular volume. Additionally, it limits the probability of overtransfusion or unneeded transfusion of blood in those whose initial status was disproportionate to the amount of blood loss. It is particularly important to distinguish the patient who is "hemodynamically stable" from one who is "hemodynamically normal." A hemodynamically stable patient may be persistently tachycardic, tachypneic, and oliguric, clearly underresuscitated and still in shock. In contrast, the hemodynamically normal patient is one who exhibits no signs of inadequate tissue perfusion. The potential response patterns can be discussed in 3 groups: rapid response, transient response, and minimal or no response to initial fluid administration.

A. Rapid Response

Patients in this group respond rapidly to the initial fluid bolus and remain hemodynamically normal when the initial fluid bolus has been completed and the fluids are slowed to maintenance rates. Such patients usually have lost minimal (less than 20%) blood volume. No further fluid bolus or immediate blood administration is indicated for this group of

Table 2—Responses to Initial Fluid Resuscitation[1]

	RAPID RESPONSE	TRANSIENT RESPONSE	NO RESPONSE
Vital signs	Return to normal	Transient improvement, recurrence of ↓ BP and ↑ HR	Remain abnormal
Estimated blood loss	Minimal (10%–20%)	Moderate and ongoing (20%–40%)	Severe (>40%)
Need for more crystalloid	Low	High	High
Need for blood	Low	Moderate to high	Immediate
Blood preparation	Type and crossmatch	Type-specific	Emergency blood release
Need for operative intervention	Possibly	Likely	Highly likely
Early presence of surgeon	Yes	Yes	Yes

[1]2000 mL Ringer's lactate solution in adults, 20 mL/kg Ringer's lactate bolus in children.

patients. Type and crossmatched blood should be kept available. **Surgical consultation and evaluation are necessary during initial assessment and treatment, as operative intervention may still be necessary.**

B. Transient Response

The second group of patients responds to the initial fluid bolus. However, some patients begin to show deterioration of perfusion indices as the initial fluids are slowed to maintenance levels, indicating either an ongoing blood loss or inadequate resuscitation. Most of these patients initially have lost an estimated 20% to 40% of their blood volume. Continued fluid administration and initiation of blood transfusion are indicated. The transient response to blood administration should identify patients who are still bleeding and require rapid surgical intervention.

C. Minimal or No Response

Failure to respond to crystalloid and blood administration in the emergency department dictates the need for immediate operative intervention to control exsanguinating hemorrhage. On very rare occasions, failure to respond may be due to pump failure as a result of blunt cardiac injury, cardiac tamponade, or tension pneumothorax. The possible diagnosis of nonhemorrhagic shock always should be entertained in this group of patients. CVP monitoring or cardiac ultrasonography helps differentiate between the various shock etiologies.

VII. BLOOD REPLACEMENT

The decision to initiate blood transfusion is based on the patient's response, as described in the previous section.

A. Crossmatched, Type-specific, and Type 0 Blood

The main purpose in transfusing blood is to restore the oxygen-carrying capacity of the intravascular volume. Volume resuscitation itself can be accomplished with crystalloids, with the added advantage of contributing to interstitial and intracellular volume restitution.

1. Fully crossmatched blood is preferable. However, the complete crossmatching process requires approximately 1 hour in most blood banks. For patients who stabilize rapidly, crossmatched

SHOCK

blood should be obtained and should be available for transfusion when indicated.

2. Type-specific blood can be provided by most blood banks within 10 minutes. Such blood is compatible with ABO and Rh blood types, but incompatibilities of other antibodies may exist. Type-specific blood is preferred for patients who are transient responders as described in the previous section. If type-specific blood is required, completion of the crossmatching should be performed by the blood bank.

3. If type-specific blood is unavailable, type O packed cells are indicated for patients with exsanguinating hemorrhage. To avoid sensitization and future complications, Rh-negative cells are preferred for females of childbearing age. For life-threatening blood loss, the use of unmatched, type-specific blood is preferred over type O blood. This is true unless multiple unidentified casualties are being treated simultaneously and the risk of inadvertently administering the wrong unit of blood to a patient is great.

B. Warming Fluids—Plasma and Crystalloid

Hypothermia must be prevented and reversed if the patient is hypothermic upon arrival at the hospital. The use of blood warmers is cumbersome yet most desirable in the emergency department. The most efficient way to prevent hypothermia in any patient receiving massive volumes of crystalloid is to heat the fluid to 39°C (102.2°F) before using it. This can be accomplished by storing crystalloids in a warmer or with the use of a microwave oven. Blood products cannot be warmed in the microwave oven but can be heated with passage through intravenous fluid warmers.

C. Autotransfusion

Adaptations of standard tube thoracostomy collection devices are commercially available that allow for sterile collection, anticoagulation (generally with sodium-citrate solutions, not heparin), and retransfusion of shed blood. Collection of shed blood for autotransfusion should be considered for any patient with a major hemothorax.

D. Coagulopathy

Coagulopathy is a rare problem in the first hour of treatment of the multiply injured patient. How-ever, massive transfusion with resultant dilution of platelets and clotting factors along with the adverse effect of hypothermia on platelet aggregation and the clotting cascade are the usual causes of coagulopathies in the injured patient. Prothrombin time, partial thromboplastin time, and platelet count are valuable baseline studies to obtain in the first hour, especially if the patient has a history of coagulation disorders, takes medications that alter coagulation (warfarin, aspirin, or nonsteroidal antiinflammatory agents), or if a reliable bleeding history cannot be obtained. Transfusion of platelets, cryoprecipitate, and fresh-frozen plasma should be guided by these coagulation parameters, including fibrinogen levels. Routine use of such products is generally not warranted unless the patient has a known coagulation disorder or has been anticoagulated pharmacologically for management of a specific medical problem. In such cases, specific factor replacement therapy is immediately indicated when there is evidence of bleeding or the potential for occult blood loss exists (eg, head injury, abdominal or thoracic injury).

Patients with major brain injury are particularly prone to the development of coagulation abnormalities as a result of substances, especially tissue thromboplastin, released by damaged neural tissue. These patients should have their coagulation parameters closely monitored.

E. Calcium Administration

Most patients receiving blood transfusions do not need calcium supplements. Excessive, supplemental calcium may be harmful.

VIII. SPECIAL CONSIDERATIONS IN THE DIAGNOSIS AND TREATMENT OF SHOCK

A. Equating Blood Pressure with Cardiac Output

Treatment of hypovolemic (hemorrhagic) shock requires correction of inadequate organ perfusion. This means increasing organ blood flow and tissue oxygenation. Increasing blood flow requires an increase in cardiac output. Ohm's law ($V = I \times R$) applied to cardiovascular physiology states that blood pressure (V) is proportional to cardiac output (I) and systemic vascular resistance (R) (afterload). An increase in blood pressure should not be equated with a concomitant increase in cardiac output. An increase in peripheral resistance, ie, vasopressor therapy, with no change in cardiac output results in increased blood pressure, but no improvement in tissue perfusion or oxygenation.

B. Age

Elderly trauma patients require special consideration. The aging process produces a relative decrease in sympathetic activity with respect to the cardiovascular system. This is thought to result from a deficit in the receptor response to catecholamines rather than from a reduction in catecholamine production. Cardiac compliance decreases with age. Older patients are unable to increase heart rate or the efficiency of myocardial contraction when stressed by blood volume loss, as are the younger patients. Atherosclerotic vascular occlusive disease makes many vital organs extremely sensitive to even the slightest reduction in blood flow. Many elderly patients have preexisting volume depletion secondary to chronic diuretic use or subtle malnutrition. For these reasons, hypotension secondary to blood loss is poorly tolerated by the elderly trauma patient. Beta-adrenergic blockade may mask tachycardia as the early indicator of shock. Other medications may adversely affect the stress response to injury or block it completely. Because the therapeutic range for volume resuscitation is relatively narrow in the elderly patient, it is prudent to consider early invasive monitoring as a means to avoid excessive or inadequate volume restoration.

The reduction in pulmonary compliance, decrease in diffusion capacity, and general weakness of the muscles of respiration limit the ability of the elderly patient to meet the increased demands for gas exchange imposed by injury. This compounds cellular hypoxia already produced by a reduction in local oxygen delivery. Glomerular and tubular senescence in the kidney reduces the ability of the elderly patient to preserve volume in response to the release of stress hormones such as aldosterone, catecholamines, vasopressin, and cortisol. The kidney also is more susceptible to the effects of reduced blood flow and nephrotoxic agents such as drugs, contrast agents, and the toxic products from cellular destruction.

Mortality and morbidity rates increase directly with age and chronic health status for mild or moderately severe injuries for the reasons listed above. Despite the adverse effects of the aging process, comorbidities from preexisting disease, and a general reduction in the "physiologic reserve" of the geriatric patient, the majority of these patients can be salvaged

and returned to their preinjury status. Treatment begins with prompt, aggressive resuscitation and careful monitoring.

C. Athletes

Rigorous training routines change the cardiovascular dynamics of this group of patients. Blood volume can increase 15% to 20%, cardiac output can increase 6-fold, stroke volume can increase 50%, and resting pulse is generally at 50. This group's ability to compensate for blood loss is truly remarkable. The usual responses to hypovolemia may not be manifested in athletes, even though significant blood loss may have occurred.

D. Pregnancy

Physiologic maternal hypervolemia requires a greater blood loss to manifest perfusion abnormalities in the mother, which also may be reflected in decreased fetal perfusion.

E. Medications

Beta-adrenergic receptor blockers and calcium channel blockers can significantly alter the patient's hemodynamic response to hemorrhage. Insulin overdosing may be responsible for hypoglycemia and may have contributed to the injury-producing event. Chronic diuretic therapy may explain unexpected hypokalemia, and nonsteroidal antiinflammatory agents may adversely affect platelet function.

F. Hypothermia

Patients suffering from hypothermia and hemorrhagic shock do not respond normally to the administration of blood and fluid resuscitation and often develop a coagulopathy. Body temperature is an important vital sign to monitor during the initial assessment phase. Esophageal or bladder temperature is an accurate clinical measurement of the core temperature. A trauma victim under the influence of alcohol and exposed to cold temperature extremes is more likely to become hypothermic as a result of vasodilatation. Rapid rewarming in a warmed environment with appropriate external warming devices, heat lamps, thermal caps, heated respiratory gases, and warmed intravenous fluids and blood generally correct the patient's hypotension and hypothermia. Core rewarming (peritoneal or thoracic cavity irrigation with crystalloid solutions warmed to 39°C [102.2°F], or extracorporeal bypass) may oc-

SHOCK

casionally be indicated. (See Chapter 9, Injuries Due to Burns and Cold.) Hypothermia is best treated by prevention.

G. Pacemaker

Patients with pacemakers are unable to respond to blood loss in the expected fashion since cardiac output is directly related to heart rate. Considering the significant number of patients with myocardial conduction defects who have such devices in place, CVP monitoring is invaluable in these patients to guide fluid therapy.

IX. REASSESSING PATIENT RESPONSE AND AVOIDING COMPLICATIONS

Inadequate volume replacement is the most common complication of hemorrhagic shock. Immediate, appropriate, and aggressive therapy that restores organ perfusion minimizes these untoward events.

A. Continued Hemorrhage

Obscure hemorrhage is the most common cause of poor patient response to fluid therapy. These patients are generally included in the transient response category as defined previously. Immediate surgical intervention may be necessary.

B. Fluid Overload and CVP Monitoring

After the patient's initial assessment and management have been completed, the risk of fluid overload is minimized by monitoring the patient carefully. Remember, the goal of therapy is restoration of organ perfusion and adequate tissue oxygenation, confirmed by appropriate urinary output, central nervous system function, skin color, and return of pulse and blood pressure toward normal.

Monitoring the response to resuscitation is best accomplished for some patients in an environment where sophisticated monitoring techniques are utilized. Early transfer of the patient to the intensive care unit should be considered for elderly patients or those with nonhemorrhagic causes of shock.

CVP monitoring is a relatively simple procedure and is used as a standard guide for assessing the ability of the right side of the heart to accept a fluid load. Properly interpreted, the response of the CVP

to fluid administration helps evaluate volume replacement. Several points to remember are:

1. The precise measure of cardiac function is the relationship between ventricular end-diastolic volume and stroke volume. Right atrial pressure (CVP) and cardiac output (as reflected by evidence of perfusion or blood pressure, or even by direct measurement) are indirect and, at best, insensitive estimates of this relationship. Remembering these facts is important to avoid overdependence on CVP monitoring.

2. The initial CVP level and the actual blood volume are not necessarily related. The initial CVP is sometimes high even with a significant volume deficit, especially in patients with chronic obstructive pulmonary disease, generalized vasoconstriction, and rapid fluid replacement. The initial venous pressure also may be high secondary to the application of the PASG or the inappropriate use of exogenous vasopressors.

3. A minimal rise in the initial, low CVP with fluid therapy suggests the need for further volume expansion (minimal or no response to fluid resuscitation category).

4. A declining CVP suggests ongoing fluid loss and the need for additional fluid or blood replacement (transient response to fluid resuscitation category).

5. An abrupt or persistent elevation in the CVP suggests volume replacement is adequate, is too rapid, or that cardiac function is compromised.

6. Pronounced elevations of the CVP may be caused by hypervolemia as a result of overtransfusion, cardiac dysfunction, cardiac tamponade, or increased intrathoracic pressure from a tension pneumothorax. Catheter malposition may produce erroneously high CVP measurements.

Aseptic techniques must be used when central venous lines are placed. Multiple sites provide access to the central circulation, and the decision as to which route to use is determined by the skill and experience level of the doctor. The ideal position for the tip of the catheter is in the superior vena cava, just proximal to the right atrium. Techniques for catheter placement are discussed in detail in Skills Station IV, Shock Assessment and Management.

The placement of central venous lines carries the risk of potentially life-threatening complications. Infections, vascular injury, nerve injury, embolization, thrombosis, and pneumothorax may result. CVP monitoring reflects right heart function. It may not be representative of the left heart function in patients with primary myocardial dysfunction or abnormal pulmonary circulation.

C. Recognition of Other Problems

When the patient fails to respond to therapy, consider cardiac tamponade, tension pneumothorax, ventilatory problems, unrecognized fluid loss, acute gastric distention, myocardial infarction, diabetic acidosis, hypoadrenalism, and neurogenic shock. **Constant reevaluation,** especially when patients deviate from expected patterns, is the key to recognizing such problems as early as possible.

X. SUMMARY

Shock management, based on sound physiologic principles, is usually successful. Hypovolemia is the cause of shock in most trauma patients. Management of these patients requires immediate hemorrhage control and fluid or blood replacement. **In patients who fail to respond to these measures, operative control of continuing hemorrhage may be necessary.** Additionally, other possible causes of the shock state must be considered in the transient responders or nonresponders. The patient's response to initial fluid therapy determines further therapeutic and diagnostic procedures. All patients who manifest signs of hypovolemic shock are potential candidates for surgical exploration. The goal of therapy is prompt restoration of organ perfusion with the delivery of oxygen and substrate to the cell for aerobic metabolism. Vasopressors are contraindicated in the management of hypovolemic shock. CVP measurement may be a valuable tool for confirming the volume status and monitoring the rate of fluid administration in selected patients.

■ BIBLIOGRAPHY

1. Abou-Khalil B, Scalea TM, Trooskin SZ, et al: Hemodynamic responses to shock in young trauma patients: Need for invasive monitoring. **Critical Care Medicine** 1994; 22(4):633–639.

2. American Heart Association and American Academy of Pediatrics: Intraosseous infusion. In: Chameides L (ed): **Textbook of Pediatric Advanced Life Support.** Dallas, American Heart Association, 1988, pp 43–44.

3. Bickell WH, Wall MJ Jr., Pepe PE, et al: Immediate versus delayed fluid resuscitation for hypotensive patients with penetrating torso injuries. **New England Journal of Medicine** 1994; 331: 1105–1109.

4. Burris D, Rhee P, Kaufmann C, et al: Controlled resuscitation for uncontrolled hemorrhagic shock. **Journal of Trauma** 1999; 46(2):216–223.

5. Carrico CJ, Canizaro PC, Shires GT: Fluid resuscitation following injury: rationale for the use of balanced salt solutions. **Critical Care Medicine** 1976; 4(2):46–54.

6. Chernow B, Rainey TG, Lake CR: Endogenous and exogenous catecholamines. **Critical Care Medicine** 1982; 10:409.

7. Cogbill TH, Blintz M, Johnson JA, et al: Acute gastric dilatation after trauma. **The Journal of Trauma** 1987; 27(10):1113–1117.

8. Cooper DJ, Walley KR, Wiggs RB, et al: Bicarbonate does not improve hemodynamics in critically ill patients who have lactic acidosis. **Annals of Internal Medicine** 1990; 112:492.

9. Counts RB, Haisch C, Simon TL, et al: Hemostasis in massively transfused trauma patients. **Annals of Surgery** 1979; 190(l):91–99.

10. Ferrara A, MacArthur JD, Wright HK, et al: Hypothermia and acidosis worsen coagulopathy in patients requiring massive transfusion. **American Journal of Surgery** 1990; 160:515.

11. Glover JL, Broadie TA: Intraoperative autotransfusion. **World Journal of Surgery** 1987; 11: 60–64.

12. Gould SA, Moore EE, Hoyt DB, et al: The first randomized trial of human polymerized hemoglobin as a blood substitute in acute trauma and emergent surgery. **Journal of the American College of Surgeons** 1998; 187(2):113–122.

13. Granger DN: Role of xanthine oxidase and granulocytes in ischemia-reperfusion injury. **American Journal of Physiology** 1988; 255: H1269–H1275.

14. Guyton AC, Lindsey AW, Kaufman BN: Effect of mean circulatory filling pressure and other peripheral circulatory factors on cardiac output. **American Journal of Physiology** 1955; 180: 463–468.

15. Harrigan C, Lucas CE, Ledgerwood AM, et al: Serial changes in primary hemostasis after massive transfusion. **Surgery** 1985; 98:836–840.

16. Jurkovich QJ: Hypothermia in the trauma patient. In: Maull KI (ed): **Advances in Trauma.** Chicago, Yearbook Medical Publishers, 1989, pp 111–140.

17. Kruse JA, Vyskocil JJ, Haupt MT: Intraosseous: A flexible option for the adult or child with delayed, difficult, or impossible conventional vascular access. **Critical Care Medicine** 1994; 22:728–735.

18. Lowry SF, Fong Y: Cytokines and the cellular response to injury and infection. In: Wilmore DW, Brennen MF, Harken AH, et al: Care of the Surgical Patient. **Scientific American**, 1990.

19. Lucas CE, Ledgerwood AM: Cardiovascular and renal response to hemorrhagic and septic shock. In: Clowes GHA Jr (ed): **Trauma, Sepsis and Shock: The Physiological Basis of Therapy.** New York, Marcel Dekker, 1988, pp 187–215.

20. Lucas CE, Ledgerwood AM, Saxe JM: Resuscitation from hemorrhagic shock. In: Ivatury RR, Cayten CG (eds): **The Textbook of Penetrating Trauma.** Baltimore, Williams & Wilkins, 1996.

21. Martin DJ, Lucas CE, Ledgerwood AM, et al: Fresh frozen plasma supplement to massive red blood cell transfusion. **Annals of Surgery** 1985; 202:505.

22. Novak L, Shackford SR, Bourguignon P, et al: Comparison of standard and alternative prehospital resuscitation in uncontrolled hemorrhagic shock and head injury. **Journal of Trauma** 1999; 47(5):834–844.

23. Pappas P, Brathwaite CE, Ross SE: Emergency central venous catheterization during resuscitation of trauma patients. **American Surgery** 1992; 58:108–111.

24. Peck KR, Altieri M: Intraosseous infusions: an old technique with modern applications. **Pediatric Nursing** 1988; 14(4):296–298.

25. Phillips GR, Rotondo MD, Schwab CW: Transfusion therapy. In: Maull IK, Rodriguez A, Wiles CE (eds): **Complications in Trauma and Critical Care.** Philadelphia, WB Saunders Company, 1996.

26. Poole GV, Meredith JW, Pennell T, et al: Comparison of colloids and crystalloids in resuscitation from hemorrhagic shock. **Surgery, Gynecology and Obstetrics** 1982; 154:577–586.

27. Rhodes M, Brader A, Lucke J, et al: A direct transport to the operating room for resuscitation of trauma patients. **Journal of Trauma** 1989; 29: 907–915.

28. Roberts JR, Hedges JR: Assessment of oxygenation. In: **Clinical Procedures in Emergency Medicine, 2nd Edition.** Philadelphia, WB Saunders Company, 1991, pp 67–83.

29. Rohrer MJ, Natale AM: Effect of hypothermia on the coagulation cascade. **Critical Care Medicine** 1992; 20:490.

30. Rotondo MF, Schwab CW, McGonigal MD, et al: "Damage control": An approach for improved survival in exsanguinating penetrating abdominal injury. **Journal of Trauma** 1993; 35:375–382.

31. Sarnoff SJ: Myocardial contractility as described by ventricular function curves: Observations on Starling's law of the heart. **Physiological Reviews** 1988; 35:107–122.

32. Sawyer RW, Bodai BI: The current status of intraosseous infusion. **Journal of the American College of Surgeons.** 1994; 179:353–361.

33. Scalea TM, Hartnett RW, Duncan AO, et al: Central venous oxygen saturation: A useful clinical tool in trauma patients. **Journal of Trauma** 1990; 30(12): 1539–1543.

34. Scalea TM, Simon HM, Duncan AO, et al: Geriatric blunt multiple trauma: Improved survival with early invasive monitoring. **Journal of Trauma** 1990; 30:129–136.

35. Schierhout G, Roberts I: Fluid resuscitation with colloid or crystalloid solutions in critically ill patients: A systematic review of randomised trials. **British Journal of Medicine** 1998; 316:961–964.

36. Schwartz SI: Hemostasis, surgical bleeding and transfusion. In: Schwartz S (ed): **Principles of Surgery, 5th Edition.** New York, McGraw-Hill, 1994, pp 95–118.

37. Shires GT: Principles and management of hemorrhagic shock. In: Shires GT (ed): **Principles of Trauma Care, 3rd Edition.** New York, McGraw-Hill, 1985, pp 3–42.

38. Velanovich V: Crystalloid versus colloid fluid resuscitation: A meta-analysis of mortality. **Surgery** 1990; 105:65–71.

39. Virgilio RW, Rice CL, Smith DE, et al: Crystalloid vs colloid resuscitation: Is one better? A randomized clinical study. **Surgery** 1979; 85(2): 129–139.

40. Werwath DL, Schwab CW, Scholter JR, et al: Microwave oven: A safe new method of warming crystalloids. **American Journal of Surgery** 1984; 12:656–659.

41. Williams JF, Seneff MG, Friedman BC, et al: Use of femoral venous catheters in critically ill adults: Prospective study. **Critical Care Medicine** 1991; 19:550–553.

42. York J, Arrilaga A, Graham R, et al: Fluid resuscitation of patients with multiple injuries and severe closed head injury: Experience with an aggressive fluid resuscitation strategy. **Journal of Trauma** 2000; 48(3):376–379.

SKILLS STATION

IV

Shock Assessment and Management

▪ OBJECTIVES:

Performance at this station will allow the participant to practice the assessment of the patient in shock, determine the cause of the shock state, institute the initial management of shock, and evaluate the patient's response to treatment. Specifically, the student will be able to:

1. Recognize the shock state.

2. Perform an evaluation of the patient to determine the extent of organ perfusion, including physical examination and the relevant adjuncts to the primary survey.

3. Identify the causes of the shock state.

4. Initiate the resuscitation of the patient in shock by identifying and controlling hemorrhage and promptly initiating volume replacement.

5. Identify the surface markings and demonstrate the techniques of vascular access for the following:
   a. Peripheral venous system
   b. Femoral vein
   c. Internal jugular vein
   d. Subclavian vein
   e. Intraosseous infusion in children

6. Utilize adjuncts in the assessment and management of the shock state, including:
   a. X-ray examination (chest and pelvic film)
   b. Diagnostic peritoneal lavage (DPL)
   c. Abdominal ultrasound
   d. Computed tomography (CT)
   e. Broselow™ Pediatric Emergency Tape

7. Identify the patients who will require operative resuscitation or transfer to the intensive care unit where extended monitoring capabilities are available.

8. Identify which additional therapeutic measures are necessary based on the patient's response to treatment and the clinical significance of the patients as classified by:
   a. Rapid responders

b. Transient responders

c. Nonresponders

■ PROCEDURES:

1. Discussion of the shock scenarios

2. Performance of vascular access procedures:
   a. Peripheral
   b. Femoral
   c. Internal jugular
   d. Subclavian
   e. Intraosseous infusion in children

3. Recognize the value of adjuncts used in the management of shock:
   a. Chest and pelvic x-rays
   b. Diagnostic peritoneal lavage
   c. Abdominal ultrasound
   d. Broselow™ Pediatric Emergency Tape

INTERACTIVE SKILLS PROCEDURES
Shock Assessment and Management

Note: A series of scenarios accompanies some of the skills procedures for this station. The scenarios are provided at the conclusion of the procedures for your review and preparation for this station. Tables pertaining to the initial assessment and management of the patient in shock also are provided for your review after the scenarios.

Note: Standard precautions are required whenever caring for the trauma patient.

I. PERIPHERAL VENOUS ACCESS

A. Select an appropriate site on an extremity, eg, antecubital, forearm, or saphenous vein.

B. Apply an elastic tourniquet above the proposed puncture site.

C. Clean the site with antiseptic solution.

D. Puncture the vein with a large-caliber, plastic over-the-needle catheter and observe for blood return.

E. Thread the catheter into the vein over the needle and then remove the needle and tourniquet.

F. Blood samples may be obtained at this time for laboratory determinations.

G. Connect the catheter to the intravenous infusion tubing and begin the infusion of warmed crystalloid solution.

H. Observe for possible infiltration of the fluids into the tissues.

I. Secure the catheter and tubing to the skin of the extremity.

II. FEMORAL VENIPUNCTURE: SELDINGER TECHNIQUE (See Figure 1, Femoral Venipuncture, page 90)

A. Place the patient in a supine position.

B. Cleanse the skin well around the venipuncture site and drape the area. Sterile gloves should be worn when performing this procedure.

C. Locate the femoral vein by palpating the femoral artery. The vein lies directly medial to the femoral artery (nerve, artery, vein, empty space). A finger should remain on the artery to facilitate anatomical location and to avoid insertion of the catheter into the artery.

D. If the patient is awake, use a local anesthetic at the venipuncture site.

E. Introduce a large-caliber needle attached to a 12-mL syringe with 0.5 to 1 mL of saline. The needle, directed toward the patient's head, should enter the skin directly over the femoral vein.

F. The needle and syringe are held parallel to the frontal plane.

G. Directing the needle cephalad and posteriorly, slowly advance the needle while gently withdrawing the plunger of the syringe.

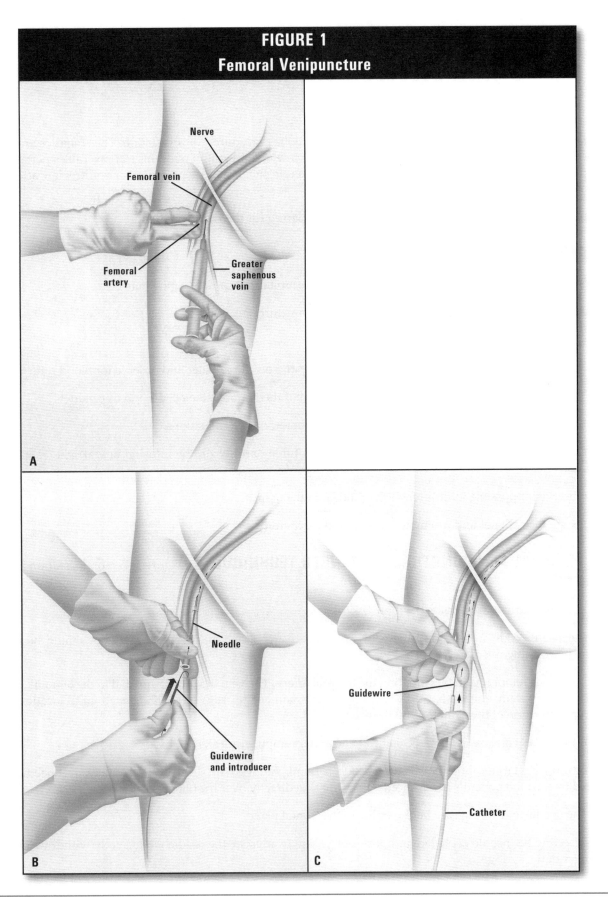

FIGURE 1
Femoral Venipuncture

A — Nerve, Femoral vein, Femoral artery, Greater saphenous vein

B — Needle, Guidewire and introducer

C — Guidewire, Catheter

Shock Assessment and Management **SHOCK**

H. When a free flow of blood appears in the syringe, remove the syringe and occlude the needle with a finger to prevent air embolism.

I. Insert the guidewire and remove the needle. Then insert the catheter over the guidewire.

J. Remove the guidewire and connect the catheter to the intravenous tubing.

K. Affix the catheter in place (ie, with suture), apply antibiotic ointment, and dress the area.

L. Tape the intravenous tubing in place.

M. Obtain chest and abdominal x-rays to identify the position and placement of the intravenous catheter.

N. The catheter should be changed as soon as practical.

Major Complications of Femoral Venous Access

1. Deep vein thrombosis

2. Arterial or neurologic injury

3. Infection

4. Arteriovenous fistula

III. SUBCLAVIAN VENIPUNCTURE: INFRACLAVICULAR APPROACH

A. Place the patient in a supine position, at least 15° head down to distend the neck veins and prevent an air embolism. Only if a c-spine injury has been excluded can the patient's head be turned away from the venipuncture site.

B. Cleanse the skin well around the venipuncture site and drape the area. Sterile gloves should be worn when performing this procedure.

C. If the patient is awake, use a local anesthetic at the venipuncture site.

D. Introduce a large-caliber needle, attached to a 12-mL syringe with 0.5 to 1 mL saline, 1 cm below the junction of the middle and medial thirds of the clavicle.

E. After the skin has been punctured, with the bevel of the needle upward, expel the skin plug that may occlude the needle.

F. The needle and syringe are held parallel to the frontal plane.

G. Direct the needle medially, slightly cephalad, and posteriorly behind the clavicle toward the posterior, superior angle to the sternal end of the clavicle (toward finger placed in the suprasternal notch).

H. Slowly advance the needle while gently withdrawing the plunger of the syringe.

I. When a free flow of blood appears in the syringe, rotate the bevel of the needle caudally, remove the syringe, and occlude the needle with a finger to prevent an air embolism.

J. Insert the guidewire while monitoring the electrocardiogram for rhythm abnormalities. Then remove the needle while holding the guidewire in place.

K. Insert the catheter over the guidewire to a predetermined depth (tip of catheter should be above the right atrium for fluid administration).

L. Connect the catheter to the intravenous tubing.

M. Affix the catheter securely to the skin (eg, with suture), apply antibiotic ointment, and dress the area.

N. Tape the intravenous tubing in place.

O. Obtain a chest film to identify the position of the intravenous line and a possible pneumothorax.

IV. INTERNAL JUGULAR VENIPUNCTURE: MIDDLE OR CENTRAL ROUTE

Note: Internal jugular catheterization is frequently difficult in the injured patient due to the precaution necessary to protect the patient's cervical spinal cord.

A. Place the patient in a supine position, at least 15° head down to distend the neck veins and to prevent an air embolism. Only if the cervical spine has been cleared radiographically can the patient's head be turned away from the venipuncture site.

B. Cleanse the skin well around the venipuncture site and drape the area. Sterile gloves should be worn when performing this procedure.

C. If the patient is awake, use a local anesthetic at the venipuncture site.

D. Introduce a large-caliber needle, attached to a 12-mL syringe with 0.5 to 1 mL of saline, into the center of the triangle formed by the 2 lower heads of the sternomastoid and the clavicle.

E. After the skin has been punctured, with the bevel of the needle upward, expel the skin plug that may occlude the needle.

F. Direct the needle caudally, parallel to the sagittal plane, at a 30° posterior angle with the frontal plane.

G. Slowly advance the needle while gently withdrawing the plunger of the syringe.

H. When a free flow of blood appears in the syringe, remove the syringe and occlude the needle with a finger to prevent air embolism. If the vein is not entered, withdraw the needle and redirect it 5° to 10° laterally.

I. Insert the guidewire while monitoring the ECG for rhythm abnormalities.

J. Remove the needle while securing the guidewire and advance the catheter over the wire. Connect the catheter to the intravenous tubing.

K. Affix the catheter in place to the skin (eg, with suture), apply antibiotic ointment, and dress the area.

L. Tape the intravenous tubing in place.

M. Obtain a chest film to identify the position of the intravenous line and a possible pneumothorax.

Complications of Central Venous Puncture

1. *Pneumo- or hemothorax*
2. *Venous thrombosis*
3. *Arterial or neurologic injury*
4. *Arteriovenous fistula*
5. *Chylothorax*
6. *Infection*
7. *Air embolism*

Shock Assessment and Management   **SHOCK**

V. INTRAOSSEOUS PUNCTURE/INFUSION: PROXIMAL TIBIAL ROUTE (See Figure 2, Intraosseous Puncture)

Note: The procedure described here is for children 6 years of age or younger for whom venous access is impossible due to circulatory collapse or for whom percutaneous peripheral venous cannulation has failed on 2 attempts. Intraosseous infusions should be limited to emergency resuscitation of the child and discontinued as soon as other venous access has been obtained. (Methylene blue dye may be mixed with the saline or water for demonstration purposes only. Provided that the needle is properly placed within the medullary canal, the methylene blue dye/saline solution seeps from the upper end of the chicken or turkey bone when the solution is injected. See item H.) (Techniques of intraosseous infusion in adults are not discussed here. See references in this chapter's bibliography for further information.)

A. Place the patient in a supine position. Selecting an uninjured lower extremity, place sufficient padding under the knee to effect an approximate 30° flexion of the knee and allow the patient's heel to rest comfortably on the gurney (stretcher).

B. Identify the puncture site—anteromedial surface of the proximal tibia, approximately 1 fingerbreadth (1 to 3 cm) below the tubercle.

C. Cleanse the skin well around the puncture site and drape the area. Sterile gloves should be worn when performing this procedure.

D. If the patient is awake, use a local anesthetic at the puncture site.

E. Initially at a 90° angle, introduce a short (threaded or smooth), large-caliber, bone-marrow aspiration needle (or a short, #18-gauge spinal needle with stylet) into the skin and periosteum with the needle bevel directed toward the foot and away from the epiphyseal plate.

F. After gaining purchase in the bone, direct the needle to 45° to 60° away from the epiphyseal plate. Using a gentle twisting or boring motion, advance the needle through the bone cortex and into the bone marrow.

G. Remove the stylet and attach to the needle a 12-mL syringe filled with approximately 6 mL of sterile saline. Gently withdraw on the plunger of the syringe. Aspiration of bone marrow into the syringe signifies entrance into the medullary cavity.

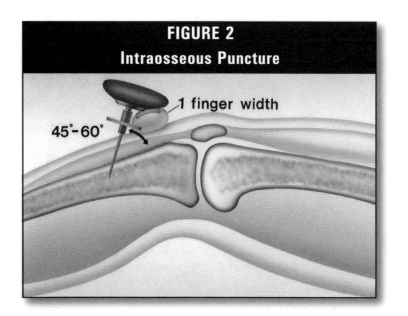

FIGURE 2
Intraosseous Puncture

1 finger width

45°-60°

H. Inject the saline into the needle to expel any clot that may occlude the needle. If the saline flushes through the needle easily and there is no evidence of swelling, the needle should be in the appropriate place. If bone marrow was not aspirated as outlined in G., but the needle flushes easily when injecting the saline without evidence of swelling, the needle should be in the appropriate place. Additionally, proper placement of the needle is indicated if the needle remains upright without support and intravenous solution flows freely without evidence of subcutaneous infiltration.

I. Connect the needle to the large-caliber intravenous tubing and begin fluid infusion. The needle is then carefully screwed further into the medullary cavity until the needle hub rests on the patient's skin and free flow continues. If a smooth needle is used, it should be stabilized at a 45° to 60° angle to the anteromedial surface of the child's leg.

J. Apply antibiotic ointment and a 3 × 3 sterile dressing. Secure the needle and tubing in place.

K. Routinely reevaluate the placement of the intraosseous needle, assuring that it remains through the bone cortex and in the medullary canal. Remember, intraosseous infusion should be limited to emergency resuscitation of the child and discontinued as soon as other venous access has been obtained.

Complications of Intraosseous Puncture

1. *Infection*
2. *Through-and-through penetration of the bone*
3. *Subcutaneous or subperiosteal infiltration*
4. *Pressure necrosis of the skin*
5. *Physeal plate injury*
6. *Hematoma*

VI. BROSELOW™ PEDIATRIC EMERGENCY TAPE

A specific skill is not outlined for the Broselow™ Pediatric Emergency Tape. However, participants need to be aware of its availability and its use when managing pediatric trauma. By measuring the height of the child, the child's estimated weight can be determined readily. One side of the tape provides drugs and their recommended doses for the pediatric patient based on weight. The other side provides equipment needs for the pediatric patient based on size. Therefore, participation at this station includes an orientation to the tape and its use.

VII. CASE SCENARIOS

A. Scenario #1

A 42-year-old woman was ejected from a vehicle during an automobile collision. En route to the emergency department, prehospital personnel report that her heart rate is 110 beats/minute, blood pressure is 88/46 mm Hg, and her respiratory rate is 26 breaths/minute. The patient is confused and her peripheral capillary refill is reduced. (See Table 3, Initial Assessment and Shock Mangement, page 95.)

B. Scenario #2

A 42-year-old woman arrives in the emergency department in full spinal protection with supplemental oxygen being administered. Her heart rate is 120 beats/minute, blood pressure is 80/46 mm Hg, and her respiratory rate is 30 breaths/minute. Her skin is pale, cool, and moist to touch. She moans when stimulated. (See Table 4, Pelvic Fractures, page 96.)

C. Scenario #3 (Continuation of previous scenario)

After the initiation of vascular access and the infusion of 1500 mL of warmed crystalloid solution, the patient's heart rate has decreased to 90 beats/minute, blood pressure is 110/80 mm Hg, and her respiratory rate is 22 breaths/minute. The patient is now able to speak, her breathing is less labored, and her peripheral perfusion has improved. (See Table 4, Pelvic Fractures, page 96.)

Table 3—Initial Assessment and Shock Management

CONDITION	ASSESSMENT (Physical Examination)	MANAGEMENT
Tension pneumothorax	• Tracheal deviation • Distended neck veins • Tympany • Absent breath sounds	• Needle decompression • Tube thoracostomy
Massive hemothorax	• ± Tracheal deviation • Flat neck veins • Percussion dullness • Absent breath sounds	• Venous access • Volume replacement • Surgical consultation • Tube thoracostomy
Cardiac tamponade	• Distended neck veins • Muffled heart tones • Ultrasound	Pericardiocentesis • Venous access • Pericardiotomy • Volume replacement • Thoracotomy
Intraabdominal hemorrhage	• Distended abdomen • Uterine lift, if pregnant • DPL/ultrasonography • Vaginal examination	• Venous access • Volume replacement • Surgical consultation • Displace uterus from vena cava
Obvious external bleeding	• Identify source of obvious external bleeding	Control external hemorrhage from all obvious sources • Direct pressure • Closure of actively bleeding • Splints scalp wounds

D. Scenario #4

The patient responds initially to the rapid infusion of 1500 mL of warmed crystalloid solution by a transient increase in her blood pressure to 110/80 mm Hg, a decrease in heart rate to 96 beats/minute, and improvements in her level of consciousness and peripheral perfusion. Fluid infusion is slowed to maintenance levels. Five minutes later, the assistant reports a deterioration in the patient blood pressure to 88/60 mm Hg, an increase in heart rate to 115 beats/minute, and a return in the delay of the peripheral capillary refill. (See Table 5, Transient Responder, page 97.)

Alternate scenario: The rapid infusion of 2000 mL of warmed crystalloid solution produces only a modest increase in the patient's blood pressure to 90/60 mm Hg and her heart rate remains at 110 beats/minute. Her urinary output since the insertion of the urinary catheter has been only 5 mL of very dark urine.

SHOCK

Table 4—Pelvic Fractures

CONDITION	IMAGE FINDINGS	SIGNIFICANCE	INTERVENTION
Pelvic fracture	Pelvic x-ray • Pubic ramus fracture	• Less blood loss than other types • Lateral compression mechanism	• Volume replacement • Possible transfusion • Avoid excessive manipulation

	• Open book	• Pelvic volume ↑	• Volume restoration
			• Probable transfusion
			• ↓ Pelvic volume
			  • Internal hip rotation
			  • PASG
			  • External fixator
			  • Angiography
			  • Skeletal traction
			• Orthopaedic consultation

	• Vertical shear	• Major source of blood loss	
Visceral organ injury	CT scan • Intraabdominal hemorrhage	• Potential for continuing blood loss • Performed only in hemodynamically normal patients	• Volume replacement • Possible transfusion • Surgical consultation

E. Scenario #5

A 42-year-old woman, ejected from her vehicle during a crash, arrives in the emergency department unconscious with a heart rate of 140 beats/minute, blood pressure of 60 mm Hg by palpation, and pale, cool, and pulseless extremities. Endotracheal intubation and assisted ventilation are initiated. Rapid volume infusion of 2000 mL of **warmed crystalloid** solution does not improve her vital signs, and she does not demonstrate evidence of improved organ perfusion. (See Table 6, Nonresponder, page 97.)

F. Scenario #6

An 18-month-old boy is brought to the emergency department by his mother who apparently is the recipient of spousal abuse. The child has evidence of multiple soft-tissue injury about the chest, abdomen, and extremities. His skin color is pale, he has a weak thready pulse rate of 160 beats/minute, and he responds only to painful stimuli with a weak cry.

Table 5–Transient Responder

ETIOLOGY	PHYSICAL EXAM	ADDITIONAL DIAGNOSTIC STEPS	INTERVENTION
Underestimation of blood loss or Continuing blood loss	• Abdominal distention • Pelvic fracture • Extremity fracture • Obvious external bleeding	• DPL or ultrasonography	• Surgical consultation • Volume infusion • Blood transfusion • Apply appropriate splints
Nonhemorrhagic • Cardiac tamponade	• Distended neck veins • ↓ Heart sounds • Normal breath sounds	• Pericardiocentesis	• Reevaluate chest • Needle decompression • Tube thoracostomy
• Recurrent/persistent tension pneumothorax	• Distended neck veins • Tracheal shift • Absent breath sounds • Hyperresonant chest percussion		

Table 6–Nonresponder

ETIOLOGY	PHYSICAL EXAM	ADDITIONAL DIAGNOSTIC STEPS	INTERVENTION
Massive blood loss (Class III or IV) • Intraabdominal bleeding	• Abdominal distention	• DPL or ultrasonography	• Immediate intervention by surgeon • Volume restoration • Operative resuscitation
Nonhemorrhagic • Tension pneumothorax	• Distended neck veins • Tracheal shift • Absent breath sounds • Hyperresonant chest percussion		• Chest decompression (needle followed by tube thoracostomy) • Recognize that invasive monitoring may be required
• Cardiac tamponade	• Distended neck veins • ↓ Heart sounds • Normal breath sounds	• Pericardiocentesis	• Reassess ABCDEs • Reevaluate cardiac status • Pericardiocentesis
• Blunt cardiac injury	• Irregular heart rate • Inadequate perfusion	• Ischemic ECG changes • Transesophageal echocardiography • Ultrasonography (pericardial)	• Prepare for OR • Invasive monitoring • Inotropic support • Consider operative intervention

SKILLS STATION

Venous Cutdown
(Optional Station)

▮ OBJECTIVES:

Performance at the station will allow the participant to practice and demonstrate on a live, anesthetized animal or fresh, human cadaver the technique of peripheral venous cutdown.

Upon completion of this station, the participant will be able to:

1. Identify and describe the surface markings and structures to be noted in performing a peripheral venous cutdown.

2. Describe the indications and contraindications for a peripheral venous cutdown.

▮ ANATOMIC CONSIDERATIONS FOR VENOUS CUTDOWN:

1. The primary site for a peripheral venous cutdown is the greater saphenous vein at the ankle, which is located at a point approximately 2 cm anterior and superior to the medial malleolus. (See Figure 3, Saphenous Venous Cutdown, page 102.)

2. A secondary site is the antecubital medial basilic vein, located 2.5 cm lateral to the medial epicondyle of the humerus at the flexion crease of the elbow.

INTERACTIVE SKILLS PROCEDURE

Venous Cutdown

Note: Standard precautions are required whenever caring for the trauma patient.

I. VENOUS CUTDOWN

A. Prepare the skin of the ankle with antiseptic solution and drape the area.

B. Infiltrate the skin over the vein with 0.5% lidocaine.

C. A full-thickness transverse skin incision is made through the area of anesthesia to a length of 2.5 cm.

D. By blunt dissection, using a curved hemostat, the vein is identified and dissected free from any accompanying structures.

E. Elevate and dissect the vein for a distance of approximately 2 cm to free it from its bed.

F. Ligate the distal mobilized vein, leaving the suture in place for traction.

G. Pass a tie around the vein, cephalad.

H. Make a small transverse venotomy and gently dilate the venotomy with the tip of a closed hemostat.

I. Introduce a plastic cannula through the venotomy and secure it in place by tying the upper ligature around the vein and cannula. The cannula should be inserted an adequate distance to prevent dislodging.

J. Attach the intravenous tubing to the cannula and close the incision with interrupted sutures.

K. Apply a sterile dressing with a topical antibiotic ointment.

Complications of Peripheral Venous Cutdown

1. *Cellulitis*
2. *Hematoma*
3. *Phlebitis*
4. *Perforation of the posterior wall of the vein*
5. *Venous thrombosis*
6. *Nerve transaction*
7. *Arterial transaction*

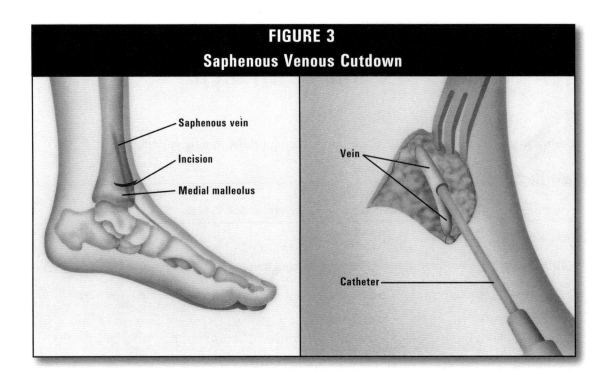

FIGURE 3
Saphenous Venous Cutdown

Saphenous vein

Incision

Medial malleolus

Vein

Catheter

FOUR

CHAPTER

Thoracic Trauma

■ OBJECTIVES:

Upon completion of this topic, the participant will be able to identify and initiate treatment of common and life-threatening thoracic injuries. Specifically, the student will be able to:

A. Identify and initiate treatment of the following injuries during the primary survey:

    1. Airway obstruction

    2. Tension pneumothorax

    3. Open pneumothorax

    4. Flail chest

    5. Massive hemothorax

    6. Cardiac tamponade

B. Identify and initiate treatment of the following injuries during the secondary survey:

    1. Simple pneumothorax

    2. Hemothorax

    3. Pulmonary contusion

    4. Tracheobronchial disruption

    5. Blunt cardiac injury

    6. Traumatic aortic disruption

    7. Traumatic diaphragmatic injury

    8. Mediastinal traversing wounds

THORACIC TRAUMA

I. INTRODUCTION

A. Incidence

Thoracic trauma is a significant cause of mortality. Many thoracic trauma patients die after reaching the hospital, and many of these deaths could be prevented with prompt diagnosis and treatment. Less than 10% of blunt chest injuries and only about 15% to 30% of penetrating chest injuries require thoracotomy. Most patients sustaining thoracic trauma may be managed by technical procedures within the capabilities of doctors who take this course.

B. Pathophysiology

Hypoxia, hypercarbia, and acidosis often result from chest injuries. Tissue hypoxia results from inadequate delivery of oxygen to the tissues because of hypovolemia (blood loss), pulmonary ventilation/perfusion mismatch (eg, contusion, hematoma, and alveolar collapse), and changes in intrathoracic pressure relationships (eg, tension pneumothorax, open pneumothorax). Hypercarbia most often results from inadequate ventilation caused by changes in intrathoracic pressure relationships and depressed level of consciousness. Metabolic acidosis is caused by hypoperfusion of the tissues (shock).

C. Initial Assessment and Management

1. Patient management must consist of:
   a. Primary survey
   b. Resuscitation of vital functions
   c. Detailed secondary survey
   d. Definitive care

2. Because hypoxia is the most serious feature of chest injury, early interventions are designed to prevent or correct hypoxia.

3. Immediately life-threatening injuries are treated as quickly and as simply as possible.

4. Most life-threatening thoracic injuries are treated by airway control or an appropriately placed chest tube or needle.

5. The secondary survey is influenced by a history of the injury and a high index of suspicion for specific injuries.

II. PRIMARY SURVEY: LIFE-THREATENING INJURIES

The primary survey of the patient with thoracic injuries begins with the airway. **Major problems should be corrected as they are identified.**

A. Airway

Major injuries affecting the airway should be recognized and addressed during the primary survey. Airway patency and air exchange should be assessed by listening for air movement at the patient's nose, mouth, and lung fields; by inspecting the oropharynx for foreign body obstruction; and by observing for intercostal and supraclavicular muscle retractions.

Laryngeal injury may accompany major thoracic trauma. Although the clinical presentation may occasionally be subtle, acute airway obstruction from laryngeal trauma is a life-threatening injury. (See Chapter 2, Airway and Ventilatory Management.)

Several unusual conditions may arise in the patient with skeletal trauma that may significantly compromise the patient's airway or breathing. Injury to the upper chest, creating a posterior dislocation or fracture dislocation of the sternoclavicular joint, can lead to acute upper airway obstruction as the displaced proximal fracture fragment or distal joint component comes to rest on the trachea. This also may be associated occasionally with vascular injury to the ipsilateral extremity as the fracture fragment compresses or lacerates the major branches of the aortic arch.

Recognition of this injury is by upper airway obstruction (stridor), a marked change in the expected voice quality (if the patient is able to talk), and obvious trauma at the base of the neck with a palpable defect in the region of the sternoclavicular joint.

Management of this injury consists of establishing a patent airway, potentially by endotracheal intubation. However, this may be difficult if there is significant pressure on the trachea. More importantly, a closed reduction of the injury may be achieved by extending the shoulders, grasping the clavicle with a pointed clamp, such as a towel clip, and manually reducing the fracture. This injury, once reduced, usually is stable if the patient is in the supine position.

Other injuries affecting the airway are addressed in Chapter 2, Airway and Ventilatory Management.

B. Breathing

The patient's chest and neck should be completely exposed to allow assessment of breathing and the neck veins. Respiratory movement and quality of respirations are assessed by observing, palpating, and listening.

Important, yet often subtle, signs of chest injury or hypoxia include an increased respiratory rate and a change in the breathing pattern, especially progressively more shallow respirations. Cyanosis is a late sign of hypoxia in the trauma patient. However, the absence of cyanosis does not necessarily indicate adequate tissue oxygenation or an adequate airway.

The major thoracic injuries affecting breathing that should be recognized and addressed during the primary survey are included herein.

1. Tension pneumothorax

A tension pneumothorax develops when a "one-way-valve" air leak occurs either from the lung or through the chest wall. Air is forced into the thoracic cavity without any means of escape, completely collapsing the affected lung. The mediastinum is displaced to the opposite side, decreasing venous return and compressing the opposite lung.

The most common cause of tension pneumothorax is mechanical ventilation with positive pressure ventilation in the patient with a visceral pleural injury. However, a tension pneumothorax can complicate a simple pneumothorax following penetrating or blunt chest trauma in which a parenchymal lung injury has failed to seal, or even after a misguided attempt at subclavian or internal jugular venous catheter insertion. Occasionally, traumatic defects in the chest wall also may cause a tension pneumothorax if incorrectly covered with occlusive dressings or if the defect itself constitutes a flap-valve mechanism. Tension pneumothorax also may occur from markedly displaced thoracic spine fractures.

Tension pneumothorax is a clinical diagnosis, and treatment should not be delayed by waiting for radiologic confirmation. A tension pneumothorax is characterized by chest pain, air hunger,

respiratory distress, tachycardia, hypotension, tracheal deviation, unilateral absence of breath sounds, neck vein distention, and cyanosis as a late manifestation. Because of the similarity in their signs, a tension pneumothorax may be confused initially with cardiac tamponade. Differentiation may be made by a hyperresonant percussion note and absent breath sounds over the affected hemithorax.

Tension pneumothorax requires **immediate decompression** and is managed initially by rapidly inserting a large-caliber needle into the second intercostal space in the midclavicular line of the affected hemithorax. This maneuver converts the injury to a simple pneumothorax. (Note: The possibility of subsequent pneumothorax as a result of the needle stick now exists.) Repeated reassessment is necessary. Definitive treatment usually requires only the insertion of a chest tube into the fifth intercostal space (usually the nipple level), just anterior to the midaxillary line.

2. Open pneumothorax (sucking chest wound)

Large defects of the chest wall, which remain open, result in an open pneumothorax or sucking chest wound. Equilibration between intrathoracic pressure and atmospheric pressure is immediate. If the opening in the chest wall is approximately two-thirds the diameter of the trachea, air passes preferentially through the chest defect with each respiratory effort, because air tends to follow the path of least resistance through the large chest-wall defect. Effective ventilation is thereby impaired, leading to hypoxia and hypercarbia.

Initial management of an open pneumothorax is accomplished by promptly closing the defect with a sterile occlusive dressing, large enough to overlap the wound's edges, that is taped securely on 3 sides. Taping the occlusive dressing on 3 sides provides a flutter-type valve effect. As the patient breathes in, the dressing occludes the wound, preventing air from entering. During exhalation the open end of the dressing allows air to escape from the pleural space. A chest tube should be placed remote from the wound as soon as possible. Securely taping all edges of the dressing can cause air to accumulate in the thoracic cavity, resulting in a tension pneumothorax unless a chest tube is in place. Any occlusive dressing (eg, plastic wrap or petrolatum gauze) may be used

THORACIC TRAUMA

as a temporary measure so rapid assessment can continue. Definitive surgical closure of the defect is frequently required.

3. Flail chest

A flail chest occurs when a segment of the chest wall does not have bony continuity with the rest of the thoracic cage. This condition usually results from trauma associated with multiple rib fractures, ie, 2 or more ribs fractured in 2 or more places. The presence of a flail chest segment results in severe disruption of normal chest wall movement. If the injury to the underlying lung is significant, serious hypoxia may result. The major difficulty in flail chest stems from the injury to the underlying lung (pulmonary contusion). Although chest wall instability leads to paradoxical motion of the chest wall during inspiration and expiration, this defect alone does not cause hypoxia. Associated pain with restricted chest wall movement and underlying lung injury contributes to the patient's hypoxia.

Flail chest may not be apparent initially because of splinting of the chest wall. The patient moves air poorly, and movement of the thorax is asymmetrical and uncoordinated. Palpation of abnormal respiratory motion and crepitus of rib or cartilage fractures aid the diagnosis. A satisfactory chest x-ray may suggest multiple rib fractures, but may not show costochondral separation. Arterial blood gas (ABG) analyses, suggesting respiratory failure with hypoxia, also may aid in diagnosing a flail chest.

Initial therapy includes adequate ventilation, administration of humidified oxygen, and fluid resuscitation. In the absence of systemic hypotension, the administration of crystalloid intravenous solutions should be carefully controlled to prevent overhydration. The injured lung in a flail chest is sensitive to both underresuscitation of shock and fluid overload. Specific measures to optimize fluid measurement must be taken for the patient with flail chest.

The definitive treatment is to reexpand the lung, ensure oxygenation as completely as possible, administer fluids judiciously, and provide analgesia to improve ventilation. Some patients can be managed without the use of a ventilator. However, prevention of hypoxia is of paramount impor-

tance for the trauma patient and a short period of intubation and ventilation may be necessary until the diagnosis of the entire injury pattern is complete. A careful assessment of the respiratory rate, arterial oxygen tension, and an estimate of the work of breathing will indicate appropriate timing for intubation and ventilation.

4. Massive hemothorax

Accumulation of blood and fluid in a hemithorax can significantly compromise respiratory efforts by compressing the lung and preventing adequate ventilation. Such massive acute accumulations of blood more dramatically present as hypotension and shock, and will be discussed further in C., Circulation.

C. Circulation

The patient's pulse should be assessed for quality, rate, and regularity. In the hypovolemic patient, the radial and dorsalis pedis pulses may be absent due to volume depletion. Blood pressure and pulse pressure should be measured and the peripheral circulation assessed by observing and palpating the skin for color and temperature. Neck veins should be assessed for distention. Remember, neck veins may not be distended in the hypovolemic patient with cardiac tamponade, tension pneumothorax, or traumatic diaphragmatic injury.

A cardiac monitor and pulse oximeter should be attached to the patient. Patients sustaining thoracic trauma—especially in the area of the sternum or from a rapid deceleration injury—are susceptible to myocardial injury, which may lead to dysrhythmias. Hypoxia and/or acidosis enhance this possibility. Premature ventricular contractions, a common dysrhythmia, may require treatment with an immediate lidocaine bolus (1 mg/kg) followed by a lidocaine drip (2 to 4 mg/minute). Pulseless electric activity (PEA, formerly known as electromechanical dissociation) is manifest by an electrocardiogram (ECG) showing a rhythm while the patient has no identifiable pulse. PEA may be present in cardiac tamponade, tension pneumothorax, profound hypovolemia, or cardiac rupture.

The major injuries affecting circulation that should be recognized and addressed during the primary survey are included herein.

1. Massive hemothorax

Massive hemothorax results from a rapid accumulation of more than 1500 mL of blood or one-third or more of the patient's blood volume in the chest cavity. It is most commonly caused by a penetrating wound that disrupts the systemic or hilar vessels. It also may be the result of blunt trauma. The blood loss is complicated by hypoxia. The neck veins may be flat secondary to severe hypovolemia. However, neck veins may be distended, if there is an associated tension pneumothorax. Rarely will the mechanical effects of massive intrathoracic blood shift the mediastinum enough to cause distended neck veins. A massive hemothorax is discovered when shock is associated with the absence of breath sounds and/or dullness to percussion on one side of the chest.

Massive hemothorax is initially managed by the simultaneous restoration of blood volume and decompression of the chest cavity. Large-caliber intravenous lines and rapid crystalloid infusion are begun and type-specific blood is administered as soon as possible. Blood from the chest tube should be collected in a device suitable for autotransfusion. A single chest tube (#38 French) is inserted usually at the nipple level, just anterior to the midaxillary line, and rapid restoration of volume continues as decompression of the chest cavity is completed. When massive hemothorax is suspected, prepare for autotransfusion. If 1500 mL is immediately evacuated, it is highly likely that the patient will require an early thoracotomy.

Some patients who have an initial volume output of less than 1500 mL but continue to bleed may require a thoracotomy. This decision is based not so much on the rate of continuing blood loss (200 mL/hour for 2 to 4 hours), but more on the patient's physiologic status. Persistent blood transfusion requirements are an indication for thoracotomy. During patient resuscitation, the volume of blood initially drained from the chest tube and the rate of continuing blood loss must be factored into the amount of intravenous fluid replacement. The color of the blood (arterial or venous) is a poor indicator of the necessity for thoracotomy.

Penetrating anterior chest wounds medial to the nipple line and posterior wounds medial to the scapula should alert the doctor to the possible need for thoracotomy, because of possible damage to the great vessels, hilar structures, and the heart, with the associated potential for cardiac tamponade. **Thoracotomy is not indicated unless a surgeon, qualified by training and experience, is present.**

2. Cardiac tamponade

Cardiac tamponade most commonly results from penetrating injuries. However, blunt injury also may cause the pericardium to fill with blood from the heart, great vessels, or pericardial vessels. The human pericardial sac is a fixed fibrous structure, and only a relatively small amount of blood is required to restrict cardiac activity and interfere with cardiac filling. Removal of small amounts of blood or fluid, often as little as 15 mL to 20 mL, by pericardiocentesis may result in immediate hemodynamic improvement if tamponade exists. The diagnosis of cardiac tamponade can be difficult. The classic diagnostic Beck's triad consists of venous pressure elevation, decline in arterial pressure, and muffled heart tones. However, muffled heart tones are difficult to assess in the noisy emergency department; distended neck veins may be absent due to hypovolemia; and hypotension is most often caused by hypovolemia. Pulsus paradoxus is a normal physiologic decrease in systolic blood pressure that occurs during spontaneous inspiration. When this change is exaggerated and exceeds 10 mm Hg, it is another sign of cardiac tamponade. However, pulsus paradoxus also may be absent in some patients or difficult to detect in the emergency setting. Additionally, tension pneumothorax, particularly on the left side, may mimic cardiac tamponade. Kussmaul's sign (a rise in venous pressure with inspiration when breathing spontaneously) is a true paradoxical venous pressure abnormality associated with tamponade. PEA in the absence of hypovolemia and tension pneumothorax suggests cardiac tamponade. Insertion of a central venous line may aid diagnosis, but can be elevated for a variety of reasons. Prompt transthoracic ultrasound (echocardiogram) may be a valuable noninvasive method of assessing the pericardium, but reports suggest it too has a significant false-negative rate of about 5% to 10%. In hemodynamically abnormal patients with blunt trauma, provided it does **not** delay patient resuscitation, an examination of the pericardial sac for the presence of fluid may be obtained as part of a focused abdominal ultrasound examination performed by the properly trained and credentialed surgical team in the emergency department. (See Chapter 5, Abdominal Trauma, V. F., Diagnostic Studies in Blunt Trauma.)

Cardiac tamponade may develop slowly, allowing a more leisurely evaluation, or may occur rapidly, requiring rapid diagnosis and treatment. Diagnostic methods include focused assessment sonogram in trauma (FAST) and/or pericardiocentesis. FAST performed in the emergency department is a rapid and accurate method of imaging the heart and pericardium. It may be 90% accurate for the presence of pericardial fluid for the experienced operator. If the FAST is positive for pericardial fluid and if the patient's diagnosis is consistent with cardiac tamponade, a subxyphoid pericardiocentesis may help to temporarily normalize the patient's hemodynamic status until the patient can be transported to the operating room for thoracotomy, pericardiotomy, and repair of the injured heart. However, not all hospitals have the ability to perform FAST. Pericardiocentesis can be diagnostic as well as therapeutic, but is not definitive treatment for cardiac tamponade. (For further information regarding FAST, see Chapter 5, Abdominal Trauma.)

Prompt diagnosis and evacuation of pericardial blood is indicated for patients who do not respond to the usual measures of resuscitation for hemorrhagic shock and have the potential for cardiac tamponade. This lifesaving maneuver should not be delayed for any diagnostic adjunct. The simplest method of performing pericardial evacuation is pericardiocentesis. A high index of suspicion coupled with a patient who is unresponsive to resuscitative efforts are all that is necessary to initiate pericardiocentesis by the subxyphoid method. Alternatively, and only if an appropriate surgeon is present, a subxyphoid pericardial window or emergency thoracotomy and pericardiotomy can be performed. These procedures are best performed in the operating room if the patient's condition allows.

Although cardiac tamponade may be strongly suspected, the initial administration of intravenous fluid raises the venous pressure and improves cardiac output transiently while preparations are made for either FAST or subxyphoid pericardiocentesis. The use of a plastic-sheathed

needle or the Seldinger technique insertion of a flexible catheter is ideal, but the urgent priority is to aspirate blood from the pericardial sac. ECG monitoring may identify current of injury (increased T-wave voltage when the pericardiocentesis needle touches the epicardium) and needle-induced dysrhythmias. Because of the self-sealing qualities of the injured myocardium, aspiration of pericardial blood alone may relieve symptoms temporarily. However, all patients with positive pericardiocentesis resulting from trauma will require open thoracotomy or median sternotomy for inspection and repair of the heart. Pericardiocentesis may not be diagnostic or therapeutic because the blood in the pericardial sac is clotted. Preparations for transfer of these patients to the appropriate facility for definitive care are necessary. Pericardiotomy via thoracotomy may be lifesaving, but is indicated **only** when a qualified surgeon is available.

III. RESUSCITATIVE THORACOTOMY

Closed heart massage for cardiac arrest or PEA is ineffective in a hypovolemic patient. Patients with **penetrating** thoracic injuries who arrive pulseless, but with myocardial electrical activity, may be candidates for immediate resuscitative thoracotomy. **A qualified surgeon must be present at the time of the patient's arrival to determine the need and potential for success of an emergency department resuscitative thoracotomy.** A left anterior thoracotomy is performed to gain access. Restoration of intravascular volume is continued, and endotracheal intubation and mechanical ventilation are essential.

Patients sustaining blunt injuries who arrive pulseless but with myocardial electrical activity are **not** candidates for resuscitative thoracotomy.

The therapeutic maneuvers that can be effectively accomplished with a resuscitative thoracotomy are (1) evacuation of pericardial blood causing tamponade, (2) direct control of exsanguinating intrathoracic hemorrhage, (3) open cardiac massage, and (4) cross-clamping of the descending aorta to slow blood loss below the diaphragm and increase perfusion to the brain and heart. Despite the value of these maneuvers, multiple reports confirm that emergency department thoracotomy for patients with blunt trauma and cardiac arrest is rarely effective.

Once these and other immediately life-threatening injuries have been treated, attention may be directed to the secondary survey.

IV. SECONDARY SURVEY: LIFE-THREATENING CHEST INJURIES

The secondary survey requires further in-depth physical examination, an upright chest x-ray if the patient's condition permits, ABG measurements, pulse oximetry monitoring, and an ECG. In addition to lung expansion and the presence of fluid, the chest film should be examined for widening of the mediastinum, a shift of the midline, or loss of anatomic detail. Multiple rib fractures and fractures of the first and/or second rib(s) suggest that a severe force has been delivered to the chest and underlying tissues.

Eight lethal injuries are considered herein:

1. Simple pneumothorax
2. Hemothorax
3. Pulmonary contusion
4. Tracheobronchial tree injury
5. Blunt cardiac injury
6. Traumatic aortic disruption
7. Traumatic diaphragmatic injury
8. Mediastinal traversing wounds

Unlike immediately life-threatening conditions that are recognized during the primary survey, the above-referenced injuries usually are not obvious on physical examination. Diagnosis requires a **high index of suspicion.** These injuries are more often missed than diagnosed during the initial posttraumatic period; however, if overlooked, lives may be lost.

A. Simple Pneumothorax

Pneumothorax results from air entering the potential space between the visceral and parietal pleura. Both penetrating and nonpenetrating trauma may cause this injury. Thoracic spine fracture dislocations also may be associated with a pneumothorax. Lung laceration with air leakage is the most common cause of trauma pneumothorax resulting from blunt trauma.

The thorax is normally and completely filled by the lung, being held to the chest wall by surface tension between the pleural surfaces. Air in the pleural

space collapses lung tissue. A ventilation/perfusion defect occurs because the blood perfusing the non-ventilated area is not oxygenated.

When a pneumothorax is present, breath sounds are decreased on the affected side. Percussion demonstrates hyperresonance. An upright, expiratory x-ray of the chest aids the diagnosis.

A pneumothorax is best treated with a chest tube usually in the fourth or fifth intercostal space, just anterior to the midaxillary line. Observation and/or aspiration of any pneumothorax are risky. Once a chest tube is inserted and connected to an underwater seal apparatus with or without suction, a chest x-ray is necessary to confirm reexpansion of the lung. General anesthesia or positive pressure ventilation should never be administered in a patient who sustains traumatic pneumothorax or who is at risk for unexpected intraoperative pneumothorax until a chest tube is inserted. A simple pneumothorax can readily convert into a life-threatening tension pneumothorax, particularly if it is initially unrecognized and positive pressure ventilation is applied. The patient's chest also should be decompressed before transporting the patient with a pneumothorax via air ambulance.

B. Hemothorax

The primary cause of hemothorax is lung laceration or laceration of an intercostal vessel or internal mammary artery due to either penetrating or blunt trauma. Thoracic spine fracture dislocations also may be associated with a hemothorax. Usually bleeding is self-limiting and does not require operative intervention.

Acute hemothorax, sufficient enough to appear on chest x-ray, is best treated with a large-caliber chest tube. The chest tube evacuates blood, reduces the risk of a clotted hemothorax, and importantly provides a method for continuous monitoring of blood loss. Evacuation of blood or fluid also will allow a better assessment of potential diaphragmatic injury. Although many factors are involved in the decision to operate on a patient with a hemothorax, the patient's physiologic status and the volume of blood drainage from the chest tube are major factors. As a guideline, if 1500 mL of blood is obtained immediately through the chest tube, if drainage of more than 200 mL/hour for 2 to 4 hours occurs, or if persistent blood transfusion is required, operative exploration should be considered.

THORACIC TRAUMA

C. Pulmonary Contusion

Pulmonary contusion is the most common potentially lethal chest injury. The respiratory failure may be subtle and develops over time rather than occurring instantaneously. The plan for definitive management may change with time, warranting careful monitoring and reevaluation of the patient.

Patients with significant hypoxia (ie, Pao_2 ≤65 mm Hg [8.6 kPa] or Sao_2 ≤90% on room air) should be intubated and ventilated within the first hour after injury. Associated medical conditions, eg, chronic pulmonary disease and renal failure, increase the likelihood of early intubation and mechanical ventilation. Some patients with stable conditions may be managed selectively without endotracheal intubation or mechanical ventilation.

Pulse oximetry monitoring, ABG determinations, ECG monitoring, and appropriate ventilatory equipment are necessary for optimal management. Any patient with the aforementioned preexisting conditions who is to be transferred should be intubated and ventilated.

D. Tracheobronchial Tree Injury

Injury to the trachea or major bronchus is an unusual and potentially fatal injury that is often overlooked on initial assessment. In blunt trauma the majority of such injuries occur within 1 inch of the carina. Most patients with this injury die at the scene. Those who reach the hospital alive have a high mortality from associated injuries.

If suspicion of a tracheobronchial injury exists, immediate surgical consultation is warranted. A patient with a tracheobronchial injury frequently presents with hemoptysis, subcutaneous emphysema, or tension pneumothorax with a mediastinal shift. A pneumothorax associated with a persistent large air leak after tube thoracostomy suggests a tracheobronchial injury. More than 1 chest tube often is necessary to overcome a very large leak and expand the lung. Bronchoscopy confirms the diagnosis of the injury. Opposite main stem bronchial intubation may be temporarily required to provide adequate oxygenation.

Intubation frequently may be difficult because of anatomic distortion from paratracheal hematoma, associated oropharyngeal injuries, or the tracheobronchial injury itself. For such patients, immediate operative intervention is indicated. In more stable patients, operative treatment of tracheobronchial injuries may be delayed until the acute inflammation and edema resolve.

E. Blunt Cardiac Injury

Blunt cardiac injury can result in myocardial muscle contusion, cardiac chamber rupture, or valvular disruption. Chamber rupture typically presents with cardiac injury tamponade, and should be recognized during the primary survey. However, occasionally the signs and symptoms of tamponade may be slow to develop with an atrial rupture.

Patients with myocardial contusion may complain of chest discomfort, but the complaints are often attributed to chest wall contusion or fractures of the sternum and/or ribs. The true diagnosis of myocardial contusion can only be established by direct inspection of the injured myocardium. The clinically important sequelae of myocardial contusion are hypotension, significant conduction abnormalities on ECG, or wall motion abnormality on 2-dimensional echocardiography. The electrocardiographic changes are variable and may even indicate frank myocardial infarction. Multiple premature ventricular contractions, unexplained sinus tachycardia, atrial fibrillation, bundle branch block (usually right), and ST segment changes are the most common electrocardiographic findings. Elevated central venous pressure in the absence of obvious cause may indicate right ventricular dysfunction secondary to contusion. It also is important to remember that the injury event may have been precipitated by a true myocardial ischemic episode.

Cardiac troponins may diagnose myocardial infarction. However, their use in diagnosing blunt cardiac injury is inconclusive and offers no additional information beyond that available by ECG. Therefore, they have no role in the evaluation and management of the patient with a myocardial contusion.

Patients with myocardial contusion diagnosed by conduction abnormalities are at risk for sudden dysrhythmias and should be monitored for the first 24 hours. After this interval, the risk of sudden dysrhythmia appears to decrease substantially.

F. Traumatic Aortic Disruption

Traumatic aortic rupture is a common cause of sudden death after an automobile collision or fall from a great height. For immediate survivors, salvage is frequently possible if aortic rupture is identified and treated early.

Patients with aortic rupture, who are potentially salvageable, tend to have an incomplete laceration near the ligamentum arteriosum of the aorta. Continuity maintained by an intact adventitial layer or contained mediastinal hematoma prevents immediate death. Many of the surviving patients die in the hospital if left untreated. Some blood may escape into the mediastinum, but 1 characteristic shared by all survivors is that this is a contained hematoma. Persistent or recurrent hypotension is usually due to a separate, unidentified bleeding site. Although free rupture of a transected aorta into the left chest does occur and causes hypotension, it usually is fatal unless the patient is operated on within a few minutes.

Specific signs and symptoms are frequently absent. A high index of suspicion prompted by a history of decelerating force and characteristic radiologic findings, followed by arteriography, are the means of making the diagnosis. Angiography should be performed liberally because the findings of the chest x-ray, especially the supine view, are unreliable. Approximately 3% of the aortograms will be positive for aortic rupture if liberal indications for angiography are employed for all patients with widened mediastinum. Adjunctive radiologic signs, which may or may not be present, indicate the likelihood of major vascular injury in the chest. They include:

1. Widened mediastinum

2. Obliteration of the aortic knob

3. Deviation of the trachea to the right

4. Obliteration of the space between the pulmonary artery and the aorta (obscuration of AP window)

5. Depression of the left main stem bronchus

6. Deviation of the esophagus (nasogastric tube) to the right

7. Widened paratracheal stripe

8. Widened paraspinal interfaces

9. Presence of a pleural or apical cap

10. Left hemothorax

11. Fractures of the first or second rib or scapula

False-positive and false-negative findings occur with each x-ray sign, and, rarely (1% to 2%), no mediastinal or initial chest x-ray abnormality is present in patients with great vessel injury. If there is the slightest suspicion of aortic injury, the patient should be evaluated at a facility capable of repairing a diagnosed injury. Aortography is the gold standard in the diagnosis of blunt aortic rupture. Transesophageal echocardiography (TEE) also appears to be a useful, less invasive diagnostic tool.

Helical contrast-enhanced computed tomography (CT) of the chest has now been shown to be an accurate screening method for patients with suspected blunt aortic injury. Generally, a patient who is hemodynamically abnormal should not be placed in a CT scanner. The sensitivity and specificity of helical contrast-enhanced CT has been shown to be 100% each, but this result is very technology dependent. If enhanced helical CT of the chest is negative for mediastinal hematoma and aortic rupture, no further diagnostic imaging of the aorta is necessary. Should the CT be positive for blunt aortic rupture, the extent of the injury can best be ascertained by aortography. The trauma surgeon caring for the patient is in the best position to determine which if any other diagnostic tests are warranted.

In hospitals lacking cardiothoracic capabilities, the decision to transfer patients with potential aortic injury may be difficult. Properly performed and interpreted helical CT, which is normal, may obviate the need for transfer to a higher level of care to exclude thoracic aortic injury.

A qualified surgeon should treat such a patient and assist in the diagnosis. The treatment is either primary repair of the aorta or resection of the injured area and grafting.

G. Traumatic Diaphragmatic Injury

A traumatic diaphragmatic rupture is more commonly diagnosed on the left side, perhaps because the liver obliterates the defect or protects it on the right side of the diaphragm, while the appearance of bowel, stomach, or nasogastric (NG) tube is more easily detected in the left chest. However, this may not be representative of the true incidence of laterality. Blunt trauma produces large radial tears that lead to herniation. Penetrating trauma produces small perforations that often take some time, even years, to develop into diaphragmatic hernias.

THORACIC TRAUMA

These injuries are missed initially if the chest film is misinterpreted as showing an elevated diaphragm, acute gastric dilatation, a loculated pneumohemothorax, or subpulmonary hematoma. If a laceration of the left diaphragm is suspected, a gastric tube should be inserted. When the gastric tube appears in the thoracic cavity on the chest film, the need for special contrast studies is eliminated. Occasionally, the diagnosis is not identified on the initial x-ray or until after chest tube evacuation of the left thorax. An upper gastrointestinal contrast study should be performed if the diagnosis is not clear. The appearance of peritoneal lavage fluid in the chest tube drainage also confirms the diagnosis. Minimally invasive endoscopic procedures (thoracoscopy) may be helpful in evaluating the diaphragm in indeterminate cases.

Right diaphragmatic ruptures are rarely diagnosed in the early postinjury period. The liver often prevents herniation of other abdominal organs into the chest. The appearance of an elevated right diaphragm on chest x-ray may be the only finding.

Operation for other abdominal injuries often reveals diaphragmatic tears. The treatment is direct repair.

H. Mediastinal Traversing Wounds

Penetrating objects that traverse the mediastinum can injure the major mediastinal structures, eg, the heart, great vessels, tracheobronchial tree, or esophagus. The diagnosis is made when careful examination and chest x-ray reveal an entrance wound in one hemithorax and an exit wound or a missile lodged in the contralateral hemithorax. Wounds in which metallic fragments from the missile are in proximity to mediastinal structures also should raise suspicion of a mediastinal traversing injury. Such wounds warrant careful consideration. **Surgical consultation is mandatory.**

Hemodynamically abnormal patients should be considered to have exsanguinating thoracic hemorrhage, tension pneumothorax, or pericardial tamponade. Bilateral tube thoracostomy should be performed to relieve hemopneumothorax and measure blood loss. Indications for urgent thoracotomy are similar to those of massive hemothorax. Preparations for thoracotomy should be made for both hemithoraces, but generally should begin on the side with the most blood loss. Patients with suspected cardiac tamponade are managed as discussed previously. Patients with mediastinal emphysema should be suspected

of having an esophageal or tracheobronchial injury. Mediastinal hematoma or a "pleural cap" suggests a great vessel injury. Consideration also should be given to neurologic function, since the missile tract may traverse the spinal cord.

Hemodynamically normal patients, even those with no clinical or chest x-ray signs of mediastinal structure injury, must nonetheless be evaluated to exclude the possibility of vascular, tracheobronchial, or esophageal injury. Tube thoracostomy is performed as indicated. If a nonoperative evaluation plan is followed, contrast-enhanced helical CT or angiography with visualization of the thoracic aorta and its major branches is required. If the helical CT or angiogram is negative, then a water-soluble contrast esophagography should be performed. Complementary esophagoscopy will increase the reliability of the esophageal evaluation. Bronchoscopy should be performed to evaluate the tracheobronchial tree. The status of the heart and pericardium is best evaluated by CT or ultrasound. If the patient becomes hemodynamically abnormal at any time during the nonoperative evaluation, other associated injuries should be considered and the patient's ABCDEs reevaluated. Immediate relief of tension pneumothorax or surgical exploration for exsanguinating hemorrhage or pericardial tamponade may be required. Identified injuries are repaired through the appropriate incision.

The overall mortality rate for mediastinal penetrating wounds is about 20%. This percentage doubles if the patient presents hemodynamically abnormal. About 50% of patients with mediastinal traversing wounds present hemodynamically abnormal, and another 30% have a positive diagnostic evaluation warranting operative intervention.

V. OTHER MANIFESTATIONS OF CHEST INJURIES

Other significant thoracic injuries should be detected during the secondary survey. While these injuries may not be immediately life threatening, they have the potential for significant harm.

A. Subcutaneous Emphysema

Subcutaneous emphysema may result from airway injury, lung injury, or, rarely, blast injury. Although it does not require treatment, the underlying injury must be addressed. If positive pressure ventilation is required, tube thoracostomy should be considered on the side of the subcutaneous emphysema in anticipation of a pneumothorax (tension) developing.

B. Crushing Injury to the Chest (Traumatic Asphyxia)

Findings associated with a crush injury to the chest include upper torso, facial, and arm plethora with petechiae secondary to acute, temporary compression of the superior vena cava. Massive swelling and even cerebral edema may be present. Associated injuries must be treated.

C. Rib, Sternum, and Scapular Fractures

The ribs are the most commonly injured component of the thoracic cage. Injuries to the ribs are often significant. Pain on motion results in splinting of the thorax, which impairs ventilation, oxygenation, and effective cough. The incidence of atelectasis and pneumonia rises significantly with preexisting lung disease.

The upper ribs (1 to 3) are protected by the bony framework of the upper limb. The scapula, humerus, and clavicle, along with their muscular attachments, provide a barrier to rib injury. Fractures of the scapula, first or second ribs, or the sternum suggest a magnitude of injury that places the head, neck, spinal cord, lungs, and the great vessels at risk for serious associated injury. Because of the severity of the associated injuries, mortality can be as high as 35%. Surgical consultation is warranted.

Sternal and scapular fractures are generally the result of a direct blow. Pulmonary contusion can accompany sternal fractures. Blunt cardiac injury should be considered with all sternal fractures. Operative repair of sternal fractures or scapular fractures occasionally is indicated. Rarely, posterior sternoclavicular dislocation results in mediastinal displacement of the clavicular heads with accompanying superior vena caval obstruction. Immediate reduction is required.

The middle ribs (4 to 9) sustain the majority of blunt trauma. Anteroposterior compression of the thoracic cage will bow the ribs outward with a fracture in the midshaft. Direct force applied to the ribs tends to fracture them and drive the ends of the bones into the thorax with potential for more intrathoracic injury, such as a pneumothorax. As a general rule, a young patient with a more flexible chest wall is less likely to sustain rib fractures. Therefore, the

presence of multiple rib fractures in young patients implies a greater transfer of force than in older patients. Fractures of the lower ribs (10 to 12) should increase suspicion for hepatosplenic injury.

Localized pain, tenderness on palpation, and crepitus are present in rib injury patients. A palpable or visible deformity suggests rib fractures. A chest x-ray should be obtained primarily to exclude other intrathoracic injuries and not just to identify rib fractures. Fractures of anterior cartilages or separation of costochondral junctions have the same significance as rib fractures, but will not be seen on the x-ray examinations. Special rib technique x-rays are expensive, may not detect all rib injuries, add nothing to treatment, require painful positioning of the patient, and are not useful. Taping, rib belts, and external splints are contraindicated. Relief of pain is important to enable adequate ventilation. Intercostal block, epidural anesthesia, and systemic analgesics may be necessary.

D. Blunt Esophageal Rupture

Esophageal trauma is most commonly penetrating. Blunt esophageal trauma, although very rare, may be lethal if unrecognized. Blunt injury of the esophagus is caused by a forceful expulsion of gastric contents into the esophagus from a severe blow to the upper abdomen. This forceful ejection produces a linear tear in the lower esophagus, allowing leakage into the mediastinum. The resulting mediastinitis and immediate or delayed rupture into the pleural space cause empyema. Esophageal trauma may be caused by mishaps of instrumentation (eg, NG tubes, endoscopes, dilators).

The clinical picture is identical to that of postemetic esophageal rupture. Esophageal injury should be considered for any patient who (1) has a left pneumothorax or hemothorax without a rib fracture, (2) has received a severe blow to the lower sternum or epigastrium and is in pain or shock out of proportion to the apparent injury, or (3) has particulate matter in the chest tube after the blood begins to clear. Presence of mediastinal air also suggests the diagnosis, which often can be confirmed by contrast studies and/or esophagoscopy.

Wide drainage of the pleural space and mediastinum with direct repair of the injury via thoracotomy is the treatment, if feasible. Repairs performed within a few hours of injury have a much better prognosis.

THORACIC TRAUMA

E. Other Indications for Chest Tube Insertion

1. Selected patients with suspected severe lung injury, especially those being transferred by air or ground vehicle

2. Individuals undergoing general anesthesia for treatment of other injuries (eg, cranial or extremity), who have suspected significant lung injury

3. Individuals requiring positive pressure ventilation who are suspected of having substantial chest injury

VI. PITFALLS

A. A simple pneumothorax in a trauma patient should not be ignored or overlooked. It can progress to a tension pneumothorax.

B. A simple hemothorax, not fully evacuated, can result in a retained, clotted hemothorax with lung entrapment or, if infected, develop into an empyema.

C. Diaphragm injuries are notorious for being overlooked in the initial trauma evaluation. An undiagnosed diaphragm injury can result in pulmonary compromise or entrapment and strangulation of peritoneal contents.

D. Delayed or extensive evaluation of the wide mediastinum without cardiothoracic surgery capabilities can result in an early inhospital rupture of the contained hematoma and rapid death from exsanguination. All patients with mechanism of injury and simple chest x-ray findings suggestive of aortic disruption should be transferred to a facility capable of rapid definitive diagnosis and treatment of this injury.

E. Underestimating severe pathophysiology of rib fractures is another common pitfall, particularly at the extremes of age. Aggressive pain control without respiratory depression is the key management principle.

F. Avoid underestimating blunt pulmonary injury severity. Pulmonary contusion can present as a wide spectrum of clinical signs, often not well correlated with chest x-ray findings. Careful monitoring of ventilation, oxygenation, and fluid status is required, often for several days. Mechanical ventilation is required frequently.

VII. SUMMARY

Thoracic trauma is common in the multiply injured patient and can be associated with life-threatening problems. These patients can usually be treated or their conditions temporarily relieved by relatively simple measures such as intubation, ventilation, tube thoracostomy, fluid resuscitation, and needle pericardiocentesis. The ability to recognize these important injuries and the skill to perform the necessary procedures can be lifesaving.

■ BIBLIOGRAPHY

1. Bertinchant JP, Robert E, Polge A, et al: Release kinetics of cardiac troponin I and cardiac troponin T in effluents from isolated perfused rabbit hearts after graded experimental myocardial contusion. **Journal of Trauma** 1999; 47(3): 474–480.

2. Brooks AP, Olson LK, Shackford SR: Computed tomography in the diagnosis of traumatic rupture of the thoracic aorta. **Clinical Radiology** 1989; 40:133–138.

3. Callaham M: Pericardiocentesis in traumatic and nontraumatic cardiac tamponade. **Annals of Emergency Medicine** 1984; 13(10):924–945.

4. Dyer DS, Moore EE, Mestek MF, et al: Can chest CT be used to exclude aortic injury? **Radiology** 1999; 213(1):195–202.

5. Esposito TJ, Jurkovich GJ, Rice CL, et al: Reappraisal of emergency room thoracotomy in a changing environment. **Journal of Trauma** 1991; 31(7):881–887.

6. Fabian TC, Richardson JD, Croce MA, et al: Prospective study of blunt aortic injury: Multicenter trial of the American Association for the Surgery of Trauma. **Journal of Trauma** 1997; 42: 374–383.

7. Gavant ML, Menke PG, Fabian TC, et al: Blunt traumatic aortic rupture: Detection with helical CT of the chest. **Radiology** 1995; 197:125–133.

8. Goldberg SP, Karalis DG, Ross JJ, et al: Severe right ventricular contusion mimicking cardiac tamponade: The value of transesophageal echocardiography in blunt chest trauma. **Annals of Emergency Medicine** 1993; 22(4):745–747.

9. Graham JG, Mattox KL, Beall AC Jr: Penetrating trauma of the lung. **Journal of Trauma** 1979; 19: 665.

10. Heniford BT, Carrillo EG, Spain DA, et al: The role of thoracoscopy in the management of retained thoracic collections after trauma. **Annals of Thoracic Surgery** 1997; 63(4):940–943.

11. Karalis DG, Victor MF, Davis GA, et al: The role of echocardiography in blunt chest trauma: A transthoracic and transesophageal echocardiography study. **Journal of Trauma** 1994; 36(l):53–58.

12. Lang-Lazdunski L, Mourox J, Pons F, et al: Role of videothoracoscopy in chest trauma. **Annals of Thoracic Surgery** 1997; 63(2):327–333.

13. Marnocha KE, Maglinte DDT, Woods J, et al: Blunt chest trauma and suspected aortic rupture: Reliability of chest radiograph findings. **Annals of Emergency Medicine** 1985; 14(7):644–649.

14. Mattox KL, Flint LM, Carrico CJ, et al: Blunt cardiac injury (editorial). **Journal of Trauma** 1994; 33(5):649–650.

15. Mattox KL, Wall MJ: Newer diagnostic measures and emergency management. **Chest Surgical Clinics of North America** 1997; 2:213–226.

16. Meyer DM, Jessen ME, Wait MA: Early evacuation of traumatic retained hemothoraces using thoracoscopy: A prospective randomized trial. **Annals of Thoracic Surgery** 1997; 64(5):1396–1400.

17. Mirvis SE, Shanmugantham K, Buell J, et al: Use of spiral computed tomography for the assessment of blunt trauma patients with potential aortic injury. **Journal of Trauma** 1999; 45:922–930.

18. Pezzella AT, Silva WE, Lancey RA: Cardiothoracic trauma. **Current Problems in Surgery** 1998; 35(8):649–650.

19. Poole G, Myers RT: Morbidity and mortality rates in major blunt trauma to the upper chest. **Annals of Surgery** 1980; 193(1):70–75.

20. Ramzy AI, Rodriguez A, Turney SZ: Management of major tracheobronchial ruptures in patients with multiple system trauma. **Journal of Trauma** 1988; 28:914–920.

21. Rozycki GS, Feliciano DV, Oschner MG, et al: The role of ultrasound in patients with possible penetrating cardiac wounds: A prospective multicenter study. **Journal of Trauma** 1999; 46(4):542–551.

22. Rozycki GS, Feliciano DV, Schmidt JA: The role of surgeon-performed ultrasound in patients with possible cardiac wounds. **Annals of Surgery** 1996; 223(6):737–744.

23. Richardson JD, Adams L, Flint LM: Selective management of flail chest and pulmonary contusion. **Annals of Surgery** 1982; 196(4):481–487.

24. Richardson JD, Flint LM, Snow NJ, et al: Management of transmediastinal gunshot wounds. **Surgery** 1981; 90(4):671–676.

25. Rosato RM, Shapiro MJ, Keegan MJ, et al: Cardiac injury complicating traumatic asphyxia. **Journal of Trauma** 1991; 31(10):1387–1389.

26. Smith MD, Cassidy JM, Souther S, et al: Transesophageal echocardiography in the diagnosis of traumatic rupture of the aorta. **New England Journal of Medicine** 1995; 332:356–362.

27. Swaaenburg JC, Klaase JM, DeJongste MJ, et al: Troponini I, troponin T, CKMB-activity and CKMG-mass as markers for the detection of myocardial contusion in patients who experienced blunt trauma. **Clinics Chim Acta** 1998; 272(2):171–181.

28. Symbas PN: Cardiothoracic trauma. **Current Problems in Surgery** 1991; 28(11):741–797.

29. Weiss RL, Brier JA, O'Connor W, et al: The usefulness of transesophageal echocardiography in diagnosing cardiac contusions. **Chest** 1996; 109(1):73–77.

30. Woodring D: Radiographic manifestations of mediastinal hemorrhage from blunt chest trauma. **Annals of Thoracic Surgery** 1984; 37(2):171–178.

31. Woodring JH: A normal mediastinum in blunt trauma rupture of the thoracic aorta and brachiocephalic arteries. **Journal of Emergency Medicine** 1990; 8:467–476.

SKILLS STATION

X-ray Identification of Thoracic Injuries

■ OBJECTIVES:

Performance at this station will allow the participant to:

1. Describe and discuss the process for viewing a chest x-ray for the purpose of identifying life-threatening and potentially life-threatening injuries.

2. Identify various thoracic injuries by using 7 specific anatomic guidelines for examining a series of chest x-rays.

    a. Trachea and bronchi

    b. Pleural spaces and lung parenchyma

    c. Mediastinum

    d. Diaphragm

    e. Bony thorax

    f. Soft tissues

    g. Tubes and lines

3. Given a series of x-rays,

    a. Diagnose fractures.

    b. Diagnose a pneumo- and hemothorax.

    c. Identify a widened mediastinum.

    d. Delineate associated injuries.

    e. Define other areas of possible injury.

INTERACTIVE SKILLS PROCEDURES

X-ray Identification of Thoracic Injuries

Note: This skills station includes a systematic method for evaluating a chest x-ray. A series of x-rays with related scenarios is then shown to the students for their evaluation and management decisions based on the findings.

I. PROCESS FOR INITIAL REVIEW OF CHEST X-RAYS

A. Confirm that the film being viewed is of your patient.

B. Quickly assess for suspected pathology.

C. Use the patient's clinical findings to focus the review of the chest x-ray, and use the x-ray findings to enhance further physical evaluation.

II. TRACHEA AND BRONCHI

A. Assess for the presence of interstitial or pleural air that may represent a large airway injury.

B. Assess for tracheal lacerations that may present as pneumomediastinum, pneumothorax, subcutaneous and interstitial emphysema of the neck, or pneumoperitoneum.

C. Assess for bronchial disruption that may present as a free pleural communication producing a massive pneumothorax with a persistent air leak that is unresponsive to tube thoracostomy.

III. PLEURAL SPACES AND LUNG PARENCHYMA

A. Pleural Space

1. Assess for abnormal collections of fluid that may represent a hemothorax.

2. Assess for abnormal collections of air that may represent a pneumothorax—usually seen as an apical lucent area without bronchial or vascular markings.

B. Lung Parenchyma

1. Assess the lung fields for infiltrates that may suggest pulmonary contusion, hematoma, aspiration, etc. Pulmonary contusion appears as air space consolidation that can be irregular and patchy, homogeneous, diffuse, or extensive.

2. Assess the parenchyma for evidence of laceration. Lacerations appear as a hematoma, vary according to the magnitude of injury, and appear as areas of consolidation.

IV. MEDIASTINUM

A. Assess for air or blood that may displace mediastinal structures, blur the demarcation between tissue planes, or outline them with radiolucency.

B. Assess for radiologic signs associated with cardiac or major vascular injury.

THORACIC TRAUMA   *X-ray Identification of Thoracic Injuries*

1. Air or blood in the pericardium may result in an enlarged cardiac silhouette. Progressive changes in the cardiac size may represent an expanding pneumopericardium or hemopericardium.

2. Aortic rupture may be suggested by:

   a. Widened mediastinum—most reliable finding

   b. Fractures of the first and second ribs

   c. Obliteration of the aortic knob

   d. Deviation of the trachea to the right

   e. Presence of a pleural cap

   f. Elevation and rightward shift of the right mainstem bronchus

   g. Depression of the left mainstem bronchus

   h. Obliteration of the space between the pulmonary artery and the aorta

   i. Deviation of the esophagus (NG tube) to the right

V. DIAPHRAGM

Diaphragmatic rupture requires a high index of suspicion, based on the mechanism of injury, the patient's signs and symptoms, and x-ray findings. Initial chest x-ray may not clearly identify a diaphragmatic injury. Sequential films or additional studies may be required.

A. Carefully evaluate the diaphragm for:

   1. Elevation (may rise to fourth intercostal space with full expiration)

   2. Disruption (stomach, bowel gas, or NG tube above the diaphragm)

   3. Poor identification (irregular or obscure) due to overlying fluid or soft-tissue masses

B. X-ray changes suggesting injury include:

   1. Elevation, irregularity, or obliteration of the diaphragm—segmental or total

   2. Masslike density above the diaphragm that may be due to a fluid-filled bowel, omentum, liver, kidney, spleen, or pancreas (may appear as a "loculated pneumothorax")

   3. Air or contrast-containing stomach or bowel above the diaphragm

   4. Contralateral mediastinal shift

   5. Widening of the cardiac silhouette if the peritoneal contents herniate into the pericardial sac

   6. Pleural effusion

C. Assess for associated injuries, eg, splenic, pancreatic, renal, and liver.

VI. BONY THORAX

A. Clavicle

Assess for evidence of:

   1. Fracture

   2. Associated injury, eg, great vessel injury

B. Scapula

Assess for evidence of:

1. Fracture

2. Associated injury, eg, airway or great vessel injury, pulmonary contusion

C. Ribs

1. Ribs 1 through 3: Assess for evidence of:
   a. Fracture
   b. Associated injury, eg, pneumothorax, major airway, or great vessel injury

2. Ribs 4 through 9: Assess for evidence of:
   a. Fracture, especially in 2 or more contiguous ribs in 2 places (flail chest)
   b. Associated injury, eg, pneumothorax, hemothorax, pulmonary contusion

3. Ribs 9 through 12: Assess for evidence of:
   a. Fracture, especially in 2 or more places (flail chest)
   b. Associated injury, eg, pneumothorax, pulmonary contusion, spleen, liver, and/or kidney

D. Sternum

1. Assess the sternomanubrial junction and sternal body for evidence of fracture or dislocation. (Sternal fractures may be confused on the AP film as a mediastinal hematoma. After the patient is stabilized, a coned-down view, overpenetrated film, lateral view, or CT may be obtained to better identify suspected sternal fracture.)

2. Assess for associated injuries, eg, myocardial contusion, great vessel injury (widened mediastinum).

VII. SOFT TISSUES

Assess for:

A. Displacement or disruption of tissue planes

B. Evidence of subcutaneous air

VIII. TUBES AND LINES

Assess for placement and positioning of:

A. Endotracheal tube

B. Chest tubes

C. Central access lines

D. Nasogastric tube

E. Other monitoring devices

THORACIC TRAUMA *X-ray Identification of Thoracic Injuries*

Table 1—Chest X-ray Suggestions

FINDINGS	DIAGNOSES TO CONSIDER
Respiratory distress without x-ray findings	CNS injury, aspiration, traumatic asphyxia
Any rib fracture	Pneumothorax, pulmonary contusion
Fracture first 3 ribs or sternoclavicular fracture–dislocation	Airway or great vessel injury
Fracture lower ribs 9 to 12	Abdominal injury
Two or more rib fractures in 2 or more places	Flail chest, pulmonary contusion
Scapular fracture	Great vessel injury, pulmonary contusion, brachial plexus injury
Sternal fracture	Blunt cardiac injury
Mediastinal widening	Great vessel injury, sternal fracture, thoracic spine injury
Persistent large pneumothorax or air leak after chest tube insertion	Bronchial tear
Mediastinal air	Esophageal disruption, tracheal injury, pneumoperitoneum
GI gas pattern in the chest (loculated air)	Diaphragmatic rupture
NG tube in the chest	Diaphragmatic rupture or ruptured esophagus
Air fluid level in the chest	Hemopneumothorax or diaphragmatic rupture
Disrupted diaphragm	Abdominal visceral injury
Free air under the diaphragm	Ruptured hollow abdominal viscus

IX. X-RAY REASSESSMENT

The patient's clinical findings should be correlated with the x-ray findings and vice versa. After careful, systematic evaluation of the initial chest film, additional x-rays or radiographic and/or imaging studies may be necessary as historical facts or physical findings dictate. Remember, neither the physical examination or the chest x-ray should be viewed in isolation. Findings on the physical examination should be used to focus the review of the chest x-ray, and findings on the chest x-ray should be used to enhance the physical examination and direct the use of ancillary diagnostic procedures. For example, review of the previous x-ray and repeat chest films may be indicated if significant changes in the patient's status develop. Thoracic CT, thoracic arteriography, or pericardial ultrasonography/echocardiography may be indicated for specificity of diagnosis.

X. REVIEW OF SCENARIO-BASED CHEST X-RAYS

A. X-ray #1 Scenario

The driver of a motor vehicle sustains blunt chest trauma when the vehicle collides with a cement bridge abutment. In the emergency department, she complains of chest pain. During the primary survey an AP chest x-ray is obtained.

X-ray Identification of Thoracic Injuries   **THORACIC TRAUMA**

B. X-ray #2 Scenario

The driver of a motor vehicle sustains blunt chest trauma when the vehicle collides with a cement bridge abutment. The patient is initially evaluated and intubated in another institution and transported to the trauma center. The patient's oxygen hemoglobin saturation level is 82% while being ventilated with 100% oxygen. A chest x-ray should be ordered to evaluate for pulmonary changes and endotracheal tube placement.

C. X-ray #3 Scenario

A young man is brought to the emergency department with a stab wound to the left posterior chest. No significant chest findings are identified during the primary survey and a chest x-ray is obtained as a resuscitation adjunct. During the secondary survey, the patient has decreased breath sounds on the left with hyperresonance to percussion.

D. X-ray #4 Scenario

A young man is brought to the emergency department with a stab wound to the left chest that occurred 4 hours ago. He delayed coming to the hospital until he became increasingly dyspneic and lightheaded. His blood pressure is 80/60 mm Hg, heart rate is 120 beats/minute, and his respiratory rate is 32 breaths/minute. Evaluation reveals markedly decreased breath sounds on the left with dullness to percussion. A chest x-ray is ordered as a resuscitation adjunct.

E. X-ray #5 Scenario

A restrained passenger in a motor vehicle sustains severe blunt chest trauma when the vehicle is struck by another car on the passenger side. In the emergency department the patient complains of severe right chest pain and dyspnea. Physical examination reveals paradoxical motion of the right chest wall. A chest x-ray is obtained as an adjunct to resuscitation.

F. X-ray #6 Scenario

A restrained passenger in a motor vehicle sustains severe blunt chest trauma when the vehicle is struck by another car on the passenger side. In the emergency department the patient complains of severe right chest pain and dyspnea. Physical examination reveals a right tension pneumothorax, which is treated by needle thoracentesis, followed by right tube thoracostomy. A chest x-ray is ordered to evaluate for lung reexpansion and chest tube placement.

G. X-ray #7 Scenario

A restrained driver of a motor vehicle sustains blunt chest trauma when the vehicle strikes a cement bridge abutment at a high rate of speed. In the emergency department, physical examination reveals a bruise across the chest. During the secondary survey, a chest x-ray is obtained.

H. X-rays #8 and #9 Scenario

An unrestrained driver of a motor vehicle sustains blunt chest and abdominal trauma when the vehicle strikes a cement bridge abutment at a high rate of speed. In the emergency department, the patient is dyspneic and complains of chest and abdominal pain. A chest x-ray is obtained before and after placement of a gastric tube.

I. X-ray #10 Scenario

An 18-month-old unrestrained passenger is injured in a single motor vehicle crash. The child strikes his chest on the dashboard of the automobile. He is tachypneic with shallow respirations. His airway is clear; breath sounds are decreased and moist sounding bilaterally.

J. X-ray #11 Scenario

An unrestrained driver of a motor vehicle sustains severe blunt chest trauma when the vehicle strikes a cement bridge abutment at a high rate of speed. The patient is treated initially in a rural hospital where a right pneumothorax is treated with tube thoracostomy. The patient is then transferred to a trauma center. In the emergency department, another chest x-ray is ordered to evaluate for changes and chest tube placement.

K. X-ray #12 Scenario

An unrestrained driver of a motor vehicle sustains severe blunt chest trauma when the vehicle strikes a cement bridge abutment at a high rate of speed. In the emergency department, the patient is dyspneic and complains of chest pain. The patient's blood pressure is 90/60 mm Hg, heart rate is 110 beats/minute, and respiratory rate is 32 breaths/minute. A chest x-ray is obtained as an adjunct to resuscitation.

SKILLS STATION

Chest Trauma Management

▮ **OBJECTIVES:**

Performance at this station will allow the student to practice and demonstrate on a live, anesthetized animal; a fresh, human cadaver; or an anatomic human body manikin the techniques of needle thoracic decompression of a tension pneumothorax, chest tube insertion for the emergency management of hemopneumothorax, and pericardiocentesis. The student also will be able to:

1. Identify the surface markings and technique for pleural decompression with needle thoracentesis, chest tube insertion, and needle pericardiocentesis.

2. Describe the underlying pathophysiology of tension pneumothorax and cardiac tamponade as a result of trauma.

3. Describe the complications of needle thoracentesis, chest tube insertion, and pericardiocentesis.

▮ **PROCEDURES:**

1. Needle thoracentesis

2. Chest tube insertion

3. Pericardiocentesis

INTERACTIVE SKILLS PROCEDURES

Chest Trauma Management

Note: Standard precautions are required whenever caring for the trauma patient.

I. NEEDLE THORACENTESIS

Note: This procedure is for the rapidly deteriorating critical patient who has a life-threatening tension pneumothorax. If this technique is used and the patient does not have a tension pneumothorax, a pneumothorax and/or damage to the lung may occur.

A. Assess the patient's chest and respiratory status.

B. Administer high-flow oxygen and ventilate as necessary.

C. Identify the second intercostal space, in the midclavicular line on the side of the tension pneumothorax.

D. Surgically prepare the chest.

E. Locally anesthetize the area if the patient is conscious or if time permits.

F. Place the patient in an upright position if a c-spine injury has been excluded.

G. Keeping the Luer-Lok in the distal end of the catheter, insert an over-the-needle catheter (2 inches or 5 cm long) into the skin and direct the needle just over (ie, superior to) the rib into the intercostal space.

H. Puncture the parietal pleura.

I. Remove the Luer-Lok from the catheter and listen for a sudden escape of air when the needle enters the parietal pleura, indicating that the tension pneumothorax has been relieved.

J. Remove the needle and replace the Luer-Lok in the distal end of the catheter. Leave the plastic catheter in place and apply a bandage or small dressing over the insertion site.

K. Prepare for a chest tube insertion, if necessary. The chest tube should be inserted, usually, at the nipple level just anterior to the midaxillary line of the affected hemithorax.

L. Connect the chest tube to an underwater-seal device or a flutter-type valve apparatus and remove the catheter used to relieve the tension pneumothorax initially.

M. Obtain a chest x-ray.

Complications of Needle Thoracentesis

1. Local hematoma
2. Pneumothorax
3. Lung laceration

THORACIC TRAUMA   *Chest Trauma Management*

II. CHEST TUBE INSERTION

A. Determine the insertion site, usually the nipple level (5th intercostal space), just anterior to the midaxillary line on the affected side. A second chest tube may be used for a hemothorax.

B. Surgically prepare and drape the chest at the predetermined site of the tube insertion.

C. Locally anesthetize the skin and rib periosteum.

D. Make a 2- to 3-cm transverse (horizontal) incision at the predetermined site and bluntly dissect through the subcutaneous tissues, just over the top of the rib.

E. Puncture the parietal pleura with the tip of a clamp and put a gloved finger into the incision to avoid injury to other organs and to clear any adhesions, clots, etc.

F. Clamp the proximal end of the thoracostomy tube and advance the thoracostomy tube into the pleural space to the desired length. The tube should be directed posteriorly along the inside of the chest wall.

G. Look for "fogging" of the chest tube with expiration or listen for air movement.

H. Connect the end of the thoracostomy tube to an underwater-seal apparatus.

I. Suture the tube in place.

J. Apply a dressing, and tape the tube to the chest.

K. Obtain a chest x-ray.

L. Obtain arterial blood gas values and/or institute pulse oximetry monitoring as necessary.

Complications of Chest Tube Insertion

1. *Laceration or puncture of intrathoracic and/or abdominal organs, all of which can be prevented by using the finger technique before inserting the chest tube*

2. *Introduction of pleural infection, eg, thoracic empyema*

3. *Damage to the intercostal nerve, artery, or vein*
   a. *Converting a pneumothorax to a hemopneumothorax*
   b. *Resulting in intercostal neuritis/neuralgia*

4. *Incorrect tube position, extrathoracic or intrathoracic*

5. *Chest tube kinking, clogging, or dislodging from the chest wall, or disconnection from the underwater-seal apparatus*

6. *Persistent pneumothorax*
   a. *Large primary leak*
   b. *Leak at the skin around the chest tube; suction on tube too strong*
   c. *Leaky underwater-seal apparatus*

7. *Subcutaneous emphysema, usually at tube site*

8. *Recurrence of pneumothorax upon removal of chest tube; seal of thoracostomy wound not immediate*

9. *Lung fails to expand due to plugged bronchus; bronchoscopy required*

10. *Anaphylactic or allergic reaction to surgical preparation or anesthetic*

Chest Trauma Management   **THORACIC TRAUMA**

III. PERICARDIOCENTESIS

A. Monitor the patient's vital signs and ECG before, during, and after the procedure.

B. Surgically prepare the xiphoid and subxiphoid areas, if time allows.

C. Locally anesthetize the puncture site, if necessary.

D. Using a #16- to #18-gauge, 6-inch (15-cm) or longer over-the-needle catheter, attach a 35-mL empty syringe with a 3-way stopcock.

E. Assess the patient for any mediastinal shift that may have caused the heart to shift significantly.

F. Puncture the skin 1 to 2 cm inferior to the left of the xiphochondral junction, at a 45° angle to the skin.

G. Carefully advance the needle cephalad and aim toward the tip of the left scapula.

H. If the needle is advanced too far, eg, into the ventricular muscle, an injury pattern known as the "current of injury" appears on the ECG monitor, eg, extreme ST-T wave changes or widened and enlarged QRS complex. This pattern indicates that the pericardiocentesis needle should be withdrawn until the previous baseline ECG tracing reappears. Premature ventricular contractions also may occur, secondary to irritation of the ventricular myocardium.

I. When the needle tip enters the blood-filled pericardial sac, withdraw as much nonclotted blood as possible.

J. During the aspiration, the epicardium reapproaches the inner pericardial surface, as does the needle tip. Subsequently, an ECG current of injury pattern may reappear. This indicates that the pericardiocentesis needle should be withdrawn slightly. Should this injury pattern persist, withdraw the needle completely.

K. After aspiration is completed, remove the syringe, and attach a 3-way stopcock, leaving the stopcock closed. Secure the catheter in place.

L. Option: Applying the Seldinger technique, pass a flexible guidewire through the needle into the pericardial sac, remove the needle, and pass a #14-gauge flexible catheter over the guidewire. Remove the guidewire and attach a 3-way stopcock.

M. Should the cardiac tamponade symptoms persist, the stopcock may be opened and the pericardial sac reaspirated. The plastic pericardiocentesis catheter can be sutured or taped in place and covered with a small dressing to allow for continued decompression en route to surgery or transfer to another care facility.

Complications of Pericardiocentesis

1. Aspiration of ventricular blood instead of pericardial blood

2. Laceration of ventricular epicardium/myocardium

3. Laceration of coronary artery or vein

4. New hemopericardium, secondary to lacerations of the coronary artery or vein, and/or ventricular epicardium/ myocardium

5. Ventricular fibrillation

6. Pneumothorax, secondary to lung puncture

7. Puncture of great vessels with worsening of pericardial tamponade

8. Puncture of esophagus with subsequent mediastinitis

9. Puncture of peritoneum with subsequent peritonitis or false-positive aspirate

FIVE

CHAPTER 5

Abdominal Trauma

■ OBJECTIVES:

Upon completion of this topic, the participant will be able to identify common patterns of abdominal trauma based on mechanism of injury and establish management priorities accordingly. Specifically, the participant will be able to:

A. Describe the anatomic regions of the abdomen.

B. Describe the differences between blunt and penetrating abdominal injury patterns.

C. Identify the clinical signs distinguishing intraperitoneal, retroperitoneal, and pelvic injury.

D. Identify and apply the diagnostic procedures useful in the assessment of abdominal trauma.

E. Identify therapeutic modalities useful in abdominal and pelvic trauma.

ABDOMINAL TRAUMA

I. INTRODUCTION

Evaluation of the abdomen is a challenging component of the initial assessment of the injured patient. The assessment of circulation during the primary survey includes early recognition of the possibility of occult hemorrhage in the abdomen and pelvis in any patient sustaining blunt trauma. Penetrating torso wounds between the nipple and perineum also must be considered as potentially causing intraabdominal injury. The mechanism of injury, injury forces, location of injury, and hemodynamic status of the patient determine the priority and best method of abdominal assessment.

Unrecognized abdominal injury continues to be a cause of preventable death after truncal trauma. It is a mistake to assume that rupture of a hollow viscus or bleeding from a solid organ can be easily recognized. The assessment of affected patients is often compromised by alcohol intoxication, use of illicit drugs, injury to the brain or spinal cord, or injury to adjacent structures such as the ribs, spine, or pelvis. Significant amounts of blood loss also may be present in the abdominal cavity without any dramatic change in appearance or dimensions and without obvious signs of peritonitis. Any patient sustaining significant blunt torso injury from a direct blow or deceleration, **or** a penetrating torso injury, must be considered to have an abdominal visceral or vascular injury.

II. EXTERNAL ANATOMY OF THE ABDOMEN

A. Anterior Abdomen

Recognizing that the abdomen is partially enclosed by the lower thorax, the anterior abdomen is defined as the area between the transnipple line superiorly, inguinal ligaments and symphysis pubis inferiorly, and the anterior axillary lines laterally.

B. Flank

This is the area between the anterior and posterior axillary lines from the sixth intercostal space to the iliac crest. The thick abdominal wall musculature in this location, rather than the much thinner aponeurotic sheaths of the anterior abdomen, acts as a partial barrier to penetrating wounds, particularly stab wounds.

C. Back

This is the area located posterior to the posterior axillary lines from the tip of the scapulae to the iliac crests. Similar to the abdominal wall muscles in the flank, the thick back, and paraspinal muscles act as a partial barrier to penetrating wounds.

III. INTERNAL ANATOMY OF THE ABDOMEN

The 3 distinct regions of the abdomen include the peritoneal cavity, the retroperitoneal space, and the pelvic cavity. The pelvic cavity in fact contains components of both the peritoneal cavity and retroperitoneal spaces.

A. Peritoneal Cavity

It is convenient to divide the peritoneal cavity into 2 parts, upper and lower. The **upper peritoneal cavity** is covered by the lower aspect of the bony thorax, and includes the diaphragm, liver, spleen, stomach, and transverse colon. This also is occasionally referred to as the thoracoabdominal component of the abdomen. As the diaphragm rises to the fourth intercostal space with full expiration, fractures of the lower ribs or penetrating wounds below the nipple line may injure abdominal viscera. The **lower peritoneal cavity** contains the small bowel, parts of the ascending and descending colon, sigmoid colon, and, in women, internal reproductive organs.

B. Pelvic Cavity

The pelvic cavity, which is surrounded by the pelvic bones, is essentially the lower part of the retroperitoneal and intraperitoneal spaces. It contains the rectum, bladder, iliac vessels, and, in women, internal reproductive organs. Similar to the thoracoabdominal area, the examination of the pelvic structures is compromised by overlying bones.

C. Retroperitoneal Space

This potential space is the area posterior to the peritoneal lining of the abdomen, and contains the abdominal aorta, inferior vena cava, most of the duodenum, the pancreas, kidneys and ureters, and the posterior aspects of the ascending and descending colon, and the retroperitoneal components of the pelvic cavity. Injuries to the retroperitoneal viscera structures are difficult to recognize because the area is remote from physical examination, and injuries do not initially present with signs or symptoms of peritonitis. Additionally, this space is not sampled by diagnostic peritoneal lavage (DPL).

IV. MECHANISM OF INJURY (See Appendix 3, Biomechanics of Injury)

A. Blunt Trauma

A direct blow, eg, contact with the lower rim of the steering wheel or an intruded door in a motor vehicular crash, may cause a compression or crushing injury to abdominal viscera. These forces deform solid or hollow organs and may cause rupture, especially of distended organs (eg, pregnant uterus), with secondary hemorrhage and peritonitis. Shearing injuries to abdominal viscera are a form of crushing that may result when a restraint device (eg, lap-type seat belt or shoulder harness component) is worn improperly. Patients injured in motor vehicular crashes also may sustain **deceleration injuries** in which there is a differential movement of fixed and nonfixed parts of the body, eg, the frequent lacerations of the liver and spleen (movable organs) at sites of supporting ligaments (fixed structures). Air bag deployment does not preclude abdominal injury. In patients undergoing celiotomy for blunt trauma, the organs most frequently injured include the spleen (40% to 55%), liver (35% to 45%), and small bowel (5% to 10%). Additionally, there is a 15% incidence of retroperitoneal hematoma in patients undergoing celiotomy for blunt trauma.

B. Penetrating Trauma

Stab wounds and low-velocity gunshot wounds cause tissue damage by laceration or cutting. High-velocity gunshot wounds transfer more kinetic energy to abdominal viscera, have an added effect of temporary cavitation, and may tumble or fragment, causing further injuries.

Stab wounds traverse adjacent abdominal structures and most commonly involve the liver (40%), small bowel (30%), diaphragm (20%), and colon (15%). Gunshot wounds cause more intraabdominal injuries based on the length of the trajectory in the body as well as greater kinetic energy and the possibility of ricochet off bony structures and the creation of secondary missiles. Gunshot wounds most commonly involve the small bowel (50%), colon (40%), liver (30%), and abdominal vascular structures (25%).

V. ASSESSMENT

In hypotensive patients, the doctor's goal is to rapidly determine if an abdominal injury is present and whether it is the cause of hypotension. Hemodynamically normal patients without signs of peritonitis may undergo a more detailed evaluation that seeks to determine whether specific injuries are present or whether signs of peritonitis or bleeding develop during a period of observation.

A. History

Pertinent historical information in assessing the patient injured in a motor vehicular crash includes speed of the vehicle, type of collision (frontal impact, lateral impact, sideswipe, rear impact, and rollover), vehicle intrusion into the passenger compartment, types of restraints, deployment of an air bag, the patient's position in the vehicle, and status of passengers. This information can be provided by the patient, other passengers, the police, or emergency medical personnel. Information about vital signs, obvious injuries, and response to prehospital treatment also should be provided by the prehospital care providers.

When assessing the patient who has sustained penetrating trauma, pertinent historical information to obtain includes the time of injury, type of weapon (knife, handgun, rifle, shotgun), distance from the assailant (important with shotgun wounds, as the likelihood of major visceral injuries decreases beyond the 10-foot or 3-meter-range), number of stab wounds or shots sustained, and the amount of external bleeding from the patient noted at the scene. If possible, important additional information to obtain from the patient includes the magnitude and location of any abdominal pain and whether this pain is referred to the shoulder.

B. Physical Examination

The abdominal examination should be conducted in a meticulous, systematic fashion in the standard sequence: inspection, auscultation, percussion, and palpation. The findings, whether positive or negative, should be documented carefully in the medical record.

1. Inspection

In most circumstances, the patient must be fully undressed. The anterior and posterior abdomen,

ABDOMINAL TRAUMA

as well as the lower chest and perineum, should be inspected for abrasions, contusions from re-straint devices, lacerations, penetrating wounds, impaled foreign bodies, evisceration of omentum or small bowel, and the pregnant state. The pa-tient should be cautiously logrolled to facilitate a complete examination.

2. Auscultation

Auscultation of the abdomen may be difficult in a noisy emergency room, but it can be used to confirm the presence or absence of bowel sounds. Free intraperitoneal blood or gastrointestinal con-tents may produce an ileus, resulting in the loss of bowel sounds. Injuries to adjacent structures, eg, ribs, spine, or pelvis, also may produce an ileus when intraabdominal injuries are not present, so absence of bowel sounds is not diagnostic of intraabdominal injuries.

3. Percussion

This maneuver causes slight movement of the peritoneum and may elicit subtle signs of perito-nitis. Percussion also may demonstrate the tym-panitic sounds over an acute gastric dilatation in the left upper quadrant or diffuse dullness when a hemoperitoneum is present.

4. Palpation

Voluntary guarding by the patient may make the abdominal examination unreliable. In contrast, involuntary muscle guarding is a reliable sign of peritoneal irritation. The goal of palpation is to elicit and localize superficial (often abdominal wall), deep, or rebound tenderness. Rebound ten-derness occurs as the palpating hand compresses the abdomen and is rapidly removed, indicat-ing peritonitis, usually due to extravasation of gastrointestinal content, and not simple, early hemoperitoneum. The presence of a pregnant uterus, as well as estimation of fetal age, also can be determined.

5. Evaluation of penetrating wounds

Most gunshot wounds to the abdomen are man-aged by exploratory celiotomy (laparotomy) as the incidence of significant intraperitoneal injury approaches 90%. Tangential gunshot wounds often are not truly tangential, and concussive or blast injury can cause intraperitoneal injury

without peritoneal penetration. Stab wounds to the abdomen are generally managed more selec-tively, but approximately 30% do cause intraperi-toneal injury. Any hemodynamically abnormal patient with a gunshot wound or stab wound to the abdomen with signs of peritonitis or abdomi-nal distention mandates immediate celiotomy (laparotomy).

When there is suspicion that a penetrating wound is superficial and it does not appear to travel be-low the abdominal musculoaponeurotic layer, an experienced surgeon may elect to explore the wound locally to determine the depth of penetra-tion. This procedure is not utilized with wounds overlying the ribs because of the risk of causing a pneumothorax, and is not indicated in the patient with peritonitis or hypotension from suspected abdominal injury. (See V., Assessment, G., Di-agnostic Studies in Penetrating Trauma, 2., Local wound exploration and serial physical exami-nations versus DPL in anterior abdominal stab wounds.) However, because 25% to 33% of stab wounds to the anterior abdomen do not penetrate the peritoneum, celiotomy for all such patients is often nonproductive. Under sterile conditions, local anesthesia is injected, and the wound track is followed through the layers of the abdominal wall or until its termination. Confirmation of penetration through the **anterior fascia** places the patient at higher risk for intraperitoneal injury, and many trauma surgeons view this as indica-tion for celiotomy. Any patient in whom the track cannot be followed because of obesity, lack of co-operation, or soft-tissue hemorrhage or distortion should be admitted for continued evaluation or surgical exploration (celiotomy).

6. Assessing pelvic stability (See Chapter 8, Musculoskeletal Trauma)

Manual compression of the anterosuperior iliac spines or iliac crests may elicit abnormal move-ment or bony pain, which suggests a pelvic frac-ture in patients who sustain blunt truncal trauma. (See VII., Special Problems, C., Pelvic Fractures and Associated Injuries.) Caution should be ex-ercised, as this maneuver may cause or aggravate bleeding.

7. Penile, perineal, and rectal examination

The presence of blood at the urethral meatus strongly suggests a urethral tear. Inspection of the scrotum and perineum also is performed to look for ecchymoses or a hematoma, also suggestive of the same injury. Goals of the rectal examination in patients sustaining blunt trauma are to assess sphincter tone, the position of the prostate (high-riding prostate indicates urethral disruption), and to determine whether fractures of the pelvic bones are present. In patients with penetrating wounds, the rectal examination is used to assess sphincter tone and look for gross blood from a bowel perforation.

8. Vaginal examination

Laceration of the vagina may occur from bony fragments from pelvic fracture(s) or from penetrating wounds. (See Chapter 11, Trauma in Women.)

9. Gluteal examination

The gluteal region extends from the iliac crests to the gluteal folds. Penetrating injuries to this area are associated with up to a 50% incidence of significant intraabdominal injuries. This includes rectal injuries below the peritoneal reflection. Intraabdominal injuries are associated with gunshot and stab wounds. These wounds mandate a search for intraabdominal injuries.

C. Intubation

The insertion of gastric and urinary catheters is frequently performed as part of the resuscitation phase, once problems with the airway, breathing, and circulation are diagnosed and treated.

1. Gastric tube

The therapeutic goal of inserting this tube early in the resuscitation process is to relieve acute gastric dilatation, decompress the stomach before performing a DPL, and remove gastric contents, thereby reducing the risk of aspiration. The presence of blood in the gastric secretions suggests an injury to the esophagus or upper gastrointestinal tract if nasopharyngeal and/or oropharyngeal sources are excluded. **Caution:** If severe facial fractures exist or there is suspicion of a basilar skull fracture, the gastric tube should be inserted through the mouth to prevent passage of the tube through the cribriform plate into the brain.

2. Urinary catheter

The goals of inserting this tube early in the resuscitation process are to relieve retention, decompress the bladder before performing a DPL, and allow for monitoring of the urinary output as an index of tissue perfusion. Hematuria is a sign of trauma to the genitourinary tract. **Caution:** The inability to void, an unstable pelvic fracture, blood at the meatus, a scrotal hematoma or perineal ecchymoses, or a high-riding prostate on rectal examination mandate a retrograde urethrogram to confirm an intact urethra before inserting a urinary catheter. A disrupted urethra detected during the primary or secondary survey may require the insertion of a suprapubic tube by an experienced doctor.

D. Blood and Urine Sampling

Blood is withdrawn from one of the initial venous access sites and sent for type and screen in the hemodynamically normal patient, or type and crossmatch in the hemodynamically abnormal patient. At the same time, blood can be sent for selected laboratory tests, which usually include complete blood count (CBC), potassium, glucose, amylase (for blunt trauma), and blood alcohol levels. Additional laboratory tests, although unnecessary in most trauma patients, may be indicated in some patients, such as those with preexisting medical conditions or those in whom additional studies using intravenous iodinated contrast material is contemplated. Urine specimens are sent for a urinalysis and a urine drug screen if indicated. A blood test or urine pregnancy test is indicated in all females of childbearing age.

E. X-ray Studies

1. Screening x-rays for blunt trauma

The lateral cervical spine x-ray, an anteroposterior (AP) chest x-ray, and a pelvic x-ray are the screening films obtained in patients with multisystem blunt trauma. Abdominal x-rays (supine, upright, or lateral decubitus) may be useful in hemodynamically normal patients to detect extraluminal air in the retroperitoneum or free air under the diaphragm, both of which mandate prompt celiotomy. Loss of a psoas shadow also suggests a retroperitoneal injury.

ABDOMINAL TRAUMA

2. Screening x-rays for penetrating trauma

The hemodynamically abnormal patient with a penetrating abdominal wound does not require any screening x-rays in the emergency department. If the patient is hemodynamically normal and has penetrating trauma above the umbilicus or a suspected thoracoabdominal injury, an upright chest x-ray is useful to exclude an associated hemo- or pneumothorax, or to document the presence of intraperitoneal air. With marker rings or clips applied to all entrance- and exit-wound sites, a supine abdominal x-ray may be obtained in the hemodynamically normal patient to determine the track of the missile or the presence of retroperitoneal air.

3. Special circumstance contrast studies

a. Urethrography

As previously noted, urethrography should be performed before inserting an indwelling urinary catheter when a urethral tear is suspected. The urethrogram is performed with a #8-French urinary catheter secured in the meatal fossa by balloon inflation to 1.5 to 2 mL. Approximately 15 to 20 mL of undiluted contrast material is instilled with gentle pressure. A radiograph is taken with an oblique projection and with slight stretch on the penis.

b. Cystography

An intra- or extraperitoneal bladder rupture is best diagnosed with a cystogram or CT cystography. A bulb syringe attached to the indwelling bladder catheter is held 40 cm above the patient, and 300 mL of water-soluble contrast is allowed to flow into the bladder or until (1) flow stops, (2) the patient voids spontaneously, or (3) the patient is in discomfort. AP, oblique, and postdrainage views are essential to definitively exclude injury. CT evaluation of the bladder and pelvis (CT cystogram) is an alternative study, and is particularly useful in providing additional information about the kidneys as well as the pelvic bones.

c. CT/IVP

Where CT scanning is available, hemodynamically normal patients with hematuria and suspected urinary system injury are best evaluated by a contrast-enhanced CT that can define the type of renal injury present. If CT is not available, an intravenous pyelogram (IVP) is an alternative.

A high-dose rapid injection of renal contrast ("screening IVP") is best performed using the recommended dosage of 200 mg of iodine/kg body weight. This involves a bolus injection of 100 mL (standard 1.5 mL/kg for a 70-kg individual) of a 60% iodine solution performed through two 50-mL syringes over 30 to 60 seconds. If only 30% iodine solution is available, the ideal dose is 3.0 mL/kg. Visualization of the calyces of the kidneys on a flat plate x-ray of the abdomen should appear 2 minutes after the injection is completed. Unilateral nonfunction indicates an absent kidney, thrombosis, or avulsion of the renal artery, or massive parenchymal disruption. Nonfunction warrants further radiologic evaluation with a contrast-enhanced CT or renal arteriogram, or surgical exploration, depending on mechanism and local availability or expertise.

d. Gastrointestinal

Isolated injuries to retroperitoneal gastrointestinal structures (duodenum, ascending or descending colon, and/or rectum) do not cause peritonitis and may not be detected on DPL. When there is suspicion of injury to 1 of these structures, CT with contrast or specific upper and lower gastrointestinal contrast studies are indicated.

F. Diagnostic Studies in Blunt Trauma

If there is early or obvious evidence that the patient will be transferred to another facility, time-consuming tests should **not** be performed. These tests include contrast urologic and gastrointestinal studies, DPL, or CT. (See Table 1, page 137, DPL Versus FAST Versus CT in Blunt Abdominal Trauma.)

1. Diagnostic peritoneal lavage

A DPL is a rapidly performed, invasive procedure that significantly alters subsequent examinations of the patient and is considered 98% sensitive for intraperitoneal bleeding. It should be performed by the surgical team caring for a hemodynamically abnormal patient with multiple blunt injuries, especially when any of these situations are present:

a. Change in sensorium — Brain injury, alcohol intoxication, and use of illicit drugs

b. Change in sensation — Injury to spinal cord

c. Injury to adjacent structures — Lower ribs, pelvis, lumbar spine

d. Equivocal physical examination

e. Prolonged loss of contact with patient anticipated — General anesthesia for extraabdominal injuries, lengthy x-ray studies, eg, angiography (hemodynamically normal or abnormal patient)

f. Lap-belt sign (abdominal wall contusion) with suspicion of bowel injury

DPL also is indicated in hemodynamically normal patients when the same situations are present, but when ultrasound or CT is not available.

The only absolute contraindication to DPL is an existing indication for celiotomy. Relative contraindications include previous abdominal operations, morbid obesity, advanced cirrhosis, and preexisting coagulopathy. Either an open or closed (Seldinger) infraumbilical technique is acceptable in the hands of trained doctors. In patients with pelvic fractures or advanced pregnancy, an open supraumbilical approach is preferred to avoid entering a pelvic hematoma or damaging the enlarged uterus. Free aspiration of blood, gastrointestinal contents, vegetable fibers, or bile through the lavage catheter in the hemodynamically abnormal patient mandates celiotomy. If gross blood (>10 mL) or gastrointestinal contents are not aspirated, lavage is performed with 1000 mL of warmed Ringer's lactate solution (10 mL/kg in a child). After ensuring adequate mixing of peritoneal contents with the lavage fluid by compressing the abdomen and logrolling the patient, the effluent is sent to the laboratory for quantitative analysis if gastrointestinal contents, vegetable fibers, or bile are not obviously present. A positive test is indicated by >100,000 RBC/mm^3, ≥ 500 WBC/mm^3, or a Gram stain with bacteria present.

Table 1—DPL Versus FAST Versus CT in Blunt Abdominal Trauma

	DPL	FAST	CT SCAN
Indication	• Document bleeding if hypotensive	• Document fluid if hypotensive	• Document organ injury if BP normal
Advantages	• Early diagnosis • All patients • Performed rapidly • 98% sensitive • Detects bowel injury • Transport: No	• Early diagnosis • All patients • Noninvasive • Performed rapidly • Repeatable • 86%–97% accurate • Transport: No	• Most specific for injury • Sensitive: 92%–98% accurate
Disadvantages	• Invasive • Specificity: Low • Misses injury to diaphragm and retroperitoneum	• Operator-dependent • Bowel gas and subcutaneous air distortion • Misses diaphragm, bowel, and pancreatic injuries	• ↑ Cost and time • Misses diaphragm, bowel, and some pancreatic injuries • Transport: Required

ABDOMINAL TRAUMA

2. FAST (Focused Assessment Sonography in Trauma)

Ultrasound can be used to detect the presence of hemoperitoneum by properly trained individuals. With specific equipment and in experienced hands, ultrasound has a sensitivity, specificity, and accuracy in detecting intraabdominal fluid comparable to DPL and abdominal computed axial tomography. Thus, ultrasound provides a rapid, noninvasive, accurate, and inexpensive means of diagnosing hemoperitoneum that can be repeated frequently. Ultrasound scanning can be done at the bedside in the resuscitation room while simultaneously performing other diagnostic or therapeutic procedures. The indications for the procedure are the same as for DPL. The only factors that compromise its utility are obesity, the presence of subcutaneous air, and previous abdominal operations.

Ultrasound scanning to detect hemoperitoneum can be accomplished rapidly. Scans are obtained of the pericardial sac, hepatorenal fossa, splenorenal fossa, and pelvis or pouch of Douglas. After the initial scan is completed, a second or "control" scan should ideally be performed after an interval of 30 minutes. The control scan is done to detect progressive hemoperitoneum in those patients with a low rate of bleeding and short intervals from injury to the initial scan.

3. Computed tomography

CT is a diagnostic procedure that requires transport of the patient to the scanner, administration of intravenous contrast, and scanning of the upper and lower abdomen, as well as the pelvis. It is time consuming and is used **only in hemodynamically normal patients** in whom there is no apparent indication for an emergency celiotomy. The CT scan provides information relative to specific organ injury and its extent, and also can diagnose retroperitoneal and pelvic organ injuries that are difficult to assess by a physical examination, FAST, or peritoneal lavage. Relative contraindications to the use of CT include delay until the scanner is available, an uncooperative patient who cannot be safely sedated, or an allergy to the contrast agent when nonionic contrast is not available. **Caution: CT may miss some gastrointestinal, diaphragmatic, and pancreatic injuries. In the absence of hepatic or splenic injuries,**

the presence of free fluid in the abdominal cavity suggests an injury to the gastrointestinal tract and/or its mesentery, and many trauma surgeons find this to be an indication for early operative intervention.

G. Diagnostic Studies in Penetrating Trauma

1. Lower chest wounds

Diagnostic options in asymptomatic patients with possible injuries to the diaphragm and upper abdominal structures include serial physical examinations, serial chest x-rays, thoracoscopy, laparoscopy, or CT (for right thoracoabdominal wounds).

Even with all the options listed, late posttraumatic left-sided diaphragmatic hernias continue to occur after thoracoabdominal stab wounds, and thus early or immediate surgical exploration (celiotomy) for such wounds also is an option. For left-sided thoracoabdominal gunshot wounds, the safest policy is celiotomy.

2. Local wound exploration and serial physical examinations versus DPL in anterior abdominal stab wounds

Approximately 55% to 60% of all patients with stab wounds penetrating the anterior peritoneum have hypotension, peritonitis, or evisceration of omentum or small bowel. These patients require an emergency celiotomy. In the remaining patients, in whom anterior peritoneal penetration can be confirmed or strongly suspected by local wound exploration, approximately half eventually require operation. Celiotomy remains a reasonable option for all such patients. Less invasive diagnostic options for the relatively asymptomatic patients (who may have pain at the site of the stab wound) include serial physical examinations over a 24-hour period, DPL, or diagnostic laparoscopy. Serial physical examinations are labor intensive, but have an overall accuracy rate of 94%. DPL allows for an earlier diagnosis of an injury in relatively asymptomatic patients and has an accuracy rate of about 90% when using the cell counts as described for blunt abdominal trauma. Diagnostic laparoscopy can confirm or exclude peritoneal penetration, but it is less useful in identifying specific injuries.

3. Serial physical examinations versus double- or triple-contrast CT in flank or back injuries

The thickness of the flank and back muscles protects the underlying viscera from injury with many stab wounds or some gunshot wounds to these areas. Again, while celiotomy is a reasonable option for all such patients, less invasive diagnostic options in patients who are initially asymptomatic include serial physical examinations, double- or triple-contrast CT, or DPL. Serial physical examination in patients who are initially asymptomatic and then become symptomatic is very accurate in detecting retroperitoneal or intraperitoneal injuries with wounds posterior to the anterior axillary line.

Double- (intravenous and oral) or triple- (intravenous, oral, and rectal) contrast-enhanced CT is time consuming and demands full study of the retroperitoneal colon on the side of the wound. The accuracy is comparable to that of serial physical examinations, but should allow for an earlier diagnosis of an injury in relatively asymptomatic patients when the CT is performed properly.

On rare occasions, these retroperitoneal injuries can be missed by serial examinations or contrast CT. Early outpatient follow-up is mandatory after the 24-hour period of inhospital observation because of the subtle presentation of certain colonic injuries.

DPL also can be used in such patients as an early screening test. A positive DPL is an indication for an urgent celiotomy.

VI. INDICATIONS FOR CELIOTOMY IN ADULTS

In individual patients, surgical judgment is required to determine the timing and need for operation. The following indications are commonly used to facilitate the surgeon's decision-making process in this regard.

1. Blunt abdominal trauma with hypotension and clinical evidence of intraperitoneal bleeding

2. Blunt abdominal trauma with positive DPL or FAST

3. Hypotension with penetrating abdominal wound

4. Gunshot wounds traversing the peritoneal cavity or visceral/vascular retroperitoneum

5. Evisceration

6. Bleeding from the stomach, rectum, or genito-urinary tract from penetrating trauma

7. Presenting or subsequent peritonitis

8. Free air, retroperitoneal air, or rupture of the hemidiaphragm after blunt trauma

9. Contrast-enhanced CT demonstrates ruptured gastrointestinal tract, intraperitoneal bladder injury, renal pedicle injury, or severe visceral parenchymal injury after blunt or penetrating trauma.

VII. SPECIAL PROBLEMS

A. Blunt Trauma

The liver, spleen, and kidney are the organs predominantly involved after blunt trauma, although the relative incidence of hollow visceral perforation, lumbar spinal injuries, and uterine rupture increases with incorrect seat belt usage. (See Table 2, Truncal and Cervical Injuries from Restraint Devices.) Difficulties in diagnosis may occur with injuries to the diaphragm, duodenum, pancreas, genitourinary system, or small bowel.

B. Specific Injuries

1. Diaphragm

Blunt tears may occur in any portion of either diaphragm; however, the left hemidiaphragm is more commonly injured. The most common injury is 5 to 10 cm in length and involves the posterolateral left hemidiaphragm. Abnormalities on the initial chest x-ray include elevation or "blurring" of the hemidiaphragm, a hemothorax, an abnormal gas shadow that obscures the hemidiaphragm, or the gastric tube positioned in the chest. However, the initial chest x-ray may be normal in a small percentage of patients.

2. Duodenum

Duodenal rupture is classically encountered in the unrestrained driver involved in a frontal-impact motor vehicular collision or in a patient with a direct blow to the abdomen, eg, from bicycle handlebars. A bloody gastric aspirate or retroperitoneal air on a flat plate x-ray of the abdomen or abdominal CT should raise suspicion for this

ABDOMINAL TRAUMA

Table 2—Truncal and Cervical Injuries from Restraint Devices

RESTRAINING DEVICE	INJURY
Lap Seat Belt • Compression	• Tear or avulsion of mesentery • Rupture of small bowel or colon • Thrombosis of iliac artery or abdominal aorta
• Hyperflexion	• Chance fracture of lumbar vertebrae
Shoulder Harness • Submarining	• Intimal tear or thrombosis in innominate, carotid, subclavian, or vertebral arteries • Fracture or dislocation of c-spine
• Compression	• Intimal tear or thrombosis in subclavian artery • Rib fractures • Pulmonary contusion • Rupture of upper abdominal viscera
Air Bag • Contact	• Corneal abrasions, keratitis • Abrasions of face, neck, chest
• Contact/deceleration	• Cardiac rupture
• Flexion (unrestrained)	• C-spine or thoracic spine fracture
• Hyperextension (unrestrained)	• C-spine fracture

injury. An upper gastrointestinal x-ray series or double-contrast CT is indicated for the high-risk patient.

3. Pancreas

Pancreatic injury most often results from a direct epigastric blow that compresses the organ against the vertebral column. An early normal serum amylase level does not exclude major pancreatic trauma. Conversely, the amylase level may be elevated from nonpancreatic sources. However, persistently elevated or rising serum amylase levels should prompt further evaluation of the pancreas and other abdominal viscera. Double-contrast CT may not identify significant pancreatic trauma in the immediate postinjury period (up to 8 hours); it should be repeated later if pancreatic injury is suspected. Should there be concern after an equivocal CT, surgical exploration of the pancreas is warranted. Alternatively, an emergent endoscopic retrograde cholangiopancreatography (ERCP) may be helpful.

4. Genitourinary

Direct blows to the back or flank resulting in contusions, hematomas, or ecchymoses are markers of potential underlying renal injury and warrant an evaluation (CT or IVP) of the urinary tract. Additional indications for evaluating the urinary tract include gross hematuria or microscopic hematuria in patients with (1) a penetrating abdominal wound, (2) an episode of hypotension (systolic blood pressure less than 90 mm Hg) in patients with blunt abdominal trauma, or (3) associated intraabdominal injuries in patients with blunt trauma. An abdominal CT scan with IV contrast documents the presence and extent of a blunt renal injury, 95% of which can be treated nonoperatively. Thrombosis of the renal artery or disruption of the renal pedicle secondary to deceleration is a rare upper tract injury in which hematuria may be absent, although the patient may have severe abdominal pain. With either injury, an IVP, CT, or renal arteriogram may be useful in diagnosis.

An anterior pelvic fracture usually is present in patients with urethral injuries. Urethral disruptions are divided into those above (posterior) or below (anterior) the urogenital diaphragm. A posterior urethral injury usually occurs in a patient with multisystem injuries and pelvic fractures. In contrast, an anterior urethral injury results from a straddle impact and may be an isolated injury.

5. Small bowel

Blunt injury to the intestines generally results from sudden deceleration with subsequent tearing near a fixed point of attachment, especially if the patient's seat belt was applied incorrectly. The appearance of transverse, linear ecchymoses on the abdominal wall (seat belt sign) or the presence of a lumbar distraction fracture (Chance fracture) on x-ray should alert the doctor to the possibility of intestinal injury. Although some patients have early abdominal pain and tenderness, diagnosis may be difficult in others, especially since minimal bleeding may result from torn intestinal organs. Early ultrasound and CT are often not diagnostic with these subtle injuries, and DPL is a better choice whenever abdominal wall ecchymoses are present.

6. Solid organ injury

Injury(ies) to the liver, spleen, or kidney that result in shock, hemodynamic instability, or evidence of continuing bleeding remain indications for urgent celiotomy. Isolated solid organ injury in the hemodynamically normal patient can often be managed nonoperatively. Such patients must be admitted to the hospital for careful observation. Evaluation by a surgeon is essential. Concomitant hollow viscus injury occurs in less than 5% of patients initially thought to have isolated solid organ injuries.

C. Pelvic Fractures and Associated Injuries

The sacrum and innominate bones (ilium, ischium, and pubis), along with a large number of ligamentous complexes, comprise the pelvis. Fractures and ligamentous disruptions of the pelvis suggest that major forces were applied to the patient. Such injuries usually result from auto-pedestrian, motor vehicle, or motorcycle crashes. Pelvic fractures have a significant association with injuries to intraperitoneal and retroperitoneal visceral and vascular struc-

tures. The incidence of tears of the thoracic aorta also appears to be significantly increased in patients with pelvic fractures, especially those of the anteroposterior type. Therefore, hypotension may or may not be related to the pelvic fracture itself when blunt trauma is the mechanism of injury. Patients with hemorrhagic shock and unstable pelvic fractures have 4 potential sources of blood loss: (1) fractured bone surfaces, (2) pelvic venous plexus, (3) pelvic arterial injury, or (4) extrapelvic source.

1. Mechanism of injury/classification

Four patterns of force leading to pelvic fractures include (1) AP compression, (2) lateral compression, (3) vertical shear, and (4) complex (combination) pattern. An AP compression injury may be caused by an auto-pedestrian collision or motorcycle crash, a direct crushing injury to the pelvis, or a fall from a height greater than 12 feet (3.6 meters). With disruption of the symphysis pubis, there often is tearing of the posterior osseous ligamentous complex (sacroiliac, sacrospinous, sacrotuberous, fibromuscular pelvic floor) represented by a sacroiliac fracture and/or dislocation or sacral fracture. With opening of the pelvic ring, there may be hemorrhage from the posterior pelvic venous complex and, occasionally, branches of the internal iliac artery.

A lateral compression injury often results from a motor vehicle crash and leads to internal rotation of the involved hemipelvis. This rotation drives the pubis into the lower genitourinary system, creating injury to the bladder and/or urethra. The pelvic volume is actually compressed in such an injury, and life-threatening hemorrhage is not common.

A high-energy shear force applied in a vertical plane across the anterior and posterior aspects of the ring disrupts the sacrospinous and sacrotuberous ligaments and leads to a major pelvic instability.

2. Assessment

The flank, scrotum, and perianal area should be inspected quickly for blood at the urethral meatus; swelling or bruising; or a laceration in the perineum, vagina, rectum, or buttocks suggestive of an open pelvic fracture. Palpation of a high-riding prostate gland also is a sign of a significant pelvic fracture.

ABDOMINAL TRAUMA

Mechanical instability of the pelvic ring is tested by manual manipulation of the pelvis. This procedure should be performed **only once** during the physical examination because repeated testing for pelvic instability may dislodge clots from coagulated vessels and result in fatal hemorrhage. The first indication of mechanical instability is leg-length discrepancy or rotational deformity (usually external) without a fracture of that extremity. As the unstable pelvis is able to rotate externally, the pelvis can be closed by pushing on the iliac crests at the level of the anterior superior iliac spine. Motion can be felt if the iliac crests are grasped and the unstable hemipelvis(es) is pushed inward and then outward (compression distraction maneuver). With posterior disruption, the involved hemipelvis can be pushed cephalad as well as pulled caudally. This translational motion can be felt by palpating the posterior iliac spine and tubercle while pushing-pulling the unstable hemipelvis. When appropriate, an AP x-ray of the pelvis confirms the clinical examination. (See Chapter 3, Shock, Skills Station IV, Shock Assessment and Management.)

3. Management

Simple techniques may be used to splint the unstable pelvic fracture and close the increased pelvic volume prior to patient transfer and during the resuscitation with crystalloid fluids and blood. These techniques include (1) a sheet wrapped around the pelvis as a sling, causing internal rotation of the lower limbs, (2) application of a vacuum-type long spine splinting device ("bean bag"), or (3) application of the pneumatic antishock garment (PASG). Reduction of an acetabular fracture by longitudinal traction of the lower extremity also can be useful. Although definitive management of patients with pelvic fractures varies, 1 treatment algorithm based on the hemodynamic status for the patient in the emergency department is provided herein. (See Algorithm 1, Management of Pelvic Fractures.) Since significant resources are required to care for the patient with a severe pelvic fracture(s), early consideration of transfer to a trauma center is essential.

VIII. SUMMARY

Early consultation with a surgeon is necessary whenever a patient with possible intraabdominal injuries is brought to the emergency department. Once the patient's vital functions have been restored, evaluation and management varies depending on the mechanism of injury as described herein.

A. Blunt Trauma

The hemodynamically abnormal patient with multiple blunt injuries is rapidly assessed for intraabdominal bleeding or contamination from the gastrointestinal tract by performing diagnostic peritoneal lavage or a focused ultrasound. The hemodynamically normal patient without peritonitis is evaluated by contrast-enhanced CT, with the decision to operate based on the specific organ involved and the magnitude of injury.

B. Penetrating Trauma

All patients with penetrating wounds in proximity to the abdomen and associated hypotension, peritonitis, or evisceration require emergent celiotomy. Patients with gunshot wounds that obviously traverse the peritoneal cavity or visceral/vascular area of the retroperitoneum on physical examination or routine x-rays also require emergent celiotomy. Asymptomatic patients with anterior abdominal stab wounds that penetrate the fascia or peritoneum on local wound exploration are evaluated by serial physical examinations or DPL. However, surgical exploration (celiotomy) remains an acceptable option. Asymptomatic patients with flank or back stab wounds that are not obviously superficial are evaluated by serial physical examinations or contrast-enhanced CT. Exploratory celiotomy is an acceptable option with these patients as well. It is safer to perform a celiotomy in patients with gunshot wounds to the flank and back.

C. Management

Management of blunt and penetrating trauma to the abdomen includes:

   1. Reestablishing vital functions and optimizing oxygenation and tissue perfusion

   2. Delineating the injury mechanism

   3. Meticulous initial physical examination, repeated at regular intervals

   4. Selecting special diagnostic maneuvers as needed, performed with a minimal loss of time

ALGORITHM 1
Management of Pelvic Fractures*

HEMODYNAMICALLY NORMAL

↓

Primary survey

↓

CT or FAST or DPL if indicated[1]

↓

Evaluate for other injuries

↓

PASG for transfer; inflate for hypotension

↓

External or internal fixation if needed for stability

HEMODYNAMICALLY ABNORMAL

↓

Primary survey

↓

Supraumbilical DPL or FAST[1]

↓

Temporary stabilization[2]

Grossly + DPL

Grossly - DPL

↓

Celiotomy

Angiography/ embolization[3]

↓

Surgical pelvic fixation[4]

* Priority order for the management of pelvic fractures depends on available resources.

[1] Differentiation of intraperitoneal hemorrhage from extraperitoneal hemorrhage in patients with a pelvic fracture may be difficult utilizing ultrasonography.

[2] Nonoperative pelvic stabilization methods include pneumatic antishock garment (PASG), pelvic sheet wrapping, and "bean bag" wrapping. These are appropriately used in select patients with unstable pelvic fractures.

[3] If angiography is not immediately available, immediate and rapid closed operative pelvic fracture stabilization may be helpful in select patients.

[4] Surgical pelvic fixation in the acute, hemodynamically abnormal patient should be performed rapidly and generally with closed techniques.

ABDOMINAL TRAUMA

5. Maintaining a high index of suspicion related to occult vascular and retroperitoneal injuries

6. Early recognition for surgical intervention and prompt celiotomy

■ BIBLIOGRAPHY

Mechanism

1. Anderson PA, Rivara FP, Maier RV, et al: The epidemiology of seat belt-associated injuries. **Journal of Trauma** 1991; 31:60–67.

2. Dischinger PC, Cushing BM, Kerns TJ: Injury patterns associated with direction of impact: Drivers admitted to trauma centers. **Journal of Trauma** 1993; 35:454–459.

3. Fabian TC, Croce MA: Abdominal trauma, including indications for celiotomy. In: Mattox LK, Felician DV, Moore EE (eds): **Trauma.** East Norwalk, CT, Appleton & Lange, 2000, pp 583–602.

4. Huizinga WK, Baker LW, Mtshali ZW: Selective management of abdominal and thoracic stab wounds with established peritoneal penetration: The eviscerated omentum. **American Journal of Surgery** 1987; 153:564–568.

5. McCarthy MC, Lowdermilk GA, Canal DF, et al: Prediction of injury caused by penetrating wounds to the abdomen, flank, and back. **Archives of Surgery** 1991; 126:962–966.

6. Nance FC, Wennar MH, Johnson LW et al: Surgical judgement in the management of penetrating wounds to the abdomen: Experience with 2,212 patients. **Annals of Surgery** 1974; 179(5): 639–646.

7. Reid AB, Letts RM, Black GB: Pediatric Chance fractures: Association with intraabdominal injuries and seat belt use. **Journal of Trauma** 1990; 30:384–391.

8. Robin AP, Andrews JR, Lange DA, et al: Selective management of anterior abdominal stab wounds. **Journal of Trauma** 1989; 29: 1684–1689.

Diagnostic Studies

9. Ballard RB, Rozycki GS, Newman PG, et al: An algorithm to reduce the incidence of false-negative FAST examinations in patients at high risk for occult injury. **Journal of the American College of Surgeons** 1999; 189(2):145–150.

10. Donohue JH, Federle MP, Griffiths BG, et al: Computed tomography in the diagnosis of blunt intestinal and mesenteric injuries. **Journal of Trauma** 1987; 27:11–17.

11. Feliciano DV, Bitondo CG, Steed G, et al: Five hundred open taps or lavages in patients with abdominal stab wounds. **American Journal of Surgery** 1984; 146:772–777.

12. Liu M, Lee C, Veng F: Prospective comparison of diagnostic peritoneal lavage, computed tomographic scanning, and ultrasonography for the diagnosis of blunt abdominal trauma. **Journal of Trauma** 1993; 35:267–270.

13. Miller KS, McAnnich JW: Radiographic assessment of renal trauma: Our 15-year experience. **Journal of Urology** 1995; 154(2 Pt 1):352–355.

14. Nordenholz KE, Rubin MA, Gularte GG, et al: Ultrasound in the evaluation and management of blunt abdominal trauma. **Annals of Emergency Medicine** 1997; 29(3):357–366.

15. Root HD: Abdominal trauma and diagnostic peritoneal lavage revisited. **American Journal of Surgery** 1990; 159:363–364.

16. Rozycki GS: Abdominal ultrasonography in trauma. **Surgical Clinics of North America** 1995; 75:175–191.

17. Rozycki GS, Ballard RB, Feliciano DV, et al: Surgeon-performed ultrasound for the assessment of truncal injuries. Lessons learned from 1540 patients. **Annals of Surgery** 1998; 228(4): 557–565.

18. Schreiber M, Gentilello L, Rhee P, et al: Limiting computed tomography to patients with peritoneal lavage — Positive results reduces cost and unnecessary celiotomies in blunt trauma. **Archives of Surgery** 1996; 131:954–959.

19. Shackford SR, Rogers FB, Osler TM, et al: Focused abdominal sonography for trauma: The learning curve of nonradiologist clinicians in detecting hemoperitoneum. **Journal of Trauma** 1999; 46(4):553–562.

20. Takishima T, Sugimota K, Hirata M, et al: Serum amylase level on admission in the diagnosis of blunt injury to the pancreas: Its significance and limitations. **Annals of Surgery** 1997; 226(1): 70–76.

21. Thal ER: Evolution of peritoneal lavage and local exploration in lower chest and abdominal stab wounds. **Journal of Trauma** 1977; 17: 642–648.

22. Zantut LF, Ivatury RR, Smith RS, et al: Diagnostic and therapeutic laparoscopy for penetrating abdominal trauma: A multicenter experience. **Journal of Trauma** 1997; 42(5):825–829.

Back, Flank, and Lower Chest Wounds

23. Boyle EM, Maier RV, Salazar JD, et al: Diagnosis of injuries after stab wounds to the back and flank. **Journal of Trauma** 1997; 42(2):260–265.

24. Demetriades D, Rabinowitz B, Sofianos C, et al: The management of penetrating injuries of the back. A prospective study of 230 patients. **Annals of Surgery** 1988; 207:72–74.

25. Fallon WF Jr, Reyna TM, Brunner RG et al: Penetrating trauma to the buttock. **Southern Medical Journal** 1988; 81(10):1236–1238.

26. Ivatury RR, Rao RM, Nallathambi M, et al: Penetrating gluteal injury. **Journal of Trauma** 1982; 23(8):706–709.

27. Meyer DM, Thal ER, Weigelt JA, et al: The role of abdominal CT in the evaluation of stab wounds to the back. **Journal of Trauma** 1989; 29:1226–1230.

28. Phillips T, Sclafani SJA, Goldstein A, et al: Use of the contrast-enhanced CT enema in the management of penetrating trauma to the flank and back. **Journal of Trauma** 1986; 26:593–601.

Pelvic Fractures

29. Agolini SF, Shah K, Jaffe J, et al: Arterial embolization is a rapid and effective technique for controlling pelvic fracture hemorrhage. **Journal of Trauma** 1997; 43(3):395–399.

30. Cryer HM, Miller FB, Evers BM, et al: Pelvic fracture classification: Correlation with hemorrhage. **Journal of Trauma** 1988; 28:973–980.

31. Dalal SA, Burgess AR, Siegel JH, et al: Pelvic fracture in multiple trauma: Classification by mechanism is key to pattern of organ injury, resuscitative requirements, and outcome. **Journal of Trauma** 1989; 29:981–1002.

32. Gylling SF, Ward RE, Holcroft JW, et al: Immediate external fixation of unstable pelvic fractures. **American Journal of Surgery** 1985; 150:721–724.

33. Koraitim MM: Pelvic fracture urethral injuries: The unresolved controversy. **Journal of Urology** 1999; 161(5):1433–1441.

34. Mendez C, Gubler KD, Maier RV: Diagnostic accuracy of peritoneal lavage in patients with pelvic fractures. **Archives of Surgery** 1994; 129(5): 477–481.

35. Routt ML Jr, Simonian PT, Swiontkowski MF: Stabilization of pelvic ring disruptions. **Orthopedic Clinics of North America** 1997; 28(3): 369–388.

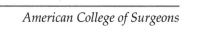

SKILLS STATION

Diagnostic Peritoneal Lavage

◼ OBJECTIVES:

Performance at this station will allow the participant to practice and demonstrate the technique of diagnostic peritoneal lavage on a live, anesthetized animal; a fresh, human cadaver; or an anatomic human body manikin. The student also will be able to:

1. Identify the indications and contraindications of peritoneal lavage.

2. Perform the Seldinger procedure and the open procedure for peritoneal lavage.

3. Describe complications of this procedure.

Note: The preferred skills procedure for peritoneal lavage is performed via the open technique method to avoid injury to underlying structures. If an individual does not routinely perform an open DPL, the method of employing the Seldinger technique is an acceptable alternative to be used by trained doctors.

INTERACTIVE SKILLS PROCEDURE

Diagnostic Peritoneal Lavage

Note: Standard precautions are required whenever caring for the trauma patient.

I. DIAGNOSTIC PERITONEAL LAVAGE: OPEN TECHNIQUE

A. Decompress the urinary bladder by inserting a urinary catheter.

B. Decompress the stomach by inserting a gastric tube.

C. Surgically prepare the abdomen (eg, costal margin to the pubic area and flank to flank, anteriorly).

D. Inject local anesthetic midline and just below the umbilicus. Use lidocaine with epinephrine to avoid blood contamination from skin and subcutaneous tissue.

E. Vertically incise the skin and subcutaneous tissues to the fascia.

F. Grasp the fascial edges with clamps, elevate and incise the fascia down to the peritoneum. Make a small nick in the peritoneum, entering the peritoneal cavity.

G. Insert a peritoneal dialysis catheter into the peritoneal cavity.

H. After inserting the catheter into the peritoneum, advance the catheter into the pelvis.

I. Connect the dialysis catheter to a syringe and aspirate.

J. If gross blood is not obtained, instill 1 liter of warmed Ringer's lactate solution/normal saline (or 10 mL/kg in a child) into the peritoneum through the intravenous tubing attached to the dialysis catheter.

K. Gentle agitation of the abdomen distributes the fluid throughout the peritoneal cavity and increases mixing with the blood.

L. If the patient's condition is stable, allow the fluid to remain a few minutes before allowing it to drain. This is done by putting the Ringer's lactate solution/normal saline container on the floor and allowing the peritoneal fluid to drain from the abdomen. Make sure the container is vented to promote flow of the fluid from the abdomen. Adequate fluid return is >30% of the infused volume.

M. After the fluid returns, send a sample to the laboratory for Gram stain, and erythrocyte and leukocyte counts (unspun). A positive test and the need for surgical intervention are indicated by 100,000 RBCs/mm^3 or more, greater than 500 WBCs/mm^3, or a positive Gram stain for food fibers or bacteria.

N. A negative lavage does not exclude retroperitoneal injuries, ie, pancreas or duodenum, or diaphragmatic tears.

II. DIAGNOSTIC PERITONEAL LAVAGE: CLOSED TECHNIQUE

A. Decompress the urinary bladder by inserting a urinary catheter.

B. Decompress the stomach by inserting a gastric tube.

C. Surgically prepare the abdomen (eg, costal margin to the pubic area and flank to flank, anteriorly).

ABDOMINAL TRAUMA   *Diagnostic Peritoneal Lavage*

D. Inject local anesthetic midline just below the umbilicus. Use lidocaine with epinephrine to avoid blood contamination from skin and subcutaneous tissue.

E. Elevate the skin on either side of the proposed needle insertion site with the fingers or forceps.

F. Insert the #18-gauge beveled needle attached to a syringe through the skin and subcutaneous tissue. Resistance is encountered when traversing the fascia and again when penetrating the peritoneum.

G. The flexible end of the guidewire is then passed through the #18-gauge needle until resistance is met or 3 cm is still showing outside the needle. The needle is then removed from the abdominal cavity so that only the guidewire remains.

H. A small skin incision is made at the entrance site of the catheter, and the peritoneal lavage catheter is inserted over the guidewire into the peritoneal cavity. The guidewire is then removed from the abdominal cavity so that only the lavage catheter remains.

I. Connect the dialysis catheter to a syringe and aspirate.

J. If gross blood is not obtained, instill 1 liter of warmed Ringer's lactate solution/normal saline (or 10 mL/kg in a child) into the peritoneum through the intravenous tubing attached to the dialysis catheter.

K. Gentle agitation of the abdomen distributes the fluid throughout the peritoneal cavity and increases mixing with the blood.

L. If the patient's condition is stable, allow the fluid to remain a few minutes before allowing it to drain. This is done by putting the Ringer's lactate solution/normal saline container on the floor and allowing the peritoneal fluid to drain from the abdomen. Make sure the container is vented to promote flow of the fluid from the abdomen.

M. After the fluid has returned, send a sample to the laboratory for Gram stain, and erythrocyte and leukocyte counts (unspun). A positive test and the need for surgical intervention are indicated by 100,000 RBCs/mm^3 or more, greater than 500 WBCs/mm^3, or a positive Gram stain for food fibers or bacteria.

Complications of Peritoneal Lavage

1. *Hemorrhage, secondary to injection of local anesthetic, incision of the skin, or subcutaneous tissues providing a false-positive study*
2. *Peritonitis due to intestinal perforation from the catheter*
3. *Laceration of urinary bladder (if bladder not evacuated prior to procedure)*
4. *Injury to other abdominal and retroperitoneal structures requiring operative care*
5. *Wound infection at the lavage site (late complication)*

SIX

CHAPTER

Head Trauma

◼ OBJECTIVES:

Upon completion of this topic, the doctor will be able to demonstrate the techniques of assessment and explain the emergency management of head trauma. Specifically, the doctor will be able to:

A. Describe the basic intracranial physiology.

B. Evaluate the head- and brain-injured patient.

C. Perform a focused neurologic examination.

D. Recognize the importance of adequate resuscitation in limiting secondary brain injury.

E. Determine the appropriate disposition of the patient.

HEAD TRAUMA

I. INTRODUCTION

Approximately 500,000 cases of brain injury occur in the United States each year. About 10% of these brain-injured patients die prior to reaching a hospital. About 80% of brain-injured patients receiving medical attention can be categorized as mild, 10% as moderate, and 10% as severe. More than 100,000 patients suffer varying degrees of disability from brain injury every year. Central nervous system (CNS) trauma accounts for more than 40% of military casualties. Therefore, even a small reduction in the mortality and morbidity resulting from brain injury should have a major impact on public health.

The primary focus of treatment for patients suspected of having a severe brain injury should be to prevent secondary brain injury. Providing adequate oxygenation and maintenance of a sufficient blood pressure to perfuse the brain are the most important ways to limit secondary brain damage and thereby improve the patient's outcome. Subsequent to managing the ABCDEs, identification of a mass lesion requiring surgical evacuation is critical, and is best achieved by immediately obtaining a computed tomography (CT) scan of the head. However, obtaining a CT scan should not delay patient transfer to a trauma center capable of immediate and definitive neurosurgical intervention.

The triage of a patient with brain injury depends on the severity of the injury and on the facilities available within a particular community. For those facilities without neurosurgical coverage, prearranged transfer agreements with higher level facilities should be in place. Consultation with a neurosurgeon early in the course of treatment is strongly recommended, especially if the patient is comatose or is otherwise suspected of having a brain injury.

In consulting a neurosurgeon about a patient with a brain injury, the doctor should relay the following information:

1. Age of patient and the mechanism and time of injury

2. Respiratory and cardiovascular status (particularly the blood pressure)

3. Results of a neurologic examination, consisting of the Glasgow Coma Scale (GCS) Score (with particular emphasis on the motor response) and pupil size and reaction to light

4. Presence and type of associated injuries

5. Results of diagnostic studies, particularly the CT scan (if available)

6. Treatment of hypotension or hypoxia

Do not delay patient transfer to obtain a CT scan or other diagnostic tests.

II. ANATOMY

A. Scalp

The scalp is made up of 5 layers of tissue (mnemonic SCALP) that cover the skull: (1) skin, (2) connective tissue, (3) aponeurosis or galea aponeurotica, (4) loose areolar tissue, and (5) pericranium. Loose areolar tissue separates the galea from the pericranium and is the site of subgaleal hematomas. Because of the scalp's generous blood supply, bleeding from a scalp laceration can result in major blood loss, especially in infants and children.

B. Skull

The skull is composed of the cranial vault (calvaria) and the base. The calvaria is especially thin in the temporal regions, but is cushioned here by the temporalis muscle. The base of the skull is irregular, and this may contribute to injury as the brain moves within the skull during acceleration and deceleration. The floor of the cranial cavity is divided into 3 distinct regions—the anterior, middle, and posterior cranial fossa. As a simplification, the anterior fossa houses the frontal lobes, the middle fossa the temporal lobes, and the posterior fossa the lower brainstem and the cerebellum.

C. Meninges

The meninges cover the brain and consist of 3 layers—the dura mater, the arachnoid, and the pia mater. The **dura mater** is a tough, fibrous membrane that adheres firmly to the internal surface of the skull. Because it is not attached to the underlying **arachnoid**, a potential space (the subdural space) exists into which hemorrhage can occur. In brain injury, the veins that travel from the surface of the brain to the superior sagittal sinus in the midline (bridging veins) may tear, leading to the formation of a subdural hematoma. At specific sites the dura splits into 2 leaves that enclose large venous sinuses that provide the major venous drainage from the brain. The midline superior sagittal sinus drains into the transverse and sigmoid sinuses. The latter are more commonly dominant on the right side. Laceration of these venous sinuses can result in massive hemorrhage.

Meningeal arteries lie between the dura and the internal surface of the skull (epidural space). Overlying skull fractures may lacerate these arteries and result in an epidural hematoma. The most commonly injured meningeal vessel is the middle meningeal artery, which is located over the temporal fossa.

Beneath the dura is a second meningeal layer, the thin transparent arachnoid membrane. The third layer, the **pia mater**, is firmly attached to the surface of the brain. Cerebrospinal fluid circulates in the subarachnoid space. Hemorrhage into this space (subarachnoid hemorrhage) is frequently caused by brain injury.

D. Brain

The brain consists of the cerebrum, the cerebellum, and the brainstem. The **cerebrum** is composed of right and left hemispheres that are separated by the falx cerebri—a dural reflection from the inferior aspect of the superior sagittal sinus. The left hemisphere contains the language centers in virtually all right-handed people and in more than 85% of left-handed people. The hemisphere that contains the language centers is referred to as the dominant hemisphere. The frontal lobe is concerned with emotions, motor function, and, on the dominant side, with expression of speech (motor speech areas). The parietal lobe is involved with sensory function and spatial orientation. The temporal lobe regulates certain memory functions. In virtually all right-handed and in the majority of left-handed persons, the left temporal lobe contains areas responsible for speech reception and integration. The occipital lobe is responsible for vision.

The **brainstem** is composed of the midbrain, the pons, and the medulla. The midbrain and upper pons contain the reticular activating system, which is responsible for the state of alertness. Vital cardio-respiratory centers reside in the medulla, which continues on to form the spinal cord. Even small lesions in the brainstem can be associated with severe neurologic deficits. The **cerebellum**, responsible mainly for coordination and balance, projects posteriorly in the posterior fossa and forms connections with the spinal cord, the brainstem, and ultimately with the cerebral hemispheres.

E. Cerebrospinal Fluid

Cerebrospinal fluid (CSF) is produced by the choroid plexus (located in the roof of the ventricles) at a rate of approximately 20 mL/hour. The CSF travels from the lateral ventricles of the brain through the foramen of Monro, third ventricle, and the aqueduct of Sylvius into the fourth ventricle. It then exits from the ventricular system into the subarachnoid space overlying the brain and spinal cord and is reabsorbed into the venous circulation through the arachnoid granulations that project into the superior sagittal sinus. The presence of blood in the CSF can occlude the arachnoid granulations, impair CSF reabsorption, and result in increased intracranial pressure (posttraumatic communicating hydrocephalus).

F. Tentorium

The tentorium cerebelli divides the head into the supratentorial compartment (comprising the anterior and middle fossae of the skull) and the infratentorial compartment (containing the posterior fossa). The midbrain connects the cerebral hemispheres to the rest of the brainstem (pons and medulla oblongata) as it passes through a large aperture in the tentorium known as the tentorial incisura. The oculomotor (IIIrd) nerve runs along the edge of the tentorium and may become compressed against it during temporal lobe herniation, which most commonly results from a supratentorial mass or edema. Parasympathetic fibers that are pupillary constrictors lie on the surface of the IIIrd nerve. Paralysis of these fibers by compression of the IIIrd nerve causes pupillary dilatation due to unopposed sympathetic activity.

The part of the brain that usually herniates through the tentorial notch is the medial part of the temporal lobe, known as the uncus. **Uncal herniation** also causes compression of the corticospinal (pyramidal) tract in the midbrain. The motor tract crosses to the opposite side at the foramen magnum, so compression at the level of the midbrain results in weakness of the opposite side of the body (contralateral hemiplegia). Ipsilateral pupillary dilatation associated with contralateral hemiplegia is the classic syndrome of uncal herniation. Infrequently, the mass lesion may push the **opposite** side of the midbrain against the tentorial edge, resulting in hemiplegia and a dilated pupil on the same side as the hematoma (Kernohan's notch syndrome).

HEAD TRAUMA

III. PHYSIOLOGY

A. Intracranial Pressure

Several pathologic processes that affect the brain can cause elevation of intracranial pressure (ICP). Elevated ICP can reduce cerebral perfusion and cause or exacerbate ischemia. Normal ICP in the resting state is approximately 10 mm Hg. Pressures greater than 20 mm Hg, particularly if sustained and refractory to treatment, are associated with poor outcomes.

B. Monro-Kellie Doctrine

This is a simple, yet vitally important concept relating to the understanding of ICP dynamics. It states that the total volume of the intracranial contents must remain constant. This is fairly obvious, because the cranium is a rigid nonexpansile container. (See Figure 1, Monro-Kellie Doctrine, and Figure 2, page 155, Volume–Pressure Curve.) Thus very early after injury a mass such as a blood clot may be enlarging while the ICP remains normal. Once the limit of displacement of CSF and intravascular blood has been reached, ICP rapidly increases.

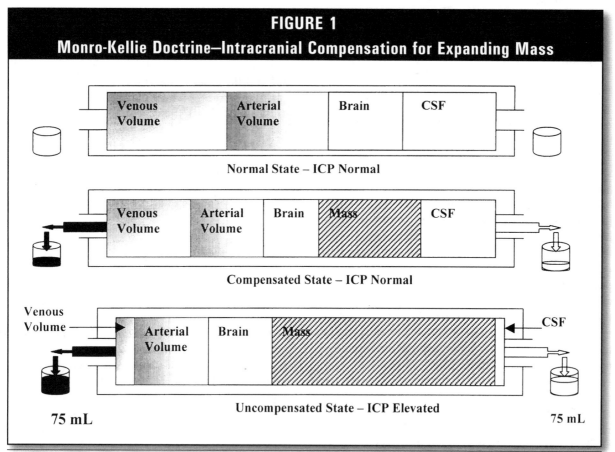

FIGURE 1
Monro-Kellie Doctrine—Intracranial Compensation for Expanding Mass

Normal State – ICP Normal

Compensated State – ICP Normal

Uncompensated State – ICP Elevated

75 mL   75 mL

Monro-Kellie doctrine: Intracranial compensation for expanding mass. The volume of the intracranial contents remains constant. If the addition of a mass such as a hematoma results in the squeezing out of an equal volume of CSF and venous blood, the ICP remains normal. However, when this compensatory mechanism is exhausted, there is an exponential increase in ICP for even a small additional increase in the volume of the hematoma, as shown in Figure 2, Volume-Pressure Curve.

Adapted with permission from Narayan RK: Head Injury, in Grossman RG, Hamilton WJ (eds): *Principles of Neurosurgery*. New York, Raven Press, 1991, p 267.

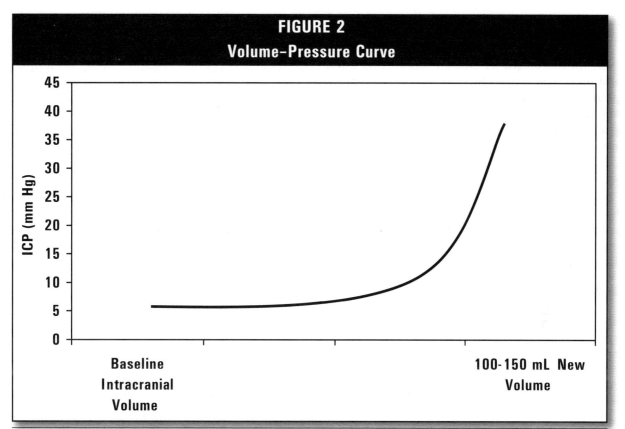

FIGURE 2
Volume-Pressure Curve

Volume-pressure curve: The intracranial contents are able to compensate for a new intracranial mass, such as a subdural or epidural hematoma, up to a point. Once the volume of this mass reaches 100 to 150 mL, there is a rapid increase in intracranial pressure that can lead to cessation of cerebral blood flow.

C. Cerebral Blood Flow

In normal adults, cerebral blood flow (CBF) is 50 to 55 mL/100 grams of brain tissue/minute. In children, CBF may be much higher depending on their age. At 1 year of age it approximates adult levels, but at 5 years of age, normal CBF is approximately 90 mL/100 grams/minute and then gradually declines to adult levels by the mid to late teens. Brain injury severe enough to cause coma can cause a 50% reduction in CBF during the first 6 to 12 hours after injury. It usually increases over the next 2 to 3 days, but for those patients who remain comatose CBF remains below normal for days or weeks after injury. There is increasing evidence that such low levels of CBF are inadequate to meet the metabolic demands of the brain early after injury and that regional, if not global, cerebral ischemia is common.

In addition, the precapillary cerebral vasculature normally has the ability to reflexively constrict or dilate in response to mean systolic blood pressures of 50 to 160 mm Hg in order to maintain a constant CBF (pressure autoregulation). These vessels also normally constrict or dilate in response to changes in the Po_2 or Pco_2 of the blood (chemical autoregulation). Severe traumatic brain injury can disrupt both of these autoregulatory mechanisms.

Consequently, the traumatized brain is vulnerable to ischemia and infarction due to a severe reduction in blood flow caused by the traumatic insult itself. This preexisting ischemia can easily be exacerbated by hypotension, hypoxia, or by hypocapnia as might be iatrogenically introduced by overly aggressive hyperventilation. **Therefore, every effort should be made to enhance cerebral perfusion and blood flow by reducing elevated ICP, maintaining normal intravascular volume, maintaining a normal mean arterial blood pressure (MAP), and restoring normal oxygenation and normocapnia.** Maintaining the cerebral perfusion pressure (MAP minus

HEAD TRAUMA

ICP) at a level of 60 to 70 mm Hg is recommended as a means of improving CBF.

Once the compensatory mechanisms are exhausted and there is an exponential increase in ICP, brain perfusion is compromised, especially in the hypotensive patient. Therefore, hematomas should be evacuated early and adequate systemic blood pressure must be maintained.

IV. CLASSIFICATION

Head injuries are classified in several ways. For practical purposes, 3 descriptions are useful: (1) mechanism, (2) severity, and (3) morphology. (See Table 1, page 157, Classifications of Brain Injury.)

A. Mechanism of Injury

Brain injury may be broadly classified as blunt or penetrating. For practical purposes, the term blunt brain injury usually is associated with automobile collisions, falls, and blunt assaults. Penetrating brain injury usually results from gunshot and stab wounds.

B. Severity of Injury

The GCS Score is used as an objective clinical measure of the severity of brain injury. Patients who open their eyes spontaneously, obey commands, and are oriented score a total of 15 points on the GCS, whereas flaccid patients who do not open their eyes or talk score the minimum (3 points). (See Table 2, page 159, Glasgow Coma Scale.) **A GCS Score of 8 or less has become the generally accepted definition of coma or a severe brain injury.** Brain-injured patients with a GCS Score of 9 to 13 are categorized as "moderate," and those with a GCS Score of 14 to 15 are designated as "mild." Note that in assessing the GCS Score, when there is right/left asymmetry **it is important to use the BEST motor response in calculating the score because this is the most reliable predictor of outcome.** However, one must record the actual response on both sides.

C. Morphology

1. Skull fractures

Skull fractures may be seen in the cranial vault or skull base, may be linear or stellate, and may be open or closed. Basal skull fractures usually require CT scanning with bone-window settings for identification. The presence of clinical signs of a basal skull fracture should increase the index of suspicion and help in its identification. These signs include periorbital ecchymosis (raccoon eyes), retroauricular ecchymosis (Battle sign), CSF leakage from the nose (rhinorrhea) or the ear (otorrhea), and VIIth and VIIIth nerve dysfunction (facial paralysis and hearing loss), which may occur immediately or a few days after the initial injury. Generally, the prognosis for the recovery of VIIth nerve function is better in the delayed onset variety, but prognosis for recovery of VIIIth nerve function is poor. Basal skull fractures that traverse the carotid canals may damage the carotid arteries (dissection, pseudoaneurysm, or thrombosis) and consideration should be given to cerebral arteriography.

Open or compound skull fractures may provide a direct communication between the scalp laceration and the cerebral surface because the dura is often torn.

The significance of a skull fracture should not be underestimated, since it takes considerable force to fracture the skull. A linear vault fracture increases the likelihood of an intracranial hematoma by about 400 times in a conscious patient and by 20 times in a comatose patient, in whom the risk of a hematoma is already much higher.

2. Intracranial lesions (See Table 1, page 157, Classifications of Brain Injury, and Figure 3, page 158, CT Scans of Intracranial Hematomas)

These lesions may be classified as focal or diffuse, although the 2 forms of intracranial lesions frequently coexist. Focal lesions include epidural hematomas, subdural hematomas, contusions, and intracerebral hematomas.

    a. Diffuse brain injuries range from mild concussions where the CT scan of the head is usually normal to severe hypoxic ischemic injuries.

    With concussions the patient has a brief loss of consciousness and may have retrograde and/or antegrade amnesia.

    Severe diffuse injury most often results from a hypoxic, ischemic insult to the brain due to prolonged shock or apnea occurring immediately after the trauma. In such cases, the CT scan may initially appear normal, or the brain

Table 1—Classifications of Brain Injury

Mechanism	• Blunt		• High velocity (automobile collision) • Low velocity (fall, assault)
	• Penetrating		• Gunshot wounds • Other penetrating injuries
Severity	• Mild • Moderate • Severe		• GCS Score 14–15 • GCS Score 9–13 • GCS Score 3–8
Morphology	• Skull fractures	• Vault	• Linear vs stellate • Depressed/nondepressed • Open/closed
		• Basilar	• With/without CSF leak • With/without VIIth nerve palsy
	• Intracranial lesions	• Focal	• Epidural • Subdural • Intracerebral
		• Diffuse	• Concussion • Multiple contusions • Hypoxic/ischemic injury

Adapted with permission from Valadka AB, Narayan RK: Emergency room management of the head-injured patient, in Narayan RK, Wilberger JE, Povlishock JT (eds): *Neurotrauma.* New York, McGraw-Hill, 1996, p 120.

may appear diffusely swollen with loss of the normal grey-white distinction. Less commonly, and particularly with high-speed rollover motor vehicle crashes, there may be multiple punctate hemorrhages throughout the cerebral hemispheres which are concentrated in the border between the grey matter and white matter. Previously, DAI (diffuse axonal injury) was used to define a clinical syndrome suggesting severe brain injury with uniformly poor outcome. Current research indicates that it is a microscopic finding in the brain and may be seen in a wide spectrum of clinical presentations.

b. Epidural hematomas

Epidural hematomas are relatively uncommon, occurring in 0.5% of all brain-injured patients and 9% of those who are comatose. These hematomas are located outside the dura but within the skull and are typically biconvex or lenticular in shape. They are most often

located in the temporal or temporoparietal region and usually result from a tear of the middle meningeal artery due to a fracture. These clots are usually arterial in origin; however, they also may result from disruption of a major venous sinus.

c. Subdural hematomas

Subdural hematomas are more common (approximately 30% of severe brain injuries) than epidural hematomas and occur most frequently from tearing of small surface vessels of the cerebral cortex. Subdural hematomas normally cover the entire surface of the hemisphere. Furthermore, the brain damage underlying an acute subdural hematoma is usually much more severe than for epidural hematomas.

d. Contusions and intracerebral hematomas

Cerebral contusions are fairly common (20% to 30% of severe brain injuries), and the majority occur in the frontal and temporal lobes,

HEAD TRAUMA

FIGURE 3
CT Scans of Intracranial Hematomas

Normal CT

Normal CT

Large frontal contusions
with shift

Subdural hematoma
with shift

Temporal epidural hematoma
with uncal herniation (arrow)

although they can occur in any part of the brain. **Contusions can, in a period of hours or days, evolve or coalesce to form an intracerebral hematoma requiring immediate surgical evacuation. This occurs in approximately 20% of patients and is best detected by repeating the head CT scan within 12 to 24 hours after the initial scan.**

V. MANAGEMENT OF MILD BRAIN INJURY (GCS 14–15) (See Algorithm 1, page 160, Management of Mild Brain Injury)

Approximately 80% of patients presenting to the emergency department with brain injury are catego-

rized as having a mild brain injury. These patients are awake but may be amnesic for events surrounding the injury. There may be a history of a brief loss of consciousness that usually is difficult to confirm. The picture often is confounded by alcohol or other intoxicants.

Most patients with mild brain injury make uneventful recoveries. However, about 3% of these patients deteriorate unexpectedly, resulting in severe neurologic dysfunction unless the decline in mental status is detected early.

A CT scan should be considered in all brain-injury patients who have a loss of consciousness of greater than 5 minutes, amnesia, severe headaches, a GCS

Score of <15, or a focal neurologic deficit attributable to the brain. X-rays of the cervical spine should be obtained if there is midline neck pain or palpation tenderness.

CT scanning is the preferred method of imaging. If CT scanning is not available, skull x-rays may be obtained for blunt or penetrating head injury. If a skull x-ray is obtained, one must look for the following features: (1) linear or depressed skull fractures, (2) midline position of the pineal gland (if calcified), (3) air-fluid levels in the sinuses, (4) pneumocephalus, (5) facial fractures, and (6) foreign bodies. **Remember, obtaining skull films should not delay transfer of the patient.**

If abnormalities are observed on the CT scan, or if the patient remains symptomatic or neurologically abnormal, the patient should be admitted to the hospital and a neurosurgeon consulted. (See Table 2, Glasgow Coma Scale.)

If the patient is asymptomatic, fully awake and alert, and neurologically normal, s/he may be observed for several hours, reexamined, and if still normal safely discharged. Ideally, the patient is discharged to the care of a companion who can stay with and observe the patient over the next 24 hours. Both the patient and his/her companion are directed according to an instruction sheet to keep the patient under close observation and to return to the emergency department if headaches develop, there is a decline in mental status, or there is development of focal neurologic deficits. In all cases, written discharge instructions should be supplied to and carefully reviewed with the patient and/or companion. (See Table 3, page 161, Head-injury Warning Discharge Instructions.) **If the patient is not alert or oriented enough to clearly understand the written and verbal instructions, the decision for discharge should be reconsidered.**

VI. MANAGEMENT OF MODERATE BRAIN INJURY (GCS SCORE 9-13) (See Algorithm 2, page 162, Management of Moderate Brain Injury)

Approximately 10% of brain-injured patients seen in the emergency department have a moderate injury.

Table 2—Glasgow Coma Scale (GCS)

ASSESSMENT AREA	SCORE
Eye Opening (E)	
Spontaneous	4
To speech	3
To pain	2
None	1
BEST Motor Response (M)	
Obeys commands	6
Localizes pain	5
Normal flexion (withdrawal)	4
Abnormal flexion (decorticate)	3
Extension (decerebrate)	2
None (flaccid)	1
Verbal Response (V)	
Oriented	5
Confused conversation	4
Inappropriate words	3
Incomprehensible sounds	2
None	1

GCS Score = (E+M+V); Best possible score = 15; Worst possible score = 3.

ALGORITHM 1
Management of Mild Brain Injury

➤ Definition: Patient is awake and may be oriented. (GCS 14–15)
➤ History

- Name, age, sex, race, occupation
- Mechanism of injury
- Time of injury
- Loss of consciousness immediately postinjury

- Subsequent level of alertness
- Amnesia: Retrograde, antegrade
- Headache: Mild, moderate, severe

➤ General examination to exclude systemic injuries
➤ Limited neurologic examination
➤ Cervical spine and other x-rays as indicated
➤ Blood-alcohol level and urine toxicology screen
➤ CT scan of the head is ideal in all patients except completely asymptomatic and neurologically normal patients

Observe in or Admit to Hospital

- No CT scanner available
- Abnormal CT scan
- All penetrating head injuries
- History of prolonged loss of consciousness
- Deteriorating level of consciousness
- Moderate to severe headache
- Significant alcohol/drug intoxication
- Skull fracture
- CSF leak: Rhinorrhea or otorrhea
- Significant associated injuries
- No reliable companion at home
- Abnormal GCS Score (<15)
- Focal neurologic deficits

Discharge from Hospital

- Patient does not meet any of the criteria for admission
- Discuss need to return if any problems develop and issue a "warning sheet"
- Schedule follow-up visit

Adapted with permission from Valadka AB, Narayan RK: Emergency room management of the head-injured patient, in Narayan RK, Wilberger JE, Povlishock JT (eds): *Neurotrauma.* New York, McGraw-Hill, 1996, p 123.

They still are able to follow simple commands but usually are confused or somnolent and may have focal neurologic deficits such as hemiparesis. Approximately 10% to 20% of these patients deteriorate and lapse into coma.

On admission to the emergency department, a brief history is obtained and cardiopulmonary stability is ensured before neurologic assessment. A CT scan of the head is obtained and a neurosurgeon is contacted. All of these patients require admission for observation in an intensive care unit (ICU) or similar unit capable of close nursing observation and frequent neurologic reassessment for the first 12 to 24 hours. A follow-up CT scan in 12 to 24 hours is recommended if the initial CT is abnormal or if there is deterioration of the patient's neurologic status.

Table 3—Head-injury Warning Discharge Instructions

We have found no evidence to indicate that your head injury was serious. However, new symptoms and unexpected complications can develop hours or even days after the injury. The first 24 hours are the most crucial and you should remain with a reliable companion at least during this period. If any of the following signs develop, call your doctor or come back to the hospital.

1. Drowsiness or increasing difficulty in awakening patient (Awaken patient every 2 hours during period of sleep.)
2. Nausea or vomiting
3. Convulsions or fits
4. Bleeding or watery drainage from the nose or ear
5. Severe headaches
6. Weakness or loss of feeling in the arm or leg
7. Confusion or strange behavior
8. One pupil (black part of eye) much larger than the other; peculiar movements of the eyes, double vision, or other visual disturbances
9. A very slow or very rapid pulse, or an unusual breathing pattern

If there is swelling at the site of the injury, apply an ice pack, making sure that there is a cloth or towel between the ice pack and the skin. If swelling increases markedly in spite of the ice pack application, call us or come back to the hospital.

You may eat and drink as usual if you so desire. However, you should NOT drink alcoholic beverages for at least 3 days after your injury.

Do not take any sedatives or any pain relievers stronger than acetaminophen, at least for the first 24 hours. Do not use aspirin-containing medicines.

If you have further questions, or in case of an emergency, we can be reached at (telephone number).

Doctor's name:_____

VII. MANAGEMENT OF SEVERE BRAIN INJURY (GCS SCORE 3-8) (See Table 4, page 163, Initial Management of Severe Brain Injury, and Table 5, page 164, Priorities for the Initial Evaluation and Triage of Patients with Severe Brain Injuries)

Patients who have sustained a severe brain injury are unable to follow simple commands even after cardiopulmonary stabilization. Although this definition includes a wide spectrum of brain injury, it identifies the patients who are at greatest risk of suffering significant morbidity and mortality. **A "wait and see" approach in such patients can be** **disastrous, and prompt diagnosis and treatment is extremely important. Do not delay patient transfer to obtain a CT scan.**

A. Primary Survey and Resuscitation

Brain injury often is adversely affected by secondary insults. Hypotension on admission in patients with severe brain injury is associated with more than double the mortality as compared with patients with no hypotension (60% vs 27%). The presence of hypoxia in addition to hypotension is associated with a mortality of approximately 75%. **Therefore, it is imperative that cardiopulmonary stabilization be achieved rapidly in patients with severe brain injury.**

HEAD TRAUMA

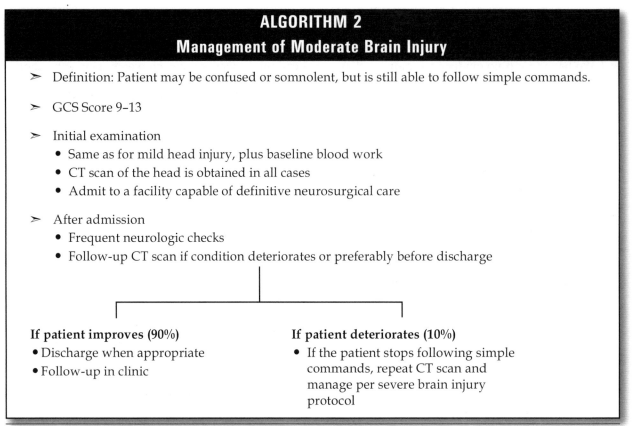

ALGORITHM 2

Management of Moderate Brain Injury

➤ Definition: Patient may be confused or somnolent, but is still able to follow simple commands.

➤ GCS Score 9–13

➤ Initial examination
- Same as for mild head injury, plus baseline blood work
- CT scan of the head is obtained in all cases
- Admit to a facility capable of definitive neurosurgical care

➤ After admission
- Frequent neurologic checks
- Follow-up CT scan if condition deteriorates or preferably before discharge

If patient improves (90%)
- Discharge when appropriate
- Follow-up in clinic

If patient deteriorates (10%)
- If the patient stops following simple commands, repeat CT scan and manage per severe brain injury protocol

Adapted with permission from Valadka AB, Narayan RK: Emergency room management of the head-injured patient, in Narayan RK, Wilberger JE, Povlishock JT (eds): *Neurotrauma.* New York, McGraw-Hill, 1996, p 125.

---

1. Airway and breathing

Transient respiratory arrest and hypoxia are common and can cause secondary brain injury. **Early endotracheal intubation should be performed for comatose patients.**

The patient is ventilated with 100% oxygen until blood gases are obtained, then appropriate adjustments to the F_{IO_2} are made. Pulse oximetry is a useful adjunct and O_2 saturations >98% are desirable. Hyperventilation should be used cautiously in patients with severe brain injury and only when acute neurologic deterioration occurs. (See VIII. B., Hyperventilation.)

2. Circulation

Hypotension usually is not due to the brain injury itself except in the terminal stages when medullary failure supervenes. Intracranial hemorrhage cannot cause hemorrhagic shock. Euvolemia should be established as soon as possible if the patient is hypotensive.

Hypotension is a marker of severe blood loss, which is not always obvious. One also must consider associated spinal cord injury (neurogenic shock), cardiac contusion or tamponade, and tension pneumothorax as possible causes.

While efforts are in progress to determine the cause of hypotension, volume replacement should be initiated. **DPL or FAST is used routinely in the hypotensive comatose patient because a clinical examination for abdominal tenderness is not possible in such patients.** (See Chapter 3, Shock, and Table 5, page 164, Priorities for the Initial Evaluation and Triage of Patients with Severe Brain Injuries.) Establishing the priority of DPL versus CT scan of the head can sometimes create conflicts between the trauma surgeons and neurosurgeons. It must be emphasized that a hypotensive patient's neurologic examination

Table 4—Initial Management of Severe Brain Injury

> ➤ Definition: Patient is unable to follow even simple commands because of impaired consciousness (GCS Score 3–8)
>
> ➤ Assessment and management
> - ABCDEs
> - Primary survey and resuscitation
> - Secondary survey and AMPLE history
> - Admit to a facility capable of definitive neurosurgical care
> - Neurologic reevaluation: GCS
>   - Eye opening
>   - Motor response
>   - Verbal response
>   - Pupillary light reaction
>
> - Therapeutic agents (usually administered after consultation with neurosurgeon)
>   - Mannitol
>   - Moderate hyperventilation (P_{CO_2} < 35 mm Hg)
>   - Anticonvulsants
>
> ➤ Diagnostic tests (in descending order of preference)
> - CT scan
> - Air ventriculogram
> - Angiogram

Modified with permission from Valadka AB, Narayan RK: Emergency room management of the head-injured patient, in Narayan RK, Wilberger JE, Povlishock JT (eds): *Neurotrauma*. New York, McGraw-Hill, 1996, p 125.

is unreliable, and that even if severe brain injury exists, hypotension is a well-known cause of secondary brain injury. Hypotensive patients who are unresponsive to any form of stimulation may revert to a near-normal neurologic examination soon after normal blood pressure is restored.

B. Neurologic Examination

As soon as the patient's cardiopulmonary status is corrected, a rapid and directed neurologic examination is performed. It consists primarily of the Glasgow Coma Scale Score and pupillary light response. In a comatose patient, motor responses may be elicited by pinching the trapezius muscle or with nail-bed pressure. If a patient demonstrates variable responses to stimulation, **the best motor response elicited is a more accurate prognostic indicator than the worst response.** Doll's eye movements (oculocephalics), ice-water calorics (oculo-vestibulars), and corneal responses are deferred to

a neurosurgeon. **Doll's eye testing should never be attempted until an unstable cervical spine injury has been ruled out.**

It is important to obtain the GCS Score and perform a pupillary examination prior to sedating or paralyzing the patient, because knowledge of the patient's clinical condition is important for deciding subsequent treatment. Long-acting paralytic agents should not be used during the primary survey. Succinylcholine or vecuronium are recommended when pharmacologic paralysis is necessary for safe endotracheal intubation, or for obtaining good quality diagnostic studies. Small repeated doses of intravenous morphine are useful for providing analgesia and sedation that is reversible.

C. Secondary Survey

Serial examinations (GCS Score, lateralization, and pupillary reaction) should be performed to detect

HEAD TRAUMA

Table 5—Priorities for the Initial Evaluation and Triage
of Patients with Severe Brain Injuries

1. All comatose, brain-injured patients should undergo resuscitation (ABCDEs) upon arrival in the emergency department (ED).

2. As soon as the BP is normalized, a neurologic exam is performed (GCS Score and pupillary reaction). If the BP cannot be normalized, the neurologic examination is still performed and the hypotension recorded.

3. If the patient's systolic BP cannot be brought up to >100 mm Hg despite aggressive fluid resuscitation, the priority is to establish the cause of the hypotension, with the neurosurgical evaluation taking second priority. In such cases the patient undergoes a DPL or ultrasound in the ED and may need to go directly to the operating room (OR) for a celiotomy. CT of the head is obtained after the celiotomy. If there is clinical evidence of an intracranial mass, an air ventriculogram, diagnostic burr holes, or craniotomy may be undertaken in the OR while the celiotomy is being performed.

4. If the patient's systolic BP is >100 mm Hg after resuscitation and the patient has clinical evidence of a possible intracranial mass (unequal pupils, asymmetric motor exam), the first priority is to obtain a CT head scan. A DPL or FAST exam may be performed in the ED, CT area, or OR, but the patient's neurologic evaluation or treatment should not be delayed.

5. In borderline cases, ie, when the systolic BP can be temporarily corrected but tends to slowly decrease, every effort should be made to get a head CT prior to taking the patient to the OR for a celiotomy or thoracotomy. Such cases call for great clinical judgment and cooperation between the trauma surgeon and the neurosurgeon.

neurologic deterioration as early as possible. A well-known early sign of temporal lobe (uncal) herniation is dilation of the pupil and loss of the pupillary response to light. Direct trauma to the eye also is a potential cause of abnormal pupillary response and may make pupil evaluation difficult. However, in the setting of brain trauma, brain injury should be considered first.

D. Diagnostic Procedures

An emergency head CT scan must be obtained as quickly as possible, after hemodynamic normalization. CT scans also should be repeated whenever there is a change in the patient's clinical status and routinely at 12 to 24 hours after injury for those with a contusion or hematoma on their initial scan.

Findings of significance on the CT images include scalp swelling or subgaleal hematomas at the region of impact. Skull fractures may be seen better with bone windows, but are often apparent even on the soft-tissue windows. The crucial findings on the CT scan are intracranial hematoma, contusions, and shift of the midline (mass effect). (See Figure 3, page 158, CT Scans of Intracranial Hematomas.) The

septum pellucidum, which lies between the 2 lateral ventricles, should be located in the midline. The midline can be determined by drawing a line from the crista galli anteriorly to the inion posteriorly. The degree of displacement of the septum pellucidum away from the side of the hematoma should be noted and the actual degree of shift should be determined by using the scale that is printed on the side of the scan. **A shift of 5 mm or greater is often indicative of the need for surgery to evacuate the blood clot or contusion causing the shift.**

Air ventriculography or cerebral arteriography for select patients with localizing neurologic signs (unilateral dilated pupil or decerebrate posturing) can be done if CT scanning is not available.

In patients whose blood pressure can be normalized, every effort should be made to get a head CT prior to taking the patient to the operating room. Such cases require good clinical judgment and cooperation between the trauma surgeon and the neurosurgeon. (See Table 4, page 163, Initial Management of Severe Brain Injury.)

VIII. MEDICAL THERAPIES FOR BRAIN INJURY

The primary aim of intensive care protocols is to prevent secondary damage to an already injured brain. The basic principle is that if an injured neuron is provided an optimal milieu in which to recover, it can go on to regain normal function. However, if the neuron is provided with a suboptimal or hostile milieu, it can die.

A. Intravenous Fluids

Intravenous fluids should be administered as required to resuscitate the patient and to maintain normovolemia. **Hypovolemia in these patients is harmful.** Care should also be taken **not** to overload the patient with fluids. **Hypotonic fluids should not be used.** Furthermore, the use of glucose-containing fluids can result in hyperglycemia, which has been shown to be harmful to the injured brain. Therefore, it is recommended that **Ringer's lactate** solution or **normal saline** be used for resuscitation. Serum sodium levels need to be very carefully monitored in head-injured patients. Hyponatremia is associated with brain edema and should be prevented.

B. Hyperventilation

In most patients, normocarbia is preferred. Hyperventilation acts by reducing $Paco_2$ and causing cerebral vasoconstriction. Aggressive and prolonged hyperventilation can actually produce cerebral ischemia by causing severe cerebral vasoconstriction and thus impaired cerebral perfusion. This is particularly true if the $Paco_2$ is allowed to fall below 30 mm Hg (4.0 kPa).

Hyperventilation should only be used in moderation and for as limited a period as possible. In general, it is preferable to keep the $Paco_2$ at 35 mm Hg or above. Brief periods of hyperventilation ($Paco_2$ 25 to 30 mm Hg) are acceptable if necessary for acute neurologic deterioration.

C. Mannitol

Mannitol is used to reduce elevated intracranial pressure. The preparation most commonly used is a 20% solution. The most widely accepted regimen is 1 g/kg administered intravenously as a bolus. Large doses of mannitol should not be given to a hypotensive patient because mannitol is a potent osmotic diuretic. A clear indication for the use of mannitol is acute neurologic deterioration, such as the development of a dilated pupil, hemiparesis, or loss of consciousness while the patient is being observed. In this setting, a bolus of mannitol (1 g/kg) should be given rapidly (over 5 minutes) and the patient transported immediately to the CT scanner or directly to the operating room if the causative lesion already has been identified by CT.

D. Furosemide (Lasix®)

This agent may be used in conjunction with mannitol in the treatment of increased ICP. A dose of 0.3 to 0.5 mg/kg of furosemide given intravenously is reasonable. The same concerns that apply to the use of mannitol also apply to the use of furosemide: it should not be used in the hypovolemic patient.

E. Steroids

Studies have not demonstrated any beneficial effect of steroids in controlling increased ICP or improving outcome from severe brain injury. Therefore, steroids are not recommended in the management of acute brain injury.

F. Barbiturates

Barbiturates are effective in reducing intracranial pressure refractory to other measures. They should not be used in the presence of hypotension or hypovolemia. Furthermore, hypotension often results from their use. Therefore, barbiturates are not indicated in the acute resuscitative phase.

G. Anticonvulsants

Posttraumatic epilepsy occurs in about 5% of all patients admitted to the hospital with closed head injuries and in 15% of those with severe head injuries. Three main factors are linked to a high incidence of late epilepsy: (1) seizures occurring within the first week, (2) an intracranial hematoma, or (3) a depressed skull fracture. A double-blind study found that phenytoin reduced the incidence of seizures in the first week of injury, but not thereafter. Phenytoin or fosphenytoin is currently the agent usually employed in the acute phase. For adults the usual loading dose is 1 g given intravenously at a rate no faster than 50 mg/minute. The usual maintenance dose is 100 mg/8 hours, with the dose titrated to achieve therapeutic serum levels. For patients

HEAD TRAUMA

with prolonged seizures diazepam or lorazepam are used in addition to phenytoin until the seizure stops. Control of continuous seizures may require general anesthesia. It is imperative that the seizure be controlled as soon as possible because prolonged seizures (30 to 60 minutes) are likely to cause secondary brain injury.

IX. SURGICAL MANAGEMENT

A. Scalp Wounds

It is important to clean the wound thoroughly before suturing. The most common cause of infected scalp wounds is inadequate cleansing and debridement. Blood loss from scalp wounds can be extensive, especially in children. In the adult patient, bleeding from the scalp alone usually is not the cause of hemorrhagic shock. Scalp hemorrhage usually can be controlled by applying direct pressure and cauterizing or ligating large vessels. Appropriate sutures, clips, or staples can then be applied. Carefully inspect the wound under direct vision for signs of a skull fracture or foreign material. The presence of a CSF leak indicates that there is an associated dural tear. A neurosurgeon should be consulted in all cases with open or depressed skull fractures. Not infrequently, a subgaleal collection of blood can feel like a skull fracture. In such cases, the presence of a fracture can be confirmed or excluded by plain x-rays of the region and/or a CT scan.

B. Depressed Skull Fractures

Generally, a depressed skull fracture needs to be elevated if the degree of depression is greater than the thickness of the adjacent skull. Less significant depressed fractures can safely be managed with closure of the overlying scalp laceration, if present. A CT scan is valuable in identifying the degree of depression, but more importantly to exclude the presence of an intracranial hematoma or contusion.

C. Intracranial Mass Lesions

These lesions typically are evacuated or cared for by a neurosurgeon. If a neurosurgeon is not available in the facility initially receiving the patient with an intracranial mass lesion, early transfer to a hospital with a neurosurgeon is essential. In very exceptional circumstances, a rapidly expanding intracranial hematoma may be imminently life-threatening and may not allow time for transfer if neurosurgical care

is some distance away. Although this circumstance is rare in urban settings, it may occur in rural areas. Under such conditions emergency craniotomy may be considered if a surgeon properly trained in the procedure is available. This procedure may be especially important in a patient whose neurologic status is rapidly deteriorating and does not respond to nonsurgical measures. Emergency craniotomy by a nonneurosurgeon should only be considered in extreme circumstances, and the procedure should be done only with the advice of a neurosurgeon.

The indications for a craniotomy performed by a nonneurosurgeon are few, and widespread use as a desperation maneuver is not recommended or supported by the Committee on Trauma. This procedure is justified only when definitive neurosurgical care is unavailable. The Committee on Trauma strongly recommends that those who anticipate the need for this procedure receive proper training from a neurosurgeon.

X. PROGNOSIS

All patients should be treated aggressively pending consultation with a neurosurgeon. This is particularly true of children, who usually have a remarkable ability to recover from seemingly devastating injuries.

XI. BRAIN DEATH

The diagnosis of "brain death" implies that there is no possibility for recovery of brain function. Most experts agree that the following criteria should be satisfied for the diagnosis of brain death.

1. Glasgow Coma Scale Score = 3
2. Nonreactive pupils
3. Absent brainstem reflexes (eg, oculocephalic, corneal, Doll's eyes, and no gag reflex)
4. No spontaneous ventilatory effort

Ancillary studies used by some in determining the diagnosis of brain death are:

1. EEG: No activity at high gain
2. CBF studies: No CBF (eg, isotope studies, Doppler studies, xenon CBF studies)
3. ICP: Exceeds MAP for 1 or more hours
4. No change in heart rate in response to atropine

Certain reversible conditions can mimic the appearance of brain death, eg, hypothermia or barbiturate coma. Therefore, diagnosis should only be considered after all physiologic parameters are normalized and CNS function is not potentially affected by medications. The remarkable ability of children to recover from seemingly devastating brain injuries should be carefully considered prior to diagnosing brain death in children.

In the United States, federal law requires that local organ procurement agencies be notified about all patients with the diagnosis or impending diagnosis of brain death prior to discontinuing artificial life support measures.

XII. SUMMARY

A. In a comatose patient, secure and maintain the airway by endotracheal intubation.

B. Prevent hypovolemia and hypoxemia. The goal in resuscitating the brain-injured patient is to prevent secondary brain injury.

C. Treat shock aggressively and look for its cause. Resuscitate with Ringer's lactate solution, normal saline, or similar isotonic solutions without dextrose. Do not use hypotonic solutions.

D. Perform a neurologic examination after normalizing the blood pressure and before paralyzing the patient. Search for associated injuries.

E. Contact a neurosurgeon as early as possible. If a neurosurgeon is not available at your facility, transfer all moderately or severely head-injured patients.

F. Frequently reassess the patient's neurologic status.

■ BIBLIOGRAPHY

1. American Association of Neurological Surgeons: **Guidelines for the Management of Severe Head Injury.** 1995.

2. Andrews BT, Chiles BW, Olsen WL, et al: The effect of intracerebral hematoma location on the risk of brainstem compression and on clinical outcome. **Journal of Neurosurgery** 1988; 69: 518-522.

3. Chestnut RM, Marshall LF, Klauber MR, et al: The role of secondary brain injury in determining outcome from severe head injury. **Journal of Trauma** 1993; 34:216-222.

4. Eisenberg HM, Frankowski RF, Contant CR, et al: High-dose barbiturates control elevated intracranial pressure in patients with severe head injury. **Journal of Neurosurgery** 1988; 69:15-23.

5. Giri BK, Krishnappa IK, Bryan RMJ, et al: Regional cerebral blood flow after cortical impact injury complicated by a secondary insult in rats. **Stroke** 2000; 31:961-967.

6. Gopinath SP, Robertson CS, Contant CF, et al: Jugular venous desaturation and outcome after head injury. **Journal of Neurology, Neurosurgery, and Psychiatry** 1994; 57:717-723.

7. Marion DW (ed): **Traumatic Brain Injury**. New York, Thieme, 1999.

8. Marion DW, Carlier PM: Problems with initial Glasgow Coma Scale assessment caused by prehospital treatment of patients with head injuries: Results of a national survey. **Journal of Trauma** 1994; 36(1):89-95.

9. Marion DW, Spiegel TP: Changes in the management of severe traumatic brain injury: 1991-1997. **Critical Care Medicine** 2000; 28:16-18.

10. Muizelaar JP, Marmarou A, Ward JD, et al: Adverse effects of prolonged hyperventilation in patients with severe head injury: A randomized clinical trial. **Journal of Neurosurgery** 1991; 75: 731-739.

11. Narayan RK, Wilberger JE, Povlishock JT (eds): **Neurotrauma.** New York, McGraw-Hill, 1996.

12. Robertson CS, Valadka AB, Hannay HJ, et al: Prevention of secondary ischemic insults after severe head injury. **Critical Care Medicine** 1999; 27:2086-2095.

13. Rosner MJ, Rosner SD, Johnson AH: Cerebral perfusion pressure management protocols and clinical results. **Journal of Neurosurgery** 1995; 83:949-962.

14. Temkin NIZ, et al: A randomized, double-blind study of phenytoin for the prevention of post-traumatic seizures. **New England Journal of Medicine** 1990; 323:497-502.

SKILLS STATION

Head and Neck Trauma Assessment and Management

■ OBJECTIVES:

Upon completion of this station, participants will be able to:

1. Demonstrate assessment and diagnostic skills in determining the type and extent of injuries with Mr. HURT (head trauma manikin).

2. Describe the importance of clinical signs and symptoms of brain trauma found through assessment.

3. Establish priorities for initial primary management of the patient with brain trauma.

4. Identify other diagnostic aids that can be used to determine the area of injury within the brain and the extent of injury.

5. Demonstrate proper helmet removal while protecting the patient's cervical spine.

6. Perform a complete secondary assessment and determine the patient's GCS Score through the use of scenarios and interactive dialogue with the instructor.

7. Determine normal versus abnormal CT scans of the head and identify injury patterns.

INTERACTIVE SKILLS PROCEDURES

Head and Neck Trauma Assessment and Management

Note: Standard precautions are required whenever caring for the trauma patient.

Note: A series of scenarios accompanies some of the skills procedures for this station. The scenarios are provided at the conclusion of the procedures for your review and preparation for this station.

I. PRIMARY SURVEY

A. ABCDEs

B. Immobilize and Stabilize the Cervical Spine

C. Perform a Brief Neurologic Examination

   1. Pupillary response

   2. GCS Score determination

II. SECONDARY SURVEY AND MANAGEMENT

A. Inspect Entire Head, Including Face

   1. Lacerations

   2. Nose and ears for presence of CSF leakage

B. Palpate Entire Head, Including Face

   1. Fractures

   2. Lacerations for underlying fractures

C. Inspect All Scalp Lacerations

   1. Brain tissue

   2. Depressed skull fractures

   3. Debris

   4. CSF leaks

D. Determine GCS Score and Pupillary Response

   1. Eye-opening response

   2. BEST limb motor response

3. Verbal response

4. Pupillary response

E. Examine Cervical Spine

1. Palpate for tenderness/pain and apply a semirigid cervical collar, if needed

2. Obtain a cross-table lateral c-spine x-ray as needed

F. Determine the Extent of Injury

G. Reassess Patient Continuously—Observe for Signs of Deterioration

1. Frequency

2. Parameters to be assessed

3. Remember, reassess ABCDEs

III. EVALUATION OF CT SCANS OF THE HEAD

Diagnosis of abnormalities seen on CT scan of the head can be very subtle and difficult. Because of the inherent complexity in interpreting these scans, early review by a neurosurgeon or radiologist is important. The steps outlined here for evaluating a CT scan of the head provide one approach to assessing for significant pathology that may be life-threatening. **Remember, obtaining a CT scan of the head should not delay resuscitation or transfer of the patient to a trauma center.**

A. Process for Initial Review of CT Scans of the Head

1. Confirm that the images being reviewed are of the correct patient.

2. Ensure that the CT scan of the head was done without intravenous contrast.

3. Use the patient's clinical findings to focus the review of the CT scan, and use the image findings to enhance further physical evaluation.

B. Scalp

Assess the scalp component for contusion or swelling that may indicate the site of external trauma.

C. Skull

Assess for skull fractures.

1. Suture lines (joining of the bones of the cranial vault) may be mistaken for fractures.

2. Depressed skull fractures (thickness of skull) require neurosurgical consultation.

3. Open fractures require neurosurgical consultation. Missile wound tracts may appear as linear areas of low attenuation.

D. Gyri and Sulci

Assess the gyri and sulci for symmetry. If asymmetry exists, consider these diagnoses.

Head and Neck Trauma Assessment and Management   **HEAD TRAUMA**

1. **Acute subdural hematomas**

    a. Typically are areas of increased density covering and compressing the gyri and sulci over the entire hemisphere

    b. Appear within the skull

    c. May cause shift of the underlying ventricles across the midline

    d. Occur more commonly than epidural hematomas

    e. May have associated cerebral contusions and intracerebral hematomas

2. **Acute epidural hematomas**

    a. Typically are lenticular or biconvex areas of increased density

    b. Appear within the skull and compress the underlying gyri and sulci

    c. May cause shift of the underlying ventricles across the midline

    d. Most often are located in the temporal or temporoparietal region

D. Cerebral and Cerebellar Hemispheres

1. Compare both cerebral and cerebellar hemispheres for similar density and symmetry.

2. Intracerebral hematomas appear as large areas of high density.

3. Cerebral contusions appear as punctate areas of high density.

4. Diffuse axonal injury may appear normal or have scattered small areas of cerebral contusion and areas of low density.

E. Ventricles

1. Assess the ventricles for size and symmetry.

2. Significant mass lesions compress and distort the ventricles, especially the lateral ventricles.

3. Significant intracranial hypertension is often associated with decreased ventricular size.

4. Intraventricular hemorrhage appears as regions of increased density (bright spots) in the ventricles.

F. Shifts

Midline shifts may occur from a hematoma or swelling that causes the septum pellucidum, between the 2 lateral ventricles, to shift away from the midline. The midline is a line extending from the crista galli anteriorly to the tent-like projection posteriorly (inion). After measuring the distance from the midline to the septum pellucidum, the actual shift is determined by correcting against the scale on the CT print. A shift of 5 mm or more is considered indicative of a mass lesion and the need for surgical decompression.

G. Maxillofacial

1. Assess the facial bones for fracture-related crepitus.

2. Assess the sinuses and mastoid air cells for air-fluid levels.

3. Facial bone fractures, sinus fractures, and sinus or mastoid air-fluid levels may indicate a basilar skull or cribriform plate fracture.

HEAD TRAUMA   *Head and Neck Trauma Assessment and Management*

H. Four Cs of Increased Density

Remember the 4 areas or Cs of increased density:

   1. Contrast

   2. Clot

   3. Cellularity (tumor)

   4. Calcification (pineal gland, choroid plexus)

IV. HELMET REMOVAL

Patients wearing a helmet who require airway management should have the head and neck held in a neutral position while the helmet is removed using the 2-person procedure. Note: A poster titled "Techniques of Helmet Removal from Injured Patients" is available from the American College of Surgeons (*http://secure.facs.org/ commerce/2004trauma.html*). This poster provides a pictorial and narrative description of helmet removal.

A. One person stabilizes the patient's head and neck by placing 1 hand on either side of the helmet with the fingers on the patient's mandible. This position prevents slippage if the strap is loose.

B. The second person cuts or loosens the helmet strap at the D-rings.

C. The second person then places 1 hand on the mandible at the angle, with the thumb on 1 side and the fingers on the other. The other hand applies pressure from under the head at the occipital region. This maneuver transfers the responsibility of inline immobilization to the second person.

D. The first person then expands the helmet laterally to clear the ears and carefully removes the helmet. If the helmet has a face cover, this device must be removed first. If the helmet provides full facial coverage, the patient's nose will impede helmet removal. To clear the nose, the helmet must be tilted backward and raised over the patient's nose.

E. Through this process, the second person must maintain inline immobilization from below to prevent head tilt.

F. After the helmet is removed, inline manual immobilization is reestablished from above and the patient's head and neck are secured during airway management.

G. If attempts to remove the helmet result in pain and paresthesia, the helmet should be removed with a cast cutter. If there is evidence of a c-spine injury on the x-rays, the helmet also should be removed utilizing a cast cutter. The head and neck must be stabilized during this procedure, which is accomplished by dividing the helmet in the coronal plane through the ears. The outer rigid layer is removed easily, and the inside Styrofoam® layer is then incised and removed anteriorly. Maintaining neutral alignment of the head and neck, the posterior portions are removed.

V. SCENARIOS

A. Scenario #1

A 17-year-old high-school football player, involved in a crushing tackle with a brief loss of consciousness, complains of neck pain and paresthesia in his left arm. He is immobilized on a long spine board with his helmet in place and transported to the emergency department. He is not in respiratory distress, talks coherently, and is awake and alert.

Head and Neck Trauma Assessment and Management **HEAD TRAUMA**

B. Scenario #2

A 25-year-old man is transported to the emergency department after a car crash while driving home from a tavern. His airway is clear, he is breathing spontaneously without difficulty, and he is hemodynamically normal. He has a scalp contusion over the left side of his head. There is a strong odor of alcohol on his breath, but he is able to answer questions appropriately. His eyes are open, but he appears confused and pushes away the examiner's hands when examined for response to pain. He is thought to have suffered a concussion and have alcohol intoxication. He is kept in the emergency department for observation.

One hour later, the patient is more somnolent, briefly opens his eyes to painful stimuli, and demonstrates an abnormal flexion response on the right and withdrawal on the left to painful stimuli. His left pupil is now 2 mm larger than his right pupil. Both pupils react sluggishly to light. His verbal response consists of incomprehensible sounds.

C. Scenario #3

A 21-year-old man was thrown from and then kicked in the face by a horse. He was initially unconscious for at least 5 minutes. He now opens his eyes to speech, moves only to painful stimuli by withdrawing his extremities, and utters inappropriate words. His blood pressure is 180/80 mm Hg and heart rate is 64 beats/minute.

D. Scenario #4

A 40-year-old motorcyclist is brought to the emergency department with obvious, isolated head trauma. The prehospital personnel report that he has unequal pupils and responds only to painful stimuli by abnormally flexing his arms, opening his eyes, and speaking incomprehensibly. When not stimulated, his respirations are very sonorous.

SEVEN

CHAPTER

7

Spine and Spinal Cord Trauma

◼ OBJECTIVES:

Upon completion of this topic, the participant will be able to demonstrate the techniques of assessment and explain the emergency management of spine and spinal cord trauma.

Specifically, the student will be able to:

A. Describe the basic spinal anatomy and physiology.

B. Evaluate a patient with suspected spinal injury.

C. Identify the common types of spinal injuries and their x-ray features.

D. Appropriately manage the spinal-injured patient during the first hour from injury.

E. Determine the appropriate disposition of the patient with spine trauma.

SPINE AND SPINAL CORD TRAUMA

I. INTRODUCTION

Vertebral column injury, with or without neurologic deficits, must always be considered in a patient with multiple injuries. Approximately 5% of brain-injured patients have an associated spinal injury, while 25% of spinal injury patients have at least a mild brain injury. Approximately 55% of spinal injuries occur in the cervical region, 15% in the thoracic region, 15% at the thoracolumbar junction, and 15% in the lumbosacral area. **Approximately 10% of patients with a c-spine fracture have a second, noncontiguous vertebral column fracture.**

The doctor and medical personnel taking care of such patients must be constantly aware that excessive manipulation and inadequate immobilization of a patient with a spinal injury can cause additional neurologic damage and worsen the patient's outcome. At least 5% of patients experience the onset of neurologic symptoms, or worsening of preexisting ones, after reaching the emergency department. This is usually due to ischemia or progression of spinal cord edema, but may also be the result of failure to provide adequate immobilization. **As long as the patient's spine is protected, evaluation of the spine and exclusion of spine injury may be safely deferred, especially in the presence of systemic instability,** eg, hypotension and respiratory inadequacy.

Excluding the presence of a spinal injury is far simpler in a patient who is awake and alert. In a neurologically normal patient, the absence of pain or tenderness along the spine virtually excludes the presence of a significant spinal injury. However, in a patient who is comatose or has a depressed level of consciousness, the process is not as simple, and it is incumbent on the treating doctor to obtain the appropriate x-rays to exclude a spinal injury. If the x-rays are inconclusive, the patient's spine should remain protected until further testing can be performed. While the dangers of inadequate immobilization have been fairly well documented, there also is some danger in prolonged immobilization of a patient on a hard surface such as a backboard. Apart from causing severe discomfort in an awake patient, prolonged immobilization can lead to the formation of serious decubitus ulcers in patients with spinal cord injuries. Therefore, the long backboard should be used only as a patient transportation device, and every effort should be made to have the patient evaluated by the appropriate specialists and removed from the spine board as quickly as possible. If this is not feasible within 2 hours, the patient should be removed from the spine board and be logrolled every 2 hours, while maintaining the integrity of the spine, to reduce the risk of decubitus ulcer formation.

II. ANATOMY AND PHYSIOLOGY

A. Spinal Column

The spinal column consists of 7 cervical, 12 thoracic, and 5 lumbar vertebrae as well as the sacrum and the coccyx. The typical vertebra consists of the anteriorly placed vertebral body, which forms the main weight-bearing column. The vertebral bodies are separated by intervertebral discs and are held together anteriorly and posteriorly by the anterior and posterior longitudinal ligaments, respectively. Posterolaterally, 2 pedicles form the pillars on which the roof of the vertebral canal (ie, the lamina) rests. The facet joints, interspinous ligaments, and paraspinal muscles all contribute to the stability of the spine.

For many reasons, the cervical spine is most vulnerable to injury. The cervical canal is wide in the upper cervical region, ie, from the foramen magnum to the lower part of C2. The majority of patients with injuries at this level who survive are neurologically intact on arrival at the hospital. However, approximately one-third of patients with upper c-spine injuries die at the injury scene from apnea caused by loss of central innervation of the phrenic nerves due to spinal cord injury at C1. Below the level of C3 the diameter of the spinal canal is much smaller relative to the diameter of the spinal cord, and vertebral column injuries are much more likely to cause spinal cord injuries.

The mobility of the thoracic spine is much more restricted. This part of the spine also has additional support from the rib cage. Hence, the incidence of thoracic fractures is much lower, with most thoracic spine fractures being wedge compression fractures not associated with spinal cord injury. However, when a fracture-dislocation in the thoracic spine does occur, it almost always results in a complete neurologic deficit because of the relatively narrow dimension of the thoracic canal. The thoracolumbar junction is a fulcrum between the inflexible thoracic region and the stronger lumbar levels. This makes it more vulnerable to injury, and 15% of all spinal injuries occur in this region.

B. Spinal Cord Anatomy

The spinal cord originates at the caudal end of the medulla oblongata at the foramen magnum. In the adult, it usually ends around the L1 bony level as the conus medullaris. Below this level is the cauda equina, which is somewhat more resilient to injury. Of the many tracts in the spinal cord, only 3 can be readily assessed clinically: (1) the corticospinal tract, (2) the spinothalamic tract, and (3) the posterior columns. Each is a paired tract that may be injured on 1 or both sides of the cord. The corticospinal tract, which lies in the posterolateral segment of the cord, controls motor power on the same side of the body and is tested by voluntary muscle contractions or involuntary response to painful stimuli. The spinothalamic tract, in the anterolateral aspect of the cord, transmits pain and temperature sensation from the opposite side of the body. Generally, it is tested by pinprick and light touch. The posterior columns carry position sense (proprioception), vibration sense, and some light-touch sensation from the same side of the body, and these columns are tested by position sense in the toes and fingers or by vibration sense using a tuning fork.

If there is no demonstrable sensory or motor function below a certain level, this is referred to as a **complete spinal cord injury.** During the first few days after injury, this diagnosis cannot be made with certainty, because of the possibility of spinal shock. (See Chapter 3, Shock, page 69, and II. E., Neurogenic Shock Versus Spinal Shock, page 181.) If any motor or sensory function remains, this is an **incomplete injury** and the prognosis for recovery is significantly better. Sparing of sensation in the perianal region (sacral sparing) may be the only sign of residual function. **Sacral sparing** may be demonstrated by preservation of some sensory perception in the perianal region and/or voluntary contraction of the rectal sphincter.

C. Sensory Examination

A dermatome is the area of skin innervated by the sensory axons within a particular segmental nerve root. Knowledge of some of the major dermatome levels is invaluable in determining the level of injury and in assessing neurologic improvement or deterioration. The sensory level is the lowest dermatome with normal sensory function and can often differ on the 2 sides of the body. For practical purposes, the upper cervical dermatomes (C1 to C4) are somewhat variable in their cutaneous distribution and are not commonly used for localization. However, it should be remembered that the supraclavicular nerves (C2 through C4) provide sensory innervation to the region overlying the pectoralis muscle (cervical cape). The presence of sensation in this region may confuse the examiner when trying to determine the sensory level in patients with lower cervical injuries. The key sensory points are (also, see Figure 1, page 180, Key Sensory Points):

1. C5 — Area over the deltoid
2. C6 — Thumb
3. C7 — Middle finger
4. C8 — Little finger
5. T4 — Nipple
6. T8 — Xiphisternum
7. T10 — Umbilicus
8. T12 — Symphysis pubis
9. L4 — Medial aspect of the calf
10. L5 — Web space between the first and second toes
11. S1 — Lateral border of the foot
12. S3 — Ischial tuberosity area
13. S4 and S5 — Perianal region

D. Myotomes

Each segmental nerve (root) innervates more than 1 muscle and most muscles are innervated by more than 1 root (usually 2). Nevertheless, for the sake of simplicity, certain muscles or muscle groups are identified as representing a single spinal nerve segment. The important key muscle(s) are:

1. C5 — Deltoid
2. C6 — Wrist extensors (biceps, extensor carpi radialis longus and brevis)
3. C7 — Elbow extensors (triceps)
4. C8 — Finger flexors to the middle finger (flexor digitorum profundus)
5. T1 — Small finger abductors (abductor digiti minimi)
6. L2 — Hip flexors (iliopsoas)
7. L3,4 — Knee extensors (quadriceps, patellar reflexes)
8. L4,5 to S1 — Knee flexion (hamstrings)
9. L5 — Ankle and big toe dorsiflexors (tibialis anterior and extensor hallucis longus)

SPINE AND SPINAL CORD TRAUMA

10. S1—Ankle plantar flexors (gastrocnemius, soleus)

In addition to bilateral testing of these muscles, the external anal sphincter should be tested by digital examination. Each muscle is graded on a 6-point scale. (See Table 1, page 181, Muscle Strength Grading.) Documentation of the power in key muscle groups helps to assess neurologic improvement or deterioration on subsequent examinations.

FIGURE 1
Key Sensory Points

• Key Sensory Points

Reprinted with permission from the American Spinal Injury Association, *International Standards for Neurological and Functional Classification of Spinal Cord Injury*, Chicago, IL, revised 2000.

E. Neurogenic Shock Versus Spinal Shock

Neurogenic shock results from impairment of the descending sympathetic pathways in the spinal cord. This condition results in loss of vasomotor tone and loss of sympathetic innervation to the heart. The former causes vasodilatation of visceral and lower extremity blood vessels, pooling of blood, and, consequently, hypotension. As a result of loss of cardiac sympathetic tone, the patient may become bradycardic or at least fail to become tachycardic in response to hypovolemia. In this condition the blood pressure may not be restored by fluid infusion alone, and massive fluid resuscitation may result in fluid overload and pulmonary edema. The blood pressure can often be restored by the judicious use of vasopressors after moderate volume replacement. Atropine may be used to counteract hemodynamically significant bradycardia.

Spinal shock refers to the flaccidity and loss of reflexes seen after spinal cord injury. The "shock" to the injured cord may make it appear completely functionless, although all areas are not necessarily destroyed. The duration of this state is variable.

F. Effect on Other Organ Systems

Hypoventilation due to paralysis of the intercostal muscles can result from an injury involving the lower cervical or upper thoracic spinal cord. If the upper or middle cervical cord is injured, the diaphragm also is paralyzed due to involvement of the C3 to C5 segments, which innervate the diaphragm via the phrenic nerve. **The inability to perceive pain may mask a potentially serious injury elsewhere in the body, such as the usual signs of an acute abdomen.**

III. CLASSIFICATIONS OF SPINAL CORD INJURIES

Spinal cord injuries can be classified according to (1) level, (2) severity of neurologic deficit, (3) spinal cord syndrome, and (4) morphology.

A. Level

The neurologic level is the most caudal segment of the spinal cord with normal sensory and motor function on both sides of the body. When the term "sensory level" is used, it refers to the most caudal segment of the spinal cord with normal sensory function. The motor level is defined similarly with respect to motor function as the lowest key muscle that has a grade of at least 3/5. (See Table 1, Muscle Strength Grading.) In complete injuries, when some impaired sensory and/or motor function is found just below the lowest normal segment, this is referred to as the zone of partial preservation. As described previously, the determination of the level of injury on both sides is important.

Table 1—Muscle Strength Grading

SCORE	RESULTS OF EXAMINATION
0	Total paralysis
1	Palpable or visible contraction
2	Full range of motion with gravity eliminated
3	Full range of motion against gravity
4	Full range of motion, but less than normal strength
5	Normal strength
NT	Not testable

Adapted with permission from the American Spinal Injury Association, *Standards for Neurological and Functional Classification of Spinal Cord Injury*, Atlanta, GA, revised 1992, p 13.

SPINE AND SPINAL CORD TRAUMA

A broad distinction can be made between lesions above and below T1. Injuries of the first 8 cervical segments of the spinal cord result in quadriplegia and lesions below the T1 level result in paraplegia. The bony level of injury is the vertebra at which the bones are damaged, causing injury to the spinal cord. The neurologic level of injury is determined primarily by clinical examination. Frequently, there is a discrepancy between the bony and the neurologic levels because the spinal nerves enter the spinal canal through the foramina and ascend or descend inside the spinal canal before actually entering the spinal cord. This discrepancy becomes more pronounced the farther caudal the injury. Apart from the initial management to stabilize the bony injury, all subsequent descriptions of the level of injury are based on the neurologic level.

B. Severity of the Neurologic Deficit

Spinal cord injury can be categorized as incomplete paraplegia, complete paraplegia, incomplete quadriplegia, and complete quadriplegia. It is important to assess for any sign of preserved long-tract function of the spinal cord. Any motor or sensory function below the level of the injury constitutes an incomplete injury. Signs of an incomplete injury may include:

1. Any sensation (including position sense) or voluntary movement in the lower extremities.

2. Sacral sparing, ie, perianal sensation, voluntary anal sphincter contraction, or voluntary toe flexion. (Sacral reflexes, such as the bulbocavernosus reflex or anal wink, do not qualify as sacral sparing.)

C. Spinal Cord Syndromes

Certain characteristic patterns of neurologic injury are frequently seen in a spinal cord-injured patient. These patterns should be recognized, since they may otherwise confuse the examiner.

Central cord syndrome is characterized by a disproportionately greater loss of motor power in the upper extremities than in the lower extremities, with varying degrees of sensory loss. Usually, it is seen after a hyperextension injury in a patient with preexisting cervical canal stenosis (often due to degenerative osteoarthritic changes). The history is commonly that of a forward fall resulting in a facial impact. It may occur with or without cervical spine

fracture or dislocation. Recovery usually follows a characteristic pattern, with the lower extremities recovering strength first, bladder function next, and the proximal upper extremities and hands last. The prognosis for recovery in central cord injuries is somewhat better than with other incomplete injuries. The central cord syndrome is thought to be due to vascular compromise of the cord in the distribution of the anterior spinal artery. This artery supplies the central portions of the cord. Because the motor fibers to the cervical segments are topographically arranged toward the center of the cord, the arms and hands are most severely affected.

Anterior cord syndrome is characterized by paraplegia and a dissociated sensory loss with loss of pain and temperature sensation. Posterior column function (position, vibration, and deep pressure sense) is preserved. Usually, anterior cord syndrome is due to infarction of the cord in the territory supplied by the anterior spinal artery. This syndrome has the poorest prognosis of the incomplete injuries.

Brown-Séquard's syndrome results from hemisection of the cord and is rarely seen. Nevertheless, variations on the classic picture are not uncommon. In its pure form, the syndrome consists of ipsilateral motor loss (corticospinal tract) and loss of position sense (posterior column) associated with contralateral loss of pain and temperature sensation beginning 1 to 2 levels below the level of injury (spinothalamic tract). Even if the syndrome is caused by a direct penetrating injury to the cord, some recovery is usually seen.

D. Morphology

Spinal injuries can be described as fractures, fracture dislocations, spinal cord injury without radiographic abnormalities (SCIWORA), or penetrating injuries. Each of these categories can be further described as stable or unstable. However, determining the stability of a particular type of injury is not always simple and, indeed, even experts may disagree. **Hence, especially in the initial management of the patient, all patients with radiographic evidence of injury and all those with neurologic deficits should be considered to have an unstable spinal injury.** These patients should be immobilized until consultation with an appropriately qualified doctor, usually a neurosurgeon or orthopaedic surgeon.

IV. SPECIFIC TYPES OF SPINAL INJURIES

Cervical spine injuries can result from 1 or a combination of these mechanisms of injury: (1) axial loading, (2) flexion, (3) extension, (4) rotation, (5) lateral bending, and (6) distraction. The injuries identified herein involve the spinal column. They are listed in anatomic sequence (not in order of frequency), progressing from the cranial to the caudal end of the spine.

A. Atlanto-occipital Dislocation

Craniocervical disruption injuries are uncommon and result from severe traumatic flexion and distraction. Most of these patients die of brainstem destruction and apnea, or are profoundly neurologically impaired (ventilator dependent and quadriplegic). An occasional patient may survive if prompt resuscitation is available at the injury scene. This injury may be identified in up to 19% of patients with fatal cervical spine injuries and is a common cause of death in cases of shaken baby syndrome where the infant dies immediately after shaking. Cervical traction is not used in patients with craniocervical dislocation. Spinal immobilization is recommended initially.

B. Atlas Fracture (C1)

The atlas is a thin bony ring with broad articular surfaces. Fractures of the atlas represent approximately 5% of acute c-spine fractures. Approximately 40% of atlas fractures are associated with fractures of the axis (C2). The most common C1 fracture is a burst fracture (Jefferson fracture). The usual mechanism of injury is **axial loading**, such as when a large load falls vertically on the head, or in a fall where the patient lands on the top of the head in a relatively neutral position. The Jefferson fracture consists of disruption of both the anterior and posterior rings of C1 with lateral displacement of the lateral masses. The fracture is best seen on an open-mouth view of the C1 to C2 region and axial CT scans. In patients that survive, these fractures usually are not associated with spinal cord injuries. However, they are unstable and should be initially treated with a cervical collar. Unilateral ring or lateral mass fractures are not uncommon and tend to be stable injuries. However, they should be treated as unstable until seen by an appropriately qualified doctor, usually a neurosurgeon or orthopaedic surgeon.

C. C1 Rotary Subluxation

This injury is most often seen in children. It may occur spontaneously, after major or minor trauma, an upper respiratory infection, or with rheumatoid arthritis. The patient appears with a persistent rotation of the head (torticollis). The injury is again best diagnosed with an open-mouth odontoid view, although the x-ray findings may be confusing. In this injury, the odontoid is not equidistant from the 2 lateral masses of C1. The patient should not be forced to overcome the rotation, but should be immobilized and referred for further specialized treatment.

D. Axis (C2) Fractures

The axis is the largest cervical vertebra and is the most unusual in shape. Therefore, it is susceptible to various fractures depending on the force and direction of the impact. Acute fractures of C2 represent approximately 18% of all c-spine injuries.

1. Odontoid fractures

Approximately 60% of C2 fractures involve the odontoid process, a peg-shaped bony protuberance that projects upward and is normally positioned in contact with the anterior arch of C1. The odontoid process is held in place primarily by the transverse ligament. Odontoid fractures are initially identified by a lateral c-spine film or on open-mouth odontoid views. However, a CT scan usually is required for further delineation. Type I odontoid fractures typically involve the tip of the odontoid and are relatively uncommon. Type II odontoid fractures occur through the base of the dens and are the most common odontoid fracture. In children younger than 6 years of age, the epiphysis may be prominent and may look like a fracture at this level. Type III odontoid fractures occur at the base of the dens and extend obliquely into the body of the axis.

2. Posterior element fractures of C2

A hangman's fracture involves the posterior elements of C2, ie, the pars interarticularis. These fractures represent approximately 20% of all axis fractures and usually are due to an extension type of injury. Patients with this fracture should be maintained in external immobilization until specialized care is available.

SPINE AND SPINAL CORD TRAUMA

Variations of a hangman's fracture include bilateral fractures through the lateral masses or pedicles. Approximately 20% of all axis fractures are nonodontoid, nonhangman's fractures. These include fractures through the body, pedicle, lateral mass, laminae, and spinous process.

E. Fractures and Dislocations (C3 through C7)

A fracture of C3 is very uncommon, possibly because it is positioned between the more vulnerable axis and the more mobile "relative fulcrum" of the c-spine, ie, C5 and C6, where the greatest flexion and extension of the c-spine occurs. In adults, the most common level of cervical vertebral fracture is C5 and the most common level of subluxation is C5 on C6. The most common injury patterns identified at these levels are vertebral body fractures with or without subluxation, subluxation of the articular processes (including unilateral or bilateral locked facets), and fractures of the laminae, spinous processes, pedicles, or lateral masses. Rarely, ligamentous disruption occurs without fractures or facet dislocations. The incidence of neurologic injury increases dramatically with facet dislocations. In the presence of unilateral facet dislocation, 80% of patients have a neurologic injury (approximately 30% root injuries only, 40% incomplete spinal cord injuries, and 30% complete spinal cord injuries). In the presence of bilateral locked facets, the morbidity is much worse, with 16% incomplete and 84% complete spinal cord injuries.

F. Thoracic Spine Fractures (T1 through T10)

Thoracic spinal fractures may be classified into 4 broad categories: (1) anterior wedge compression injuries, (2) burst injuries, (3) Chance fractures, and (4) fracture-dislocations. (Also see Chance fractures in G., Thoracolumbar Junction Fractures.)

Axial loading with flexion produces an **anterior wedge compression** injury. The amount of wedging usually is quite small and the anterior portion of the vertebral body rarely is more than 25% shorter than the posterior body. Because of the rigidity of the rib cage, most of these fractures are stable. The second type of thoracic fracture is the **burst injury** caused by vertical-axial compression. **Chance fractures** are transverse fractures through the vertebral body. They are caused by flexion about an axis anterior to the vertebral column and are most frequently seen following motor vehicle crashes in which the patient was restrained only by a lap belt. Chance fractures

may be associated with retroperitoneal and abdominal visceral injuries. **Fracture-dislocations** are relatively uncommon in the thoracic and lumbar spine because of the orientation of the facet joints. These injuries almost always are due to extreme flexion or severe blunt trauma to the spine which causes disruption of the posterior elements (pedicles, facets, lamina) of the vertebra. The thoracic spinal canal is narrow in relation to the spinal cord, so fracture subluxations in the thoracic spine commonly result in complete neurologic deficits.

Simple compression fractures are usually stable and often treated with a rigid brace. Burst fractures, Chance fractures, and fracture-dislocations are extremely unstable and almost always require internal fixation.

G. Thoracolumbar Junction Fractures (T11 through L1)

Fractures at this level are due to the relative immobility of the thoracic spine compared with the lumbar spine. They most often result from a combination of acute hyperflexion and rotation, and, consequently, they are usually unstable. Patients who fall from a height and restrained drivers who sustain severe flexion energy transfer are at particular risk for this type of injury.

The spinal cord terminates as the conus medullaris at approximately the level of L1, and injury to this part of the cord commonly results in bladder and bowel dysfunction, as well as decreased sensation and strength in the lower extremities. Patients with thoracolumbar fractures are particularly vulnerable to rotational movement. Therefore, modified logrolling should be performed with extreme care.

H. Lumbar Fractures

The radiographic signs associated with a lumbar fracture are similar to those of thoracic and thoracolumbar fractures. However, because only the cauda equina is involved, the probability of a complete neurologic deficit is much less in these injuries.

I. Penetrating Injuries

The most common types of penetrating injuries are those caused by gunshot wounds or stabbings. It is important to determine the path of the bullet or knife. This can be done by combining information from the history, clinical examination (entry and exit sites), plain x-rays, and CT scans. If the path of injury passes directly through the vertebral canal, a complete neurologic deficit usually results. Complete deficits also can result from energy transfer associated with a high velocity missile (ie, bullet) passing close to the spinal cord rather than through it. Penetrating injuries of the spine usually are stable injuries unless the missile destroys a large portion of the vertebra.

V. X-RAY EVALUATION

A. Cervical Spine

Cervical spine radiographs are indicated for all trauma patients who have midline neck pain, palpation tenderness, neurologic deficits referable to the cervical spine, an altered level of consciousness, or who are suspected of being intoxicated. Lateral AP and open-mouth odontoid views should be obtained.

On the lateral view, the base of the skull, all 7 cervical vertebrae, and the first thoracic vertebra must be visualized. The patient's shoulders may have to be pulled down when obtaining the lateral c-spine x-ray to avoid missing fractures or fracture dislocations in the lower c-spine. If all 7 cervical vertebrae are not visualized with the lateral x-ray, a swimmer's view of the lower cervical and upper thoracic area should be obtained.

The open-mouth odontoid view should include the entire odontoid process and the right and left C1, C2 articulations. The AP view of the c-spine assists in the identification of a unilateral facet dislocation in instances where there is little or no dislocation identified on the lateral film. Axial CT scans at 3-mm intervals also should be obtained through suspicious areas identified on the plain films or through the lower cervical spine if it is not adequately visualized on the plain films. Axial CT images through C1 and C2 may also be more sensitive than plain films for detection of fractures of these vertebrae. If these films are of good quality and are properly interpreted, unstable cervical spine injuries will be detected with a sensitivity of greater than 97%. **The complete series of cervical spine radiographs must be reviewed by a doctor experienced in the proper interpretation of these films before they are considered normal and the cervical collar is removed.**

If the screening radiographs described previously are normal, **flexion-extension x-rays of the c-spine** may be obtained in injured patients without an al-

tered level of consciousness, or those who complain of neck pain, to detect occult instability or to determine the stability of a known fracture, eg, a laminar or compression fracture. It is possible for patients to have a purely ligamentous spine injury that results in instability without any associated fracture, although recent studies suggest that if plain 3-view cervical spine radiographs with CT supplementation are truly normal (eg, no anterior soft-tissue swelling, no abnormal angulation), significant instability is unlikely. In some patients with significant soft-tissue injury, paraspinal muscle spasm may severely limit the degree of flexion and extension that the patient allows. In such cases, the patient is treated with a semirigid cervical collar for 2 to 3 weeks before another attempt is made to obtain flexion-extension views. Under no circumstances should the patient's neck be forced into a position that elicits pain. All movements should be voluntary. These films should be obtained under the direct supervision and control of a doctor experienced in the interpretation of such films. **Approximately 10% of patients with a c-spine fracture have a second noncontiguous vertebral column fracture.** This warrants a complete radiographic screening of the entire spine in patients with a c-spine fracture. Such screening also is advisable in all comatose trauma patients.

In the presence of neurologic deficits, magnetic resonance imaging (MRI) is recommended to detect any soft-tissue compressive lesion such as a spinal epidural hematoma or traumatic herniated disc, which cannot be detected with plain films. MRI will also detect spinal cord contusions or disruption, and paraspinal ligamentous and soft tissue injury. However, MRI is frequently not feasible in a hemodynamically abnormal patient. When MRI is not available or appropriate, CT myelography may be used to exclude the presence of acute spinal cord compression caused by a traumatic herniated disc or epidural hematoma. These specialized studies usually are performed at the discretion of a spine surgery consultant. Guidelines for screening trauma patients for c-spine injury are included in Table 2, page 186, Guidelines for Screening Patients with Suspected C-spine Injury, and may serve as a model for the development of hospital policies.

B. Thoracic and Lumbar Spine

The indications for thoracic and lumbar screening radiographs are the same as those for the cervical spine. AP and lateral plain radiographs with axial CT scans at 3-mm intervals through suspicious areas

SPINE AND SPINAL CORD TRAUMA

Table 2—Guidelines for Screening Patients with Suspected C-spine Injury

1. **The presence of paraplegia or quadriplegia is presumptive evidence of spinal instability.**

2. **Patients who are awake, alert, sober, and neurologically normal, and have no neck pain or midline tenderness:** These patients are extremely unlikely to have an acute c-spine fracture or instability. With the patient in a supine position, remove the c-collar and palpate the spine. If there is no significant tenderness, ask the patient to voluntarily move his or her neck from side to side. **Never force the patient's neck.** When performed voluntarily by the patient, these maneuvers are generally safe. If there is no pain, have the patient voluntarily flex and extend his or her neck. Again, if there is no pain, c-spine films are not necessary.

3. **Patients who are awake and alert, neurologically normal, cooperative, and able to concentrate on their spine but do have neck pain or midline tenderness:** The burden of proof is on the doctor to exclude a spinal injury. All such patients should undergo lateral, AP, and open-mouth odontoid x-rays of the c-spine with axial CT images of suspicious areas or of the lower cervical spine if not adequately visualized on the plain films. **Assess the c-spine films for** (a) bony deformity, (b) fracture of the vertebral body or processes, (c) loss of alignment of the posterior aspect of the vertebral bodies (anterior extent of the vertebral canal), (d) increased distance between the spinous processes at 1 level, (e) narrowing of the vertebral canal, and (f) increased prevertebral soft-tissue space. If these films are normal, remove the c-collar. Under the care of a knowledgeable doctor, obtain flexion and extension, lateral cervical spine films with the patient voluntarily flexing and extending his/her neck. If the films show no subluxation, the patient's c-spine can be cleared and the c-collar removed. However, if any of these films are suspicious or unclear, replace the collar and obtain consultation from a spine specialist.

4. **Patients who have an altered level of consciousness or are too young to describe their symptoms:** Lateral, AP, and open-mouth odontoid films with CT supplementation through suspicious areas (eg, C1 and C2, and through the lower cervical spine if areas are not adequately visualized on the plain films) should be obtained on all such patients. In children, CT supplementation is optional. If the entire c-spine can be visualized and is found to be normal, the collar can be removed after appropriate evaluation by a doctor/consultant skilled in the evaluation/management of spine-injured patients. Clearance of the c-spine is particularly important if the pulmonary or other care of the patient is compromised by inability to mobilize the patient.

5. **When in doubt, leave the collar on.**

6. **Consult:** Doctors who are skilled in the evaluation and management of the spine-injured patient should be consulted in all cases where a spine injury is detected or suspected.

7. **Backboards:** Patients who have neurologic deficits (quadriplegia or paraplegia) should be evaluated quickly and taken off the backboard as soon as possible. **A paralyzed patient who is allowed to lie on a hard board for more than 2 hours is at high risk for developing serious decubiti.**

8. **Emergency situations:** Trauma patients who require emergent surgery before a complete work-up of the spine can be accomplished should be transported and moved carefully with the assumption that an unstable spine injury is present. The c-collar should be left on and the patient logrolled when moved to and from the operating table. The patient should not be left on a rigid backboard during surgery. The surgical team should take particular care to protect the neck as much as possible during the operation. The anesthesiologist should be informed of the status of the work-up.

will detect more than 99% of unstable injuries. On the AP views, the vertical alignment of the pedicles and distance between pedicles of each thoracic and lumbar vertebra should be observed. Unstable fractures commonly cause widening of the interpedicular distance. The lateral films detect subluxations, compression fractures, and Chance fractures. CT scanning is particularly useful for detecting fractures of the posterior elements (pedicles, lamina, and spinous processes) and for determining the degree of canal compromise caused by burst fractures. Sagittal reconstructions of axial CT images or plain tomography may be needed to adequately characterize Chance fractures. **As with the cervical spine, a complete series of good quality radiographs must be properly interpreted as normal by an experienced doctor before spine precautions are discontinued.**

VI. GENERAL MANAGEMENT

A. Immobilization

Prehospital care personnel usually immobilize patients before their transport to the emergency department. Any patient with a suspected spine injury should be immobilized above and below the suspected injury site until a fracture is excluded by x-rays. **Remember,** spinal protection should be maintained until a c-spine injury is excluded. Proper immobilization is achieved with the patient in the neutral position, ie, supine without rotating or bending the spinal column. No effort should be made to reduce an obvious deformity. Children may have torticollis, and the elderly may have severe degenerative spine disease that cause them to have a nontraumatic kyphotic or angulation deformity of their spine. Such patients should be immobilized on a backboard in a position of comfort. Supplemental padding is often necessary. **Attempts to align the spine for the purpose of immobilization on the backboard are not recommended if they cause pain.**

Immobilization of the neck with a semirigid collar does not assure complete stabilization of the c-spine. Immobilization using a spine board with appropriate bolstering devices is more effective in limiting certain neck motions. The use of long spine boards is recommended. **Cervical spine injury requires continuous immobilization of the entire patient with a semirigid cervical collar, head immobilization, backboard, tape, and straps before and during transfer to a definitive-care facility.** Extension

or flexion of the neck should be avoided. The airway is of critical importance in spinal cord-injured patients, and early intubation should be accomplished if there is evidence of respiratory compromise. During intubation, the neck must be maintained in a neutral position.

Of special concern is the maintenance of adequate immobilization of the restless, agitated, or violent patient. This condition may be due to pain, confusion associated with hypoxia or hypotension, alcohol or drugs, or simply a personality disorder. The doctor should search for and correct the cause, if possible. If necessary, a sedative or paralytic agent may be administered, keeping in mind the need for adequate airway protection, control, and ventilation. The use of sedatives or paralytic agents in this setting requires considerable clinical judgment, skill, and experience. The use of short-acting, reversible agents is advised.

Once the patient arrives at the emergency department, every effort should be made to get the patient off the rigid spine board as early as possible to reduce the risk of decubitus ulcer formation. Removal of the board is often done as part of the secondary survey when the patient is logrolled for inspection and palpation of the back. It should not be delayed solely for the purpose of obtaining definitive spine radiographs, particularly if radiographic evaluation may not be completed for several hours.

The safe movement, or logrolling, of a patient with an unstable or potentially unstable spine, requires preplanning and the assistance of 4 or more individuals, depending on the size of the patient. Neutral anatomic alignment of the entire vertebral column must be maintained while rolling or lifting the patient. One person is assigned to maintain inline immobilization of the head and neck. Individuals positioned on the same side of the patient's torso manually prevent segmental rotation, flexion, extension, lateral bending, or sagging of the chest or abdomen during transfer of the patient. A fourth person is responsible for moving the legs and removing the spine board and examining the patient's back.

B. Intravenous Fluids

In the patient suspected of having a spine injury, intravenous fluids are administered as they would usually be for resuscitation of the trauma patient. If active hemorrhage is not detected or suspected, persistent hypotension despite 2 liters or more of

SPINE AND SPINAL CORD TRAUMA

Table 3—Guidelines for Screening Patients with Suspected Thoracolumbar Spine Injuries

1. **The presence of paraplegia or a level of sensory loss on the chest or abdomen is presumptive evidence of spinal instability.**

2. **Patients who are awake, alert, sober, neurologically normal, and have no midline thoracic or lumbar back pain or tenderness:** The entire extent of the spine should be palpated and inspected. If there is no palpation tenderness or ecchymosis over the spinous processes, an unstable spine fracture is unlikely and thoracolumbar radiographs may not be necessary.

3. **Patients who have spine pain or palpation tenderness, neurologic deficits, an altered level of consciousness, or are suspected of being intoxicated:** AP and lateral radiographs should be obtained of the entire thoracic and lumbar spine. Axial CT images at 3-mm intervals should be obtained through suspicious areas identified on the plain films. **All images must be of good quality and interpreted as normal by an experienced doctor before discontinuing spine precautions.**

4. **Consult** a doctor skilled in the evaluation and management of spine injuries if a spine injury is detected or suspected.

fluid replacement should raise the suspicion of neurogenic shock. Patients with hypovolemic shock are usually tachycardic, while those with neurogenic shock are classically bradycardic. If the blood pressure does not improve after a fluid challenge, the judicious use of vasopressors may be indicated. Phenylephrine hydrochloride, dopamine, or norepinephrine are recommended. Overzealous fluid administration may cause pulmonary edema in a patient with neurogenic shock. When the fluid status is uncertain, the use of invasive monitoring may be helpful. A urinary catheter is inserted to monitor urinary output and prevent bladder distention.

C. Medications

High-dose methylprednisolone may be administered to the patient with **nonpenetrating** spinal cord injury within the **first 8 hours** of injury. Methylprednisolone is given in doses of 30 mg/kg within the first 15 minutes, followed by 5.4 mg/kg/hour. For patients in whom the drug is administered within 3 hours of injury, the intravenous infusion should be given for 24 hours. If therapy is started between 3 to 8 hours after injury, it should be continued for 48 hours unless there are complicating medical factors. Studies have been inconclusive in demonstrating benefit from this or other steroids in spinal cord injury management.

D. Transfer

Patients with spine fractures or a neurologic deficit should be transferred to a definitive-care facility. The safest procedure is to transfer the patient after telephone consultation with a spine specialist. Avoid unnecessary delay. The patient's condition should be stabilized, and the necessary splints, backboard, and/or semirigid cervical collar applied. **Remember, cervical spine injuries above C6 can result in partial or total loss of respiratory function.** If there is any concern about the adequacy of ventilation, the patient should be intubated prior to transfer.

VII. SUMMARY

A. Attend to life-threatening injuries first, minimizing any movement of the spinal column.

B. Establish and maintain proper immobilization of the patient until vertebral fractures or spinal cord injuries have been excluded.

C. Obtain lateral, AP, and open-mouth odontoid c-spine x-rays, when indicated, as soon as life-threatening injuries are controlled.

D. Document the patient's history and physical examination so as to establish a baseline for any changes in the patient's neurologic status.

E. Obtain early consultation with a neurosurgeon and/or orthopaedic surgeon whenever a spinal injury is suspected or detected.

F. Transfer patients with vertebral fractures or spinal cord injuries to a definitive-care facility.

■ BIBLIOGRAPHY

1. Bachulis BL, Long WI, Hynes GD, et al: Clinical indications for cervical spine radiographs in the traumatized patient. **American Journal of Surgery** 1987; 153:473–477.

2. Bracken MB, Shepard MJ, Collins WF, et al: A randomized, controlled trial of methylprednisolone or naloxone in the treatment of spinal cord injury. Results of the second National Spinal Cord Injury Study. **New England Journal of Medicine** 1990; 322:1405–1411.

3. Bracken MB, Shepard MJ, Holford TR, et al: Methylprednisolone or tirlazad mesylate administration after acute spinal cord injury: 1-year follow up. Results of the third national Acute Spinal Cord Injury Randomized Controlled Trial. **Journal of Neurosurgery** 1998; 89: 699–706.

4. Cooper C, Dunham CM, Rodriguez A: Falls and major injuries are risk factors for thoracolumbar fractures: Cognitive impairment and multiple injuries impede the detection of back pain and tenderness. **Journal of Trauma** 1995; 38(5):692–696.

5. Hadley MN, Fitzpatrick B, Browner C, et al: Facet fracture-dislocation injuries of the cervical spine. **Journal of Neurosurgery** 1992; 30: 661–666.

6. **International Standards for Neurological and Functional Classification of Spinal Cord Injury.** American Spinal Injury Association and International Medical Society of Paraplegia (ASIA/IMSOP), Atlanta, GA, revised 1996.

7. Macdonald RL, Schwartz ML, Mirich D, et al: Diagnosis of cervical spine injury in motor vehicle crash victims: How many x-rays are enough? **Journal of Trauma** 1990; 30:392–397.

8. Marion DW, Pryzybylski G: Injury to the Vertebrae and Spinal Cord. In: Mattox KL, Feliciano DV, Moore EE (eds): **Trauma.** New York, McGraw-Hill, 2000, p 451–471.

9. McGuire RA, Neville S, Green BA, et al: Spine instability and the log-rolling maneuver. **Journal of Trauma** 1987; 27:525–531.

10. Michael DB, Guyot DR, Darmody WR: Coincidence of head and cervical spine injury. **Journal of Neurotrauma** 1989; 6:177–189.

11. Narayan RK, Wilberger JE, Povlishock JT (eds): **Neurotrauma.** New York, McGraw-Hill, 1996.

12. Pasquale M, Marion DW, Domeier R, et al: Practice management guidelines for trauma: Identifying cervical spine instability after trauma. **Journal of Trauma** 1998; 44:945–946.

13. Tator CH: Spinal cord syndromes: Physiologic and anatomic correlations. In: Menezes AH, Sonntag VKH (eds): **Principles of Spinal Surgery.** New York, McGraw-Hill, 1995.

14. Tator CH, Fehlings MG: Review of the secondary injury theory of acute spinal cord trauma with special emphasis on vascular mechanisms. **Journal of Neurosurgery** 1991; 75:15–26.

SKILLS STATION

X-ray Identification of Spine Injuries

■ OBJECTIVES:

Performance at this station will allow the participant to do the following:

1. Identify various spine injuries by using specific anatomic guidelines for examining a series of spine x-rays.

2. Given a series of spine x-rays and scenarios,
   a. Define limitations of examination.
   b. Diagnose fractures.
   c. Delineate associated injuries.
   d. Define other areas of possible injury.

INTERACTIVE SKILLS PROCEDURES
X-ray Identification of Spine Injuries

I. C-SPINE X-RAY ASSESSMENT

A. Identify Presence of All 7 Cervical Vertebrae and Superior Aspect of T1

B. Anatomic Assessment

1. **Alignment** — Identify and assess the 4 lordotic curves/lines.
    a. Anterior vertebral bodies
    b. Anterior spinal canal
    c. Posterior spinal canal
    d. Spinous process tips

2. **Bone** — Assess for
    a. Vertebral body contour and axial height
    b. Lateral bony mass
        1) Pedicles
        2) Facets
        3) Laminae
        4) Transverse processes
    c. Spinous processes

3. **Cartilage** — Assess for
    a. Intervertebral discs
    b. Posterolateral facet joints

4. **Soft-tissue spaces** — Assess for
    a. Prevertebral space
    b. Prevertebral fat stripe
    c. Space between spinous processes

C. Assessment Guidelines for Detecting Abnormalities

1. **Alignment** — Assess for
    a. Loss of alignment of the posterior aspect of the vertebral bodies (anterior extent of the vertebral canal) — dislocation
    b. Narrowing of the vertebral canal — spinal cord compression

2. **Bone** — Assess for
    a. Bony deformity — compression fracture
    b. Fracture of the vertebral body or processes

SPINE AND SPINAL CORD TRAUMA   *X-ray Identification of Spine Injuries*

3. Soft-tissue spaces—Assess for

a. Increased prevertebral soft-tissue space (>5 mm opposite C3)—hemorrhage accompanying spinal injury

b. Increased distances between the spinous processes at one level—torn interspinous ligaments and likely spinal-canal fracture anteriorly

II. THORACIC AND LUMBAR X-RAY ASSESSMENT

A. Anteroposterior View—Assess for

1. Alignment

2. Symmetry of pedicles

3. Contour of bodies

4. Height of disc spaces

5. Central position of spinous processes

B. Lateral View—Assess for

1. Alignment of bodies/angulation of spine

2. Contour of bodies

3. Presence of disc spaces

4. Encroachment of body on canal

III. REVIEW SPINE X-RAYS

SKILLS STATION

Spinal Cord Injury Assessment and Management

■ OBJECTIVES:

Performance at this skills station will allow the participant to:

1. Demonstrate the assessment techniques for examining a patient suspected of having spine and/or spinal cord injuries.

2. Discuss the principles for immobilizing and logrolling the patient with neck and/or spinal injuries, as well as indications for removing protective devices.

3. Perform a neurologic examination and determine the level of spinal cord injury.

4. Determine the need for neurosurgical consultation.

5. Determine the need for inter- or intrahospital transfer and how the patient should be properly immobilized for transfer.

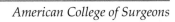

INTERACTIVE SKILLS PROCEDURES

Spinal Cord Injury Assessment and Management

Note: **Standard precautions are required whenever caring for the trauma patient.**

Note: This skills station includes scenarios and related x-rays for use in making evaluation and management decisions based on the findings. (See VI. Case Scenarios.)

I. PRIMARY SURVEY AND RESUSCITATION–ASSESSING SPINE INJURIES

Note: The patient should be maintained in a supine, neutral position using proper immobilization techniques.

A. Airway

Assess the airway while protecting the c-spine. Establish a definitive airway as needed.

B. Breathing

Assess and provide adequate oxygenation and ventilatory support as needed.

C. Circulation

1. If hypotensive, differentiate hypovolemic shock (decreased blood pressure, increased heart rate, and cool extremities) from neurogenic shock (decreased blood pressure, decreased heart rate, and warm extremities).

2. Replace fluids for hypovolemia.

3. If spinal cord injury is present, fluid resuscitation should be guided by CVP monitoring. (Note: Some patients may need inotropic support.)

4. When performing a rectal examination before inserting the urinary catheter, assess for rectal sphincter tone and sensation.

D. Disability–Brief Neurologic Examination

1. Determine level of consciousness and assess pupils.

2. Determine GCS Score.

3. Recognize paralysis/paresis.

II. SECONDARY SURVEY–NEUROLOGIC ASSESSMENT

A. Obtain AMPLE History

1. History and mechanism of injury

2. Medical history

SPINE AND SPINAL CORD TRAUMA *Spinal Cord Injury Assessment and Management*

3. Identify and record drugs given prior to patient's arrival and during assessment and management phases

B. Reassess Level of Consciousness and Pupils

C. Reassess GCS Score

D. Spine Assessment (See Section III, Examination for Level of Spinal Cord Injury in this skills station)

1. Palpation

Palpate the entire spine posteriorly by carefully logrolling the patient, assessing for:

   a. Deformity and/or swelling

   b. Grating crepitus

   c. Increased pain with palpation

   d. Contusions and lacerations/penetrating wounds

2. Pain, paralysis, paresthesia

   a. Presence/absence

   b. Location

   c. Neurologic level

3. Sensation

Test sensation to pinprick in all dermatomes and record the most caudal dermatome that feels the pinprick.

4. Motor function

5. Deep tendon reflexes (least informative in the emergency setting)

6. Document and repeat

Record the neurologic examination and repeat motor and sensory examinations regularly until consultation is obtained.

E. Reevaluate–Assess for Associated/Occult Injuries

III. EXAMINATION FOR LEVEL OF SPINAL CORD INJURY

A patient with a spinal cord injury may have varying levels of neurologic deficit. The level of motor function and sensation must be reassessed frequently and carefully documented because changes in the level of function may occur.

A. Best Motor Examination

1. Determining the level of quadriplegia, nerve-root level

   a. Raises elbow to level of shoulder—Deltoid, C5

   b. Flexes forearm—Biceps, C6

   c. Extends forearm—Triceps, C7

   d. Flexes wrist and fingers, C8

   e. Spreads fingers, T1

Spinal Cord Injury Assessment and Management **SPINE AND SPINAL CORD TRAUMA**

2. Determining the level of paraplegia, nerve-root level

   a. Flexes hip—Iliopsoas, L2

   b. Extends knee—Quadriceps, L3,4

   c. Flexes knee—Hamstrings, L4,5 to S1

   d. Dorsiflexes big toe—Extensor hallucis longus, L5

   e. Plantar flexes ankle—Gastrocnemius, S1

B. Sensory Examination

Determining the level of sensation is done primarily by assessing the dermatomes. (See Chapter 7, Spine and Spinal Cord Trauma, Figure 1, Key Sensory Points, page 180.) Remember, the cervical sensory dermatomes of C2 through C4 form a cervical cape or mantle that may extend down as far as the nipples. Because of this unusual pattern, the examiner should not depend on presence or absence of sensation in the neck and clavicular area, and the level of sensation must be correlated with the motor response level.

IV. TREATMENT PRINCIPLES FOR PATIENTS WITH SPINAL CORD INJURIES

A. Protection from Further Injury

Patients with suspected spine injury must be protected from further injury. Such protection includes the application of a semirigid cervical collar and a long backboard, performing a modified logroll to ensure neutral alignment of the entire spine, and removing the patient from the long spine board as soon as possible. Paralyzed patients, immobilized on a long spine board, are at particular risk of developing pressure points and decubitus ulcers. Therefore, paralyzed patients should be removed from the long spine board as soon as possible after a spine injury is diagnosed, eg, within 2 hours.

B. Fluid Resuscitation and Monitoring

1. CVP monitoring

Intravenous fluids usually are limited to maintenance levels unless specifically needed for the management of shock. A central venous catheter should be inserted to carefully monitor fluid administration.

2. Urinary catheter

A urinary catheter should be inserted during the primary survey and resuscitation phases to monitor urinary output and prevent bladder distention.

3. Gastric catheter

A gastric catheter should be inserted in all patients with paraplegia and quadriplegia to prevent gastric distention and aspiration.

C. Steroid Administration

Corticosteroids may be administered to patients with neurologic deficits from nonpenetrating spinal cord injury within the first 8 hours of injury. The drug of choice is methylprednisolone (30 mg/kg), administered intravenously over approximately 15 minutes. This initial dose is followed by a maintenance dose of 5.4 mg/kg/hour for the next 24 hours if initiated within 3 hours of the injury, or for 48 hours if initiated between 3 and 8 hours of injury, unless there are complicating factors.

SPINE AND SPINAL CORD TRAUMA *Spinal Cord Injury Assessment and Management*

V. PRINCIPLES OF SPINE IMMOBILIZATION AND LOGROLLING

A. Adult Patient

Four people are needed to perform the modified logrolling procedure and immobilize the patient, eg, on a long spine board: (1) 1 to maintain manual, inline immobilization of the patient's head and neck; (2) 1 for the torso (including the pelvis and hips); (3) 1 for the pelvis and legs; and (4) 1 to direct the procedure and move the spine board. This procedure maintains the patient's entire body in neutral alignment, thereby minimizing any untoward movement of the spine. This procedure assumes that any extremity suspected of being fractured has already been immobilized.

1. The long spine board with straps is placed next to the patient's side. The straps are positioned for fastening later across the patient's thorax, just above the iliac crests, thighs, and just above the ankles. Straps or tape may be used to secure the patient's head and neck to the long board.

2. Apply gentle, inline manual immobilization to the patient's head and apply a semirigid cervical collar.

3. The patient's arms are gently straightened and placed (palm in) next to the torso.

4. The patient's leg's are carefully straightened and placed in neutral alignment with the patient's spine. The ankles are tied together with a roller-type dressing or cravat.

5. Alignment of the patient's head and neck is maintained while another person reaches across and grasps the patient at the shoulder and wrist. A third person reaches across and grasps the patient's hip just distal to the wrist with 1 hand and with the other hand firmly grasps the roller bandage or cravat that is securing the ankles together.

6. At the direction of the person who is maintaining immobilization of the patient's head and neck, the patient is cautiously logrolled as a unit toward the 2 assistants at the patient's side, but only to the minimal degree necessary to position the board under the patient. Neutral alignment of the entire body must be maintained during this procedure.

7. The spine board is placed beneath the patient and the patient is carefully logrolled as a unit onto the spine board. Remember, the spine board is used only for transferring the patient and should not be left under the patient for any length of time.

8. Padding may be required under the patient's head to avoid hyperextension of the neck and for patient comfort.

9. Padding, rolled blankets, or similar bolstering devices are placed on either side of the patient's head and neck, and the patient's head is secured firmly to the board. Tape also is placed over the cervical collar, further securing the patient's head and neck to the long board.

B. Pediatric Patient

1. A pediatric-sized long spine board is preferable when immobilizing a small child. If only an adult-sized board is available, blanket rolls are placed along the entire sides of the child to prevent lateral movement.

2. A child's head is proportionately larger than an adult's. Therefore, padding should be placed under the shoulders to elevate the torso so that the large occiput of the child's head does not produce flexion of the cervical spine, thereby maintaining neutral alignment of the child's spine. Such padding extends from the child's lumbar spine to the top of the shoulders and laterally to the edges of the board.

C. Complications

If left immobilized for any length of time (approximately 2 hours or longer) on the long spine board, the patient may develop pressure sores at the occiput, scapulae, sacrum, and heels. Therefore, padding should be applied under these areas as soon as possible, and the patient should be removed from the long spine board as soon as the patient's condition permits.

D. Removal from a Long Spine Board

Movement of a patient with an unstable vertebral spine injury may cause or worsen a spinal cord injury. To reduce the risk of spinal cord damage, mechanical protection is necessary for all patients at risk. Such protection should be maintained until an unstable spine injury has been excluded.

1. As previously described, properly securing the patient to a long spine board is the basic technique for splinting the spine. Generally, this is done in the prehospital setting and the patient arrives at the hospital already immobilized. The long spine board provides an effective splint and permits safe transfers of the patient with a minimal number of assistants. However, the unpadded spine board may soon become uncomfortable for a conscious patient and poses a significant risk for pressure sores on posterior bony prominences (occiput, scapulae, sacrum, and heels). Therefore, the patient should be transferred from the spine board to a firm, well-padded gurney or equivalent surface as soon as it can be done safely. Before removing the patient from the spine board, c-spine, chest, and pelvis x-rays should be obtained as indicated, because the patient can be easily lifted and the x-ray plates placed beneath the spine board.

While the patient is immobilized on the spine board, it is very important to maintain immobilization of the head and the body continuously as a unit. The straps used to immobilize the patient to the board should not be removed from the body while the head remains taped to the upper portion of the spine board.

2. The patient should be removed from the spine board as early as possible. Preplanning is required. A good time to remove the board from under the patient is when the patient is logrolled to evaluate the back.

3. Safe movement of a patient with an unstable or potentially unstable spine requires continuous maintenance of anatomic alignment of the vertebral column. Rotation, flexion, extension, lateral bending, and shearing-type movements in any direction must be avoided. Manual, inline immobilization best controls the head and neck. No part of the patient's body should be allowed to sag as the patient is lifted off the supporting surface. The transfer options listed herein may be used, depending on available personnel and equipment resources.

4. Modified logroll technique

The modified logroll technique, previously outlined, is reversed to remove the patient from the long spine board. Four assistants are required: (1) 1 to maintain manual, in-line immobilization of the patient's head and neck; (2) 1 for the torso (including the pelvis and hips); (3) 1 for the pelvis and legs; and (4) 1 to direct the procedure and remove the spine board.

5. Scoop stretcher

An alternative to using the modified logrolling techniques is use of the scoop stretcher for patient transfer. The proper use of this device can provide rapid, safe transfer of the patient from the long spine board onto a firm, padded patient gurney. For example, this device may be used to transfer the patient from 1 transport device to another or to a designated place, eg, x-ray table.

Remember, the patient must remain securely immobilized until a spine injury is excluded. After the patient is transferred from the backboard to the gurney (stretcher) and the scoop stretcher is removed, the patient **must be reimmobilized securely** to the gurney (stretcher). The scoop stretcher is **not** a device on which the

SPINE AND SPINAL CORD TRAUMA *Spinal Cord Injury Assessment and Management*

patient is immobilized. Additionally, the scoop stretcher is not used to transport the patient, nor should the patient be transferred to the gurney by picking up only the foot and head ends of the scoop stretcher. Without firm support under the stretcher it can sag in the middle, resulting in loss of neutral alignment of the spine.

E. Immobilization of the Patient with Possible Spine Injury

Patients frequently arrive in the emergency department with spinal protective devices in place. These devices should cause the examiner to suspect that a c-spine and/or thoracolumbar spine injury may exist, based on mechanism of injury. In the multiply injured patient with a diminished level of consciousness, protective devices should be left in place, until a spine injury is excluded by clinical examination and x-rays. (See Chapter 7, Spine and Spinal Cord Trauma, Table 2, Guidelines for Screening Patients with Suspected C-spine Injury, page 186.)

If a patient is immobilized on a spine board and is paraplegic, spinal instability should be presumed and all appropriate x-rays obtained to determine the site of spinal injury. However, if the patient is awake, alert, sober, neurologically normal, is not experiencing neck or back pain, and does not have tenderness to spine palpation, spine x-rays or immobilization devices are not needed.

Patients who sustain multiple trauma and are comatose should be kept immobilized on a padded gurney (stretcher) and logrolled to obtain the necessary x-rays to exclude a fracture. Then, using one of the aforementioned procedures, they can be transferred carefully to a bed for better ventilatory support.

VI. CASE SCENARIOS

A. Scenario #1

A 15-year-old boy is riding his bicycle through a parking lot. While not being alert to his surroundings, he hits a car at low speed when it backs out of a parking space. He is thrown from his bicycle across the trunk of the car and sustains a mild abrasion and an angled deformity of the left wrist. He is brought to the emergency department immobilized on a long spine board and with a semirigid cervical collar in place. He is alert, cooperative, and hemodynamically normal.

B. Scenario #2

A 75-year-old man, walking to the store, trips and falls forward, striking his chin on a parked car. He is transported to the emergency department immobilized on a long spine board with a semirigid cervical collar applied. He has an abrasion on his chin and is alert and appropriately responsive. Physical examination reveals paralysis of his hands, with very little finger motion. He has some upper extremity movement (grade 2/5), but is clearly weak bilaterally. Examination of the lower extremities reveals weakness, but he is able to flex and extend both his legs at the hip and knee. He has various areas of hypesthesia over his body.

C. Scenario #3

A 25-year-old male passenger sustains multiple injuries in a car collision. The driver died at the scene of the injury. The patient is transported to the emergency department immobilized on a long spine board with a semirigid cervical collar applied. Oxygen is being administered, and 2 large-caliber intravenous lines with warmed crystalloid fluids are initiated. His blood pressure is 85/40 mm Hg, heart rate is 130 beats/minute, and respiratory rate is 40 breaths/minute. His respirations are shallow and there is a contusion over the chest wall. His eyes are open and his verbal response is appropriate. He is able to shrug his shoulders, but is unable to raise his elbow to the shoulder level and move his legs.

D. Scenario #4

This scenario is essentially the same as Scenario #3, but the instructor will make changes in the patient's neurologic status as the student examines the patient. A 25-year-old passenger sustains multiple injuries in a

Spinal Cord Injury Assessment and Management SPINE AND SPINAL CORD TRAUMA

car collision. The driver died at the scene of the injury. The passenger is transported to the emergency department immobilized on a long spine board with a semirigid cervical collar applied. Oxygen is being administered, and 2 large-caliber intravenous lines with warmed crystalloid fluids are initiated.

E. Scenario #5

A 6-year-old boy fell off his bicycle and hit the back of his head. In the emergency department, his head and neck are in a flexed position, and he complains of pain in his neck. He is immobilized on an unpadded long spine board without a cervical collar.

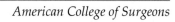

EIGHT

CHAPTER

Musculoskeletal Trauma

8

■ OBJECTIVES:

Upon completion of this topic, the participant will be able to initially assess and manage the patient with life- and limb-threatening musculoskeletal injuries. Specifically, the participant will be able to:

A. Recognize and describe the significance of musculoskeletal injuries in the multiply injured patient.

B. Outline priorities in the assessment of musculoskeletal trauma to identify life- and limb-threatening injuries.

C. Outline the proper principles of initial management for musculoskeletal injuries.

MUSCULOSKELETAL TRAUMA

I. INTRODUCTION

Injuries to the musculoskeletal system often appear dramatic and occur in 85% of patients who sustain blunt trauma, but rarely cause an immediate threat to life or limb. However, musculoskeletal injuries must be assessed and managed properly and appropriately so life and limb are not jeopardized. The doctor must learn to recognize the presence of such injuries, define the anatomy of the injury, protect the patient from further disability, and anticipate and prevent complications.

Major musculoskeletal injuries indicate significant forces sustained by the body. The patient with long-bone fractures above and below the diaphragm has an increased likelihood of associated internal torso injuries. Unstable pelvic fractures and open femur fractures may be accompanied by brisk bleeding. Severe crush injuries cause the release of myoglobin that can precipitate in the renal tubules and result in renal failure. Swelling into an intact musculofascial space can cause an acute compartment syndrome that, if not diagnosed and treated, may lead to lasting impairment and loss of extremity use. Fat embolism, an uncommon but highly lethal complication of long-bone fractures, may lead to pulmonary failure and impaired cerebral function.

Musculoskeletal trauma does not warrant a reordering of the priorities of resuscitation (ABCDEs). However, the presence of significant musculoskeletal trauma does pose a challenge to the treating doctor. Musculoskeletal injuries cannot be ignored and treated at a later time. The doctor must treat the whole patient, including musculoskeletal injuries, to assure optimal outcome. Despite careful assessment and management of the multiply injured patient, fractures and soft-tissue injuries may not be initially recognized. **Remember, continued reevaluation of the patient is necessary to identify all injuries.**

II. PRIMARY SURVEY AND RESUSCITATION

During the primary survey, it is imperative to recognize and control hemorrhage from musculoskeletal injuries. Deep soft-tissue lacerations may involve major vessels and lead to exsanguinating hemorrhage. Hemorrhage control is best effected by direct pressure.

Hemorrhage from long-bone fractures can be significant. Certain femoral fractures may result in up to 3 to 4 units of blood loss into the thigh, producing Class III shock. Appropriate splinting of the fracture can significantly decrease bleeding by reducing motion and enhancing a tamponade effect of the muscle. If the fracture is open, application of a sterile pressure dressing usually controls hemorrhage. Aggressive fluid resuscitation is an important supplement to these mechanical measures.

III. ADJUNCTS TO PRIMARY SURVEY

A. Fracture Immobilization

The goal of **initial** fracture immobilization is to realign the injured extremity in as close an anatomic position as possible and to prevent excessive fracture-site motion. This realignment is accomplished by the application of in-line traction to realign the extremity and is maintained by an immobilization device. The proper application of a splint helps control blood loss, reduces pain, and prevents further soft-tissue injury. If an open fracture is present, the doctor need not be concerned about pulling exposed bone back into the wound because all open fractures require surgical debridement.

Joint dislocations usually require splinting in the position in which they are found. If a closed reduction has successfully relocated the joint, immobilization in an anatomic position can be accomplished in a number of different ways: prefabricated splints, pillows, or plaster. These devices will maintain the extremity in its unreduced position.

Application of splints should be applied as soon as possible, but they must not take precedence over resuscitation. However, the use of splints may be very helpful during this phase to control hemorrhage and pain.

B. X-rays

X-ray examination of most skeletal injuries occurs as the part of the secondary survey. Which x-rays to obtain and when to obtain them are determined by the patient's initial and obvious clinical findings, the patient's hemodynamic status, and the mechanism of injury. An anteroposterior (AP) view of the pelvis should be obtained early for all multiply injured patients who are hemodynamically abnormal and for whom a source of bleeding has not been identified.

IV. SECONDARY SURVEY

A. History

1. Mechanism of injury

Information obtained from the transport personnel, patient, relatives, and bystanders at the scene of the injury should be documented and included as a part of the patient's medical record. It is particularly important to determine the mechanism of injury, which raises suspicion of injuries that may not be immediately apparent. (See Appendix 3, Biomechanics of Injury.) The doctor should mentally reconstruct the injury scene, identify other potential injuries that the patient may have sustained, and determine as much of the following information as possible.

a. What was the precrash location of the patient in the vehicle, ie, driver or passenger? This may indicate the type of fracture, eg, lateral compression fracture of the pelvis resulting from a side impact in a vehicle collision.

b. What was the postcrash location of the patient, eg, inside the vehicle or ejected? This may indicate patterns of injury. If the patient was ejected, determine the distance the patient was thrown. Ejection generally results in increased injury severity and unpredictable patterns of injury.

c. Was there external damage to the vehicle, eg, deformation to the front of the vehicle from a head-on collision? This information raises the suspicion of a hip dislocation.

d. Was there internal damage to the vehicle, eg, bent steering wheel, deformation to the dashboard, damage to the windscreen? These findings indicate a greater likelihood of sternal, clavicular, or spinal fractures, or hip dislocation.

e. Was the patient wearing a restraint; if so, what type (lap or 3-point safety belt), and was it applied properly? Faulty application of safety restraints may cause spinal fractures and associated intraabdominal visceral injuries. Was an air bag deployed?

f. Did the patient fall; if so, what was the distance of the fall and how did the patient land? This information helps identify the spectrum of injuries. Landing on the feet may cause foot and ankle injuries with associated spinal fractures.

g. Was the patient crushed by an object? If so, identify the weight of the crushing object, the site of the injury, and duration of weight applied to the site. Depending on whether a subcutaneous bony surface or a muscular area was crushed, different degrees of soft-tissue damage may occur, ranging from a simple contusion to a severe degloving extremity injury with compartment syndrome and tissue loss.

h. Did an explosion occur? If so, what was the magnitude of the blast and what was the patient's distance from the blast? A person close to the explosion may sustain primary blast injury from the force of the blast wave. A secondary blast injury may occur from debris and other objects accelerated by the blast effect (eg, fragments), leading to penetrating wounds, lacerations, and contusions. The patient also may be violently thrown to the ground or against other objects by the blast effect, leading to blunt musculoskeletal and other injuries (tertiary blast effect).

i. Was the patient involved in a vehicle-pedestrian collision? Musculoskeletal injuries may follow predicted patterns (bumper injury to leg) based on the size and age of the patient.

2. Environment

Prehospital care personnel should be asked about (1) patient exposure to temperature extremes, (2) patient exposure to toxic fumes or agents, (3) broken glass fragments (which also may injure the examiner), and (4) sources of bacterial contamination (eg, dirt, animal feces, fresh or salt water). This information helps the doctor anticipate potential problems and determine the initial antibiotic treatment.

3. Preinjury status and predisposing factors

It is important to determine the patient's baseline condition prior to injury. This information may alter the understanding of the patient's condition, treatment regimen, and outcome. The AMPLE history also should include information about the patient's (1) exercise tolerance and activity level, (2) ingestion of alcohol and/or other drugs, (3) emotional problems or illnesses, and (4) previous musculoskeletal injuries.

MUSCULOSKELETAL TRAUMA

4. Prehospital observations and care

Findings at the incident site that may help the doctor identify potential injuries include (1) the position in which the patient was found, (2) bleeding or pooling of blood at the scene and the estimated amount, (3) bone or fracture ends that may have been exposed, (4) open wounds in proximity to obvious or suspected fractures, (5) obvious deformity or dislocation, (6) presence or absence of motor and/or sensory function in each extremity, and (7) delays in extrication procedures or transport. Time of the injury should be noted, especially if there is ongoing bleeding and delay in reaching the hospital.

Prehospital observations and care must be reported and documented. Other information that may be important includes (1) changes in limb function, perfusion, or neurologic state, especially after immobilization or during transfer to the hospital; (2) reduction of fractures or dislocations during extrication or splinting at the scene; and (3) dressings and splints applied with special attention to excessive pressure over bony prominences that may result in peripheral nerve compression injuries, compartment syndromes, or crush syndromes.

B. Physical Examination

The patient must be completely undressed for adequate examination. Obvious extremity injuries should be splinted prior to the patient's arrival in the emergency department. Assessment of the trauma patient's extremities has three goals: (1) identification of life-threatening injury (primary survey), (2) identification of limb-threatening injuries (secondary survey), and (3) systematic review to avoid missing any other musculoskeletal injury (continuous reevaluation).

Assessment of musculoskeletal trauma can be achieved by looking at and talking to the patient, and should include palpation of the patient's extremities and performing a logical systematic review of each extremity. The 4 components that must be assessed are (1) skin, which protects the patient from excessive fluid loss and infection; (2) neuromuscular function; (3) circulatory status; and (4) skeletal and ligamentous integrity. This evaluation process reduces the risk of missing an injury.

1. Look and ask

Visually assess the extremities for (1) color and perfusion, (2) wounds, (3) deformity (angulation, shortening), (4) swelling, and (5) discoloration or bruising.

A rapid visual inspection of the entire patient is necessary to identify sites of major external bleeding. A pale or white distal extremity is indicative of a lack of arterial inflow. The extremity that is swollen in the region of major muscle groups may represent a crush injury with an impending compartment syndrome. Swelling in or around a joint and/or over the subcutaneous surface of a bone is a sign of a musculoskeletal injury. Extremity deformity is an obvious sign of major extremity injury. (See Table 1, page 209, Common Joint Dislocation Deformities.) Inspection of the patient's entire body for lacerations and abrasions is accomplished in the secondary survey. Open wounds are obvious unless on the dorsum of the body. The patient must be carefully logrolled to assess for an injury or skin laceration. If a bone protrudes or is visualized in the wound, an open fracture exists. Any open wound to a limb with an associated fracture also is considered an open fracture until proven otherwise by a surgeon.

Observation of the patient's spontaneous extremity motor function helps identify any neurologic and/or muscular impairment. If the patient is unconscious, absent spontaneous extremity movement may be the only sign of impaired function. With a cooperative patient, active voluntary muscle and peripheral nerve function can be assessed by asking the patient to contract major muscle groups. The ability to move all major joints through a full range of motion usually indicates that the nerve-muscle unit is intact and the joint is stable.

2. Feel

The extremities should be palpated to determine sensation to the skin (neurologic function) and areas of tenderness (fracture or deep muscle injury). Loss of sensation to pain and touch demonstrates the presence of a spinal or peripheral nerve injury. Areas of tenderness or pain over muscles may indicate a muscle contusion or a fracture. Pain, tenderness, swelling, and deformity over a subcutaneous bony surface usually confirm the diagnosis of a fracture. If pain or tenderness is as-

Table 1—Common Joint Dislocation Deformities

JOINT	DIRECTION	DEFORMITY
Shoulder	Anterior Posterior	Squared off Locked in internal rotation
Elbow	Posterior	Olecranon prominent posteriorly
Hip	Anterior Posterior	Flexed, abducted, externally rotated Flexed, adducted, internally rotated
Knee	Anteroposterior	Loss of normal contour, extended
Ankle		Externally rotated, prominent medial malleous
Subtalar joint	Lateral is most common	Laterally displaced os calcis

sociated with painful abnormal motion through the bone, the diagnosis of a fracture is made. However, attempts to elicit crepitus or demonstrate abnormal motion are not recommended. At the time of logrolling, the patient's back must be palpated to identify any lacerations, palpable gaps between the spinous processes, hematomas, or defects in the posterior pelvic region that are indicative of unstable axial skeletal injuries.

Closed soft-tissue injuries are more difficult to evaluate. Soft-tissue avulsion may shear the skin from the deep fascia, allowing for significant accumulation of blood. Alternatively, the skin may be sheared from its blood supply and undergo necrosis over a few days. This area may show local abrasions or bruised skin that are clues to a more severe degree of muscle damage and potential compartment syndromes or crush syndromes. These soft-tissue injuries are best evaluated by knowing the mechanism of injury and by palpation of the specific involved component.

Joint stability can be determined only by clinical examination. Any abnormal motion through a joint segment is indicative of a ligamentous rupture. The joint is palpated to identify any swelling and tenderness of the ligaments as well as intraarticular fluid. Following this, cautious stressing of the specific ligaments can be performed. Excessive pain may mask abnormal ligament motion because of guarding of the joint by muscular contraction or spasm and may need to be reassessed later.

3. Circulatory evaluation

The distal pulses in each extremity are palpated and capillary refill of the digits is assessed. If hypotension limits digital examination of the pulse, the use of a Doppler probe can detect blood flow to an extremity. The Doppler signal must have a triphasic quality to assure no proximal lesion. Loss of sensation in a stocking or glove distribution is an early sign of vascular impairment.

In the hemodynamically normal patient, pulse discrepancies, coolness, pallor, paresthesia, and even motor function abnormalities are suggestive of an arterial injury. Open wounds and fractures in proximity to arteries may be a clue to an arterial injury. The Doppler ankle/brachial index of less than 0.9 is indicative of an abnormal arterial flow secondary to injury or peripheral vascular disease. The ankle/brachial index is determined by taking the systolic blood pressure value as measured by the Doppler at the ankle of the injured leg and dividing it by the Doppler-determined systolic blood pressure of the uninjured arm. Auscultation may reveal a bruit with an associated palpable thrill. Expanding hematomas or pulsatile hemorrhage from an open wound also are indicative of arterial injury.

4. X-rays

The clinical examination often suggests the need for x-rays. Any area over a bone that is tender and deformed probably represents a fracture. If the patient is hemodynamically normal, an x-ray

MUSCULOSKELETAL TRAUMA

should be obtained. Joint effusions, abnormal joint tenderness, or joint deformity represent a joint injury or dislocation that also must be x-rayed. The only reason for not obtaining an x-ray prior to treatment of a dislocation or a fracture is related to a vascular compromise or impending skin breakdown. This is seen commonly with fracture dislocations of the ankle. Immediate reduction or realignment of the extremity should be performed to reestablish the arterial blood supply and reduce the pressure on the skin if there is going to be a delay in obtaining x-rays. Alignment can be maintained by appropriate immobilization techniques.

V. POTENTIALLY LIFE-THREATENING EXTREMITY INJURIES

A. Major Pelvic Disruption with Hemorrhage

1. Injury

Pelvic fractures associated with hemorrhage commonly exhibit disruption of the posterior osseous-ligamentous (sacroiliac, sacrospinous, sacrotuberous, and the fibromuscular pelvic floor) complex from a sacroiliac fracture and/or dislocation, or from a sacral fracture. The force vector opens the pelvic ring, tears the pelvic venous plexus, and occasionally disrupts the internal iliac arterial system (anterior-posterior compression injury). This mechanism of pelvic ring injury can be caused by motorcycle crashes or pedestrian-vehicle collisions, direct crushing injury to the pelvis, and falls from heights greater than 12 feet (3.6 meters).

In motor vehicle collisions, the more common mechanism of pelvic fracture is a force applied to the lateral aspect of the pelvis that tends to rotate the involved hemipelvis internally, closing down the pelvic volume and relieving any tension on the pelvic vascular system (lateral compression injury). This rotational motion drives the pubis into the lower genitourinary system, creating injury to the bladder and/or urethra. This injury rarely kills the patient from hemorrhage or its sequelae, as does the completely unstable pelvic injury.

2. Assessment

Major pelvic hemorrhage occurs rapidly and the diagnosis must be made quickly to initiate ap-

propriate resuscitative treatment. Unexplained hypotension may be the only initial indication of major pelvic disruption with instability in the posterior ligamentous complex. The most important physical signs are progressive flank, scrotal, or perianal swelling and bruising. This is associated with failure to respond to initial fluid resuscitation. Open fracture wounds about the pelvis (especially if the open area is in the perineum, rectum, or buttocks), a high-riding prostate gland, blood at the urethral meatus, and demonstrable mechanics instability are signs of unstable pelvic ring injury.

Mechanical instability of the pelvis ring is tested by manual manipulation of the pelvis. This procedure should be performed only once during the physical examination. Repeated testing for pelvic instability may result in further hemorrhage. The first indication of mechanical instability is leg-length discrepancy or rotational deformity (usually external) without a fracture of that extremity. The unstable hemipelvis migrates cephalad due to muscular pull and rotates outward secondary to the effect of gravity on the unstable hemipelvis. As the unstable pelvis is able to rotate externally, the pelvis can be closed by pushing on the iliac crests at the level of the anterior superior iliac spine. Motion can be felt if the iliac crests are grasped and the unstable hemipelvis(es) is pushed inward and then outward (compression-distraction maneuver). With posterior disruption, the involved hemipelvis can be pushed cephalad as well as pulled caudally. This translational motion can be felt by palpating the posterior iliac spine and tubercle while pushing-pulling the unstable hemipelvis. The identification of neurologic abnormalities or open wounds in the flank, perineum, and rectum may be evidence of pelvic ring instability. When appropriate, an AP x-ray of the pelvis confirms the clinical examination. (See Skills Station IV, Shock Assessment and Management.)

3. Management

Initial management of a major pelvic disruption associated with hemorrhage requires hemorrhage control and rapid fluid resuscitation. Hemorrhage control is achieved through mechanical stabilization of the pelvic ring and external counter pressure (pneumatic antishock garment). Patients with these injuries may be initially assessed and treated in hospitals that do not have the resources to definitively manage the degree of associated hemorrhage. Simple techniques may be employed to stabilize the pelvis before patient transfer. Longitudinal traction applied through the skin or the skeleton is a first-line method. Because these injuries externally rotate the hemipelvis(es), internal rotation of the lower limbs also reduces the pelvic volume. This procedure can be supplemented by applying a support directly to the pelvis. A sheet wrapped around the pelvis as a sling, a vacuum-type long-spine splinting device, or the pneumatic antishock garment (PASG) can apply sufficient stability for the unstable hemipelvis(es). These temporary methods are suitable to gain early pelvic stabilization. Definitive care of the hemodynamically abnormal patient demands the cooperative efforts of a team that must include a trauma surgeon and an orthopaedic surgeon, as well as any other surgeon whose expertise is required because of the patient's injuries. (See Chapter 5, Abdominal Trauma.)

Open pelvic fractures with obvious bleeding require pressure dressings to control hemorrhage, which is done by packing the open wounds. Early surgical consultation is essential.

B. Major Arterial Hemorrhage

1. Injury

Penetrating wounds of an extremity can result in major arterial vascular injury. Blunt trauma resulting in an extremity fracture or joint dislocation in close proximity to an artery also may disrupt the artery. These injuries may lead to significant hemorrhage through the open wound or into the soft tissues.

2. Assessment

An injured extremity should be assessed for external bleeding, loss of a previously palpable pulse or changes in pulse quality, and changes in Doppler tone and ankle/brachial index. A cold, pale, pulseless extremity indicates an interruption in arterial blood supply. A rapidly expanding hematoma suggests a significant vascular injury.

3. Management

If a major arterial injury exists or is suspected, immediate consultation with a surgeon is warrant-

ed. Management of major arterial hemorrhage includes application of direct pressure to the open wound and aggressive fluid resuscitation.

The judicious use of a pneumatic tourniquet may be helpful and lifesaving. The application of vascular clamps into bleeding open wounds in the emergency department is not recommended, unless a superficial vessel is clearly identified. If a fracture is associated with an open hemorrhaging wound, the fracture should be realigned and splinted while direct pressure is applied to the open wound. A joint dislocation simply requires immobilization because joint reduction may be extremely difficult, and therefore should be managed by emergency surgical intervention. The use of arteriography or other investigations are indicated only in the resuscitated, hemodynamically normal patient. Urgent consultation with a surgeon skilled in vascular and extremity trauma is necessary.

C. Crush Syndrome (Traumatic Rhabdomyolysis)

1. Injury

Crush syndrome refers to the clinical effects caused by injured muscle that, if untreated, may lead to acute renal failure. This condition is seen in individuals who have sustained a crush injury of a significant muscle mass, most often a thigh or calf. The muscular insult is a combination of direct muscle injury, muscle ischemia, and cell death with release of myoglobin.

2. Assessment

The myoglobin produces dark amber urine that tests positive for hemoglobin. The myoglobin assay must be specifically requested to confirm its presence. Rhabdomyolysis may lead to hypovolemia, metabolic acidosis, hyperkalemia, hypocalcemia, and disseminated intravascular coagulation (DIC).

3. Management

The initiation of intravenous fluid therapy during the period of resuscitation is critical to protecting the kidney and preventing renal failure. Myoglobin-induced renal failure may be prevented by intravascular fluid expansion and osmotic diuresis to maintain a high tubular volume and urine flow. Alkalization of the urine with sodium

MUSCULOSKELETAL TRAUMA

bicarbonate reduces intratubular precipitation of myoglobin and is indicated in most patients. It is recommended to maintain the patient's urinary output at 100 mL/hour until the myoglobinuria is cleared.

VI. LIMB-THREATENING INJURIES

A. Open Fractures and Joint Injuries

1. Injury

Open fractures represent a communication between the external environment and the bone. Muscle and skin must be injured for this to occur. The degree of soft-tissue injury is proportional to the energy applied. This damage, along with bacterial contamination, makes open fractures prone to problems with infection, healing, and function.

2. Assessment

Diagnosis is based on the history of the incident and physical examination of the extremity that demonstrates an open wound with or without significant muscle damage, contamination, and associated fracture. Management decisions should be based on a complete history of the incident and assessment of the injury.

Documentation of the open wound commences in the prehospital phase with the initial description of the injury and any treatment rendered at the scene. No further inspection of the open wound is warranted, providing documentation is adequate. If documentation or history is inadequate, the dressing should be removed under as sterile conditions as possible to visually examine the wound. A sterile dressing is then reapplied. At no time should the wound be probed. If a fracture and an open wound exist in the same limb segment, the fracture is considered open until disproved.

If an open wound exists over or near a joint, it should be assumed that this injury connects with or enters the joint, and surgical consultation should be obtained. The insertion of dye, saline, or any other material into the joint to determine whether the joint cavity communicates with the wound is not recommended. The only safe way to determine communication between an open

wound and a joint is to surgically explore and debride the wound.

3. Management

The presence of an open fracture or a joint injury should be promptly recognized. Appropriate immobilization should be applied after an accurate description of the wound is made and associated soft-tissue, circulatory, and neurologic involvement is determined. Prompt surgical consultation is necessary. The patient should be adequately resuscitated and hemodynamic stability achieved if possible. Wounds then may be operatively debrided and fractures stabilized. Tetanus prophylaxis should be administered. Antibiotics are used only after consultation with a surgeon.

B. Vascular Injuries, Including Traumatic Amputation

1. History and assessment

A vascular injury should be strongly suspected if there is presence of vascular insufficiency associated with a history of blunt, crushing, twisting, or penetrating injury to an extremity. The limb may initially appear viable because extremities often have some collateral circulation that provides enough retrograde flow. Partial vascular injury results in the distal part of the extremity being cool and having prolonged capillary refill, diminished peripheral pulses, and an abnormal ankle/brachial index. Alternatively, the distal extremity may have a complete disruption of flow and be cold, pale, and pulseless.

2. Management

An acutely avascular extremity must be recognized promptly and treated emergently. Muscle does not tolerate a lack of arterial blood flow for longer than 6 hours before necrosis commences. Nerves also are very sensitive to an anoxic environment. Therefore, early operative revascularization is required to restore arterial flow to the impaired distal extremity. If there is an associated fracture deformity, it can be corrected quickly by gently realigning and splinting the injured extremity.

If an arterial injury is associated with a dislocation of a joint, a doctor, skilled in joint reduction, may attempt **one** gentle reduction maneuver.

Otherwise, splinting of the dislocated joint and emergency surgical consultation is necessary. Arteriography must not delay reestablishing arterial blood flow and is indicated only after surgical consultation.

The potential for vascular compromise also exists whenever an injured extremity is splinted or placed in a cast. This may be identified by the loss or change in distal pulse exam, but excessive pain after cast application also must be investigated. The splint, cast, or any circumferential dressings must be released promptly and the vascular supply reassessed.

Amputation is a traumatic event for the patient both physically and emotionally. A traumatic amputation is a severe form of open fracture that results in loss of the extremity and requires consultation with and intervention by a surgeon. Certain open fractures with prolonged ischemia, neurologic injury, and muscle damage may require amputation. Amputation of an injured extremity may be lifesaving in the hemodynamically abnormal patient who is difficult to resuscitate.

Although the potential for replantation should be considered, it must be put into perspective with the patient's other injuries. **Remember, a patient with multiple injuries who requires intensive resuscitation and emergency surgery is not a candidate for replantation.** Replantation usually is performed with an isolated extremity injury. A patient with clean, sharp amputations of fingers or of a distal extremity, below the knee or elbow, should be transported to an appropriate surgical team skilled in the decision making and management of replantation procedures.

The amputated part should be thoroughly washed in isotonic solution (eg, Ringer's lactate solution) and wrapped in sterile gauze soaked in aqueous penicillin (100,000 units in 50 mL Ringer's lactate solution). The amputated part is then wrapped in a similarly moistened sterile towel, placed in a plastic bag, and transported with the patient in an insulated cooling chest with crushed ice. Care must be taken not to freeze the amputated part.

C. Compartment Syndrome

1. Injury

A compartment syndrome may occur in any site

in which muscle is contained within a closed fascial space. **Remember,** the skin also may act as a restricting membrane in certain circumstances. Common areas where compartment syndrome occurs are the lower leg, forearm, foot, hand, the gluteal region, and the thigh. Compartment syndrome develops when the pressure within an osteofascial compartment of muscle causes ischemia and subsequent necrosis. This ischemia can be caused by an increase in compartment size, eg, swelling secondary to revascularization of an ischemic extremity or by decreasing the compartment size, eg, constricting dressing. The end-stage of this neuromuscular injury is called Volkmann's ischemic contracture.

2. Assessment

Any injury to an extremity has the potential to cause a compartment syndrome. However, certain injuries as listed herein are considered as high-risk injuries.

  a. Tibial and forearm fractures

  b. Injuries immobilized in tight dressings or casts

  c. Severe crush injury to muscle

  d. Localized, prolonged external pressure to an extremity

  e. Increased capillary permeability secondary to reperfusion of ischemic muscle

  f. Burns

  g. Excessive exercise

A high degree of awareness is important, especially if the patient has an altered mental sensorium and is unable to respond appropriately to pain.

The signs and symptoms of compartment syndrome are (1) pain greater than expected and that typically increases by passive stretching of involved muscles, (2) paresthesia in the distribution of the involved peripheral nerve, (3) decreased sensation or functional loss of the nerves that traverse the involved compartment, and (4) tense swelling of the involved region. **A palpable distal pulse usually is often present in a compartment syndrome.** Weakness or paralysis of involved muscles and loss of pulses (because the compartment pressure exceeds the systolic pressure) in the affected limb are **late signs** of compartment syndrome.

MUSCULOSKELETAL TRAUMA

Remember, changes in distal pulses or capillary refill times are **not** reliable in diagnosing a compartment syndrome. Clinical diagnosis is based on the history of injury and physical signs coupled with a high index of suspicion. Intracompartmental pressure measurements may be helpful in diagnosing a suspected compartment syndrome. Tissue pressures that are greater than 35 to 45 mm Hg suggest decreased capillary blood flow that results in increased muscle and nerve anoxic damage. Systemic blood pressure is important. The lower the systemic pressure, the lower the compartment pressure that causes a compartment syndrome. Pressure measurement is indicated in all patients who have an altered response to pain.

3. Management

All constricting dressings, casts, and splints applied over the affected extremity must be released. The patient must be carefully monitored and reassessed clinically for the next 30 to 60 minutes. If no significant changes occur, fasciotomy is required. Compartment syndrome is a time-dependent condition. The higher the compartment pressure and the longer it remains elevated, the greater the degree of resulting neuromuscular damage and functional deficit. Delay in performing a fasciotomy may result in **myoglobinuria**, which may cause decreased renal function. **Surgical consultation of diagnosed or suspected compartment syndrome must be obtained early.**

D. Neurologic Injury Secondary to Fracture Dislocation

1. Injury

A fracture or, in particular, a dislocation may cause significant neurologic injury due to the anatomic relationship or proximity of the nerve to the joint, eg, sciatic nerve compression from posterior hip dislocation or axillary nerve injury from anterior shoulder dislocation. Optimum functional outcome is jeopardized unless this injury is recognized and treated early.

2. Assessment

A thorough examination of the neurologic system is essential in a patient with a musculoskeletal injury. Determination of neurologic impairment is important and progressive changes must be documented.

Assessment usually demonstrates a deformity of the extremity. Assessment of nerve function usually requires a cooperative patient. For each significant peripheral nerve, voluntary motor function and sensation must be confirmed systematically. (See Table 2, Peripheral Nerve Assessment of Upper Extremities, and Table 3, page 215, Peripheral Nerve Assessment of Lower Extremities.) Muscle testing must include palpation of the contracting muscle.

Table 2—Peripheral Nerve Assessment of Upper Extremities

NERVE	MOTOR	SENSATION	INJURY
Ulnar	Index finger abduction	Little finger	Elbow injury
Median distal	Thenar contraction with opposition	Index finger	Wrist dislocation
Median, anterior interosseous	Index tip flexion		Supracondylar fracture of humerus (children)
Musculocutaneous	Elbow flexion	Lateral forearm	Anterior shoulder dislocation
Radial	Thumb, finger MCP extension	1st dorsal web space	Distal humeral shaft, anterior shoulder dislocation
Axillary	Deltoid	Lateral shoulder	Anterior shoulder dislocation, proximal humerus fracture

Table 3—Peripheral Nerve Assessment of Lower Extremities

NERVE	MOTOR	SENSATION	INJURY
Femoral	Knee extension	Anterior knee	Pubic rami fractures
Obturator	Hip adduction	Medial thigh	Obturator ring fractures
Posterior tibial	Toe flexion	Sole of foot	Knee dislocation
Superficial peroneal	Ankle eversion	Lateral dorsum of foot	Fibular neck fracture, knee dislocation
Deep peroneal	Ankle/toe dorsiflexion	Dorsal 1st to 2nd web space	Fibular neck fracture, compartment syndrome
Sciatic nerve	Plantar dorsiflexion	Foot	Posterior hip dislocation
Superior gluteal	Hip abduction		Acetabular fracture
Inferior gluteal	Gluteus maximus hip extension		Acetabular fracture

In most multiply injured patients, it is difficult to initially assess nerve function. However, it must be repeated on an ongoing basis, especially after the patient is stabilized. Progression is indicative of continued nerve compression. The most important aspect of any neurologic assessment is the documentation of progression. It also is an important aspect of surgical decision making.

3. Management

The injured extremity should be immobilized in the dislocated position and surgical consultation obtained immediately. If indicated and if the treating doctor is knowledgeable, a careful reduction of the dislocation may be attempted. After reducing a dislocation, neurologic function should be reevaluated and the limb splinted.

VII. OTHER EXTREMITY INJURIES

A. Contusions and Lacerations

Simple contusions and/or lacerations should be assessed to exclude vascular and/or neurologic injury. In general, lacerations require debridement and closure. If a laceration extends below the fascial level, it requires operative intervention to more formally debride the wound and assess for damage to underlying structures.

Contusions usually are recognized by pain in the area and decreased function of the extremity. Palpa-

tion confirms localized swelling and tenderness. The patient usually cannot use the muscle or decreased function occurs from pain in the affected extremity. Contusions are treated by limiting function of the injured part and applying cold packs, if the patient is seen early.

Beware of small wounds, especially those resulting from crush injuries. When a very strong force is applied very slowly over an extremity, significant devascularization and crushing of muscle can occur with only a small skin wound. Crush and degloving injuries can be very subtle and must be suspected based on mechanism of injury.

The risk of tetanus is increased with wounds that (1) are more than 6 hours old, (2) are contused and/or abraded, (3) are more than 1 cm in depth, (4) result from high velocity missiles, (5) are due to burn or cold, and (6) have significant contamination (especially burn wounds and wounds with denervated or ischemic tissue). (See Appendix 4, Tetanus Immunization.)

B. Joint Injuries

1. Injury

Joint injuries that are not dislocated (the joint is within its normal anatomic configuration but has sustained significant ligamentous injury) usually are not limb threatening. However, such joint injuries can decrease the function of the limb.

MUSCULOSKELETAL TRAUMA

2. Assessment

The patient usually relates some form of abnormal stress to the joint, eg, impact to the anterior tibia pushing the knee back, an impact to the lateral aspect of the leg that results in a valgus strain to the knee, or a fall onto an outstretched arm that causes a hyperflexion injury to the elbow.

Physical examination reveals tenderness throughout the affected ligament. A hemarthrosis usually is present unless the joint capsule is disrupted and the bleeding diffuses into the soft tissues. Passive ligamentous testing of the affected joint reveals instability. X-rays usually demonstrate no significant injury. However, some small avulsion fractures from ligamentous insertions or origins may be present radiographically.

3. Management

Joint injuries should be immobilized. Vascular and neurologic status of the limb, distal to the injury, should be reassessed. Surgical consultation usually is warranted.

C. Fractures

1. Injury

Fractures are defined as a break in the continuity of the bone cortex leading to abnormal motion associated with crepitus and pain. Fractures usually are associated with some form of soft-tissue injury, whether the fracture is closed or open.

2. Assessment

Examination of the extremity demonstrates pain, swelling, deformity, tenderness, crepitus, and abnormal motion at the fracture site. The evaluation for crepitus and abnormal motion at the fracture site may occasionally be necessary to make the diagnosis, but this is painful and potentially can increase soft-tissue damage. These diagnostic tests must not be done routinely or repetitively. Usually the swelling, tenderness, and deformity are sufficient to confirm a fracture. It is important to periodically reassess the neurovascular status of a limb, especially if a splint is in place.

X-rays taken at right angles to each other confirm the history and physical examinations. Depending on the hemodynamic status of the patient, x-rays may have to be delayed until the patient is stabilized. X-rays through the joint above and below the suspected fracture site must be included to exclude occult dislocation and concomitant injury.

3. Management

a. Immobilization must include the joint above and below the fracture. After splinting, the neurologic and vascular status of the extremity must be reassessed.

b. Surgical consultation is required for further treatment.

VIII. PRINCIPLES OF IMMOBILIZATION

Splinting of extremity injuries, unless associated with life-threatening injuries, usually can be left until the secondary survey. However, all such injuries must be splinted before patient transport. Assess the limb's neurovascular status after applying splints or realigning a fracture.

Specific types of splints can be applied for specific fracture needs. The PASG is not generally recommended as a lower extremity splint. However, it may be temporarily useful for patients with life-threatening hemorrhage from pelvic injuries or severe lower extremity injuries with soft-tissue injury. Prolonged inflation (>2 hours) of the leg components in hypotensive patients may lead to compartment syndrome.

A long spine board provides a total body splint for multiply injured patients with possible or confirmed unstable spine injuries. However, its hard, unpadded surface may cause pressure sores on the patient's occiput, scapulae, sacrum, and heels. Therefore, as soon as possible, the patient should be moved carefully to an equally supportive padded surface, using a scoop-style stretcher or appropriate logrolling maneuver to facilitate the transfer. The patient should be fully immobilized and an adequate number of personnel should be available during this transfer. (See Chapter 7, Spine and Spinal Cord Trauma Skills Station XI, Spinal Cord Injury Assessment and Management, pages 200–202, V. Principles of Spine Immobilization and Logrolling.)

A. Femoral Fractures

Femoral fractures are immobilized temporarily with traction splints. The traction splint's force is applied distally at the ankle or through the skin. Proximally, the splint is pushed into the thigh and hip areas by a ring that applies pressure to the buttocks, perineum, and groin. Excessive traction may cause skin damage to the foot, ankle, or perineum. Neurovascular compromise may result from stretching the peripheral nerves. Hip fractures can be similarly immobilized with a traction splint, but are more suitably immobilized with skin traction or a foam boot traction with the knee in slight flexion. A simple method of splinting is to bind the injured leg to the opposite leg.

B. Knee Injuries

The use of commercially available knee immobilizers or the application of a long-leg splint of plaster is very helpful in maintaining comfort and stability. The leg should not be immobilized in complete extension, but should be immobilized with about 10° of flexion to take pressure off the neurovascular structures.

C. Tibia Fractures

Tibia fractures are best immobilized with a well-padded cardboard or metal gutter long-leg splint. If readily available, plaster splints immobilizing the lower leg, the knee, and the ankle may be used.

D. Ankle Fractures

Ankle fractures may be immobilized with a pillow splint or padded cardboard splint, thereby avoiding pressure over bony prominences.

E. Upper Extremity and Hand Injuries

The **hand** can be **temporarily** splinted in an anatomic, functional position, with the wrist slightly dorsiflexed and the fingers gently flexed 45° at the metacarpal phalangeal joints. This position usually can be achieved by gently immobilizing the hand over a large roll of gauze and using a short-arm splint.

The **forearm and wrist** are immobilized flat on padded or pillow splints. The **elbow** usually is immobilized in a flexed position, either by using padded splints or by direct immobilization to the body with a sling and swath device. The **upper arm** usually is immobilized by splinting it to the body or by applying a sling or swath, which can be augmented by a thoracobrachial bandage. **Shoulder** injuries are managed by a sling and swath device or a Velcro-type of dressing.

IX. PAIN CONTROL

Analgesics are generally indicated for a joint injury or a fracture. However, the administration of pain medications must be tempered by the patient's clinical situation. The appropriate use of splints significantly decreases the patient's discomfort by controlling the amount of motion that occurs at the injured site.

Patients who do not appear to have significant pain and discomfort from a major fracture may have other associated injuries, eg, intracranial lesions, hypoxia, or may be under the influence of alcohol and/or other drugs.

Effective pain relief usually requires administration of narcotics, which should be given in small doses intravenously and repeated as needed. Muscle relaxants and sedatives should be administered cautiously in the patient with an isolated extremity injury, eg, reduction of a dislocation. Whenever analgesics, muscle relaxants, or sedatives are administered to an injured patient, the potential exists for respiratory arrest. Consequently, appropriate resuscitative equipment must be immediately available.

X. ASSOCIATED INJURIES

Certain musculoskeletal injuries, because of their common mechanism of injury, are often associated with a second injury that is not immediately apparent or may be missed. (See Table 4, page 218, Associated Injuries.) Steps to ensure recognition and management of these injuries include:

A. Review the injury history, especially the mechanism of injury, to determine if another injury may be present.

B. Thoroughly reexamine all extremities, placing special emphasis on the hands, wrists, feet, and the joint above and below a fracture or dislocation.

C. Visually examine the patient's dorsum, including the spine and pelvis. Open injuries and closed soft-tissue injuries that may be indicative of an unstable injury must be documented.

D. Review the x-rays obtained in the secondary survey to identify subtle injuries that may be associated with more obvious trauma.

MUSCULOSKELETAL TRAUMA

Table 4—Associated Injuries

INJURY	MISSED/ASSOCIATED INJURY
Clavicular fracture Scapular fracture Fracture and/or dislocation of shoulder	Major thoracic injury, especially pulmonary contusion and rib fractures
Displaced thoracic spine fracture	Thoracic aortic rupture
Spine fracture	Intraabdominal injury
Fracture/dislocation of elbow	Brachial artery injury Median, ulnar, and radial nerve injury
Major pelvic disruption (motor vehicle occupant)	Abdominal, thoracic, or head injury
Major pelvic disruption (motorcyclist or pedestrian)	Pelvic vascular hemorrhage
Femur fracture	Femoral neck fracture Posterior hip dislocation
Posterior knee dislocation	Femoral fracture Posterior hip dislocation
Knee dislocation or displaced tibial plateau fracture	Popliteal artery and nerve injuries
Calcaneal fracture	Spine injury or fracture Fracture-dislocation of hind foot Tibial plateau fracture
Open fracture	70% incidence of associated nonskeletal injury

XI. OCCULT SKELETAL INJURIES

Remember, not all injuries can be diagnosed during the initial assessment and management of the patient. Joints or bones that are covered or well padded within muscular areas may contain occult injuries. It may be difficult to identify nondisplaced fractures or joint ligamentous injuries, especially if the patient is unresponsive or there are other severe injuries. It is important to recognize that injuries are commonly discovered days after the injury incident, eg, when the patient is being mobilized. Therefore, is it important to reassess the patient routinely and to relate this possibility to other members of the trauma team and the patient's family.

XII. PITFALLS

A. Musculoskeletal injuries are a potential source of occult blood loss in the hemodynamically abnormal patient. Occult sites of hemorrhage are the retroperitoneum from unstable pelvic ring injuries, the thigh from femoral fractures, and any open fracture with major soft-tissue involvement where blood loss may be serious and occur before the patient reaches the hospital.

B. A compartment syndrome is limb-threatening. Clinical findings must be recognized and surgical consultation obtained early. These may be normal in patients with hypotension.

C. Despite a thorough examination, occult associated injuries may not be appreciated during the initial evaluation of the patient. It is imperative to repeatedly reevaluate the patient to assess for these injuries.

XIII. SUMMARY

The goal of initial assessment and management of musculoskeletal trauma is to identify injuries that pose a threat to life and/or limb. Although uncommon, life-threatening musculoskeletal injuries must be properly assessed and managed. Most extremity injuries are appropriately diagnosed and managed during the secondary survey. It is essential to recognize and manage in a timely manner pelvic fractures, arterial injuries, compartment syndrome, open fractures, crush injuries, and fracture-dislocations. Knowledge of the mechanism of injury and history of the injury-producing event enables the doctor to be aware of what associated conditions potentially exist with the injured extremity. Early splinting of fractures and dislocations can prevent serious complications and late sequelae. Additionally, an awareness of the patient's tetanus immunization status, particularly in cases of open fractures or significantly contaminated wounds, can prevent serious complications. Armed with the proper knowledge and skills, as outlined in this chapter, the doctor can satisfactorily provide the initial management for most musculoskeletal trauma.

■ BIBLIOGRAPHY

1. American Academy of Orthopaedic Surgeons: **Emergency Care and Transportation of the Sick and Injured, 8th Edition.** Sudbury, MA, Jones and Bartlett Publishers, 2002.

2. Bone LB, Johnson KD, Weigelt J, et al: Early versus delayed stabilization of femoral fractures: A prospective, randomized study. **Journal of Bone and Joint Surgery** 1989; 71A:336–340.

3. Browner BD (ed): Controversies and perils. **Techniques in Orthopedics** 1994; 9(4):258.

4. Browner BD, Jupiter JB, Levine AM, et al (eds): **Skeletal Trauma.** Philadelphia, WB Saunders, 1991.

5. Carter PR: Common hand injuries and infections. In: **A Practical Approach to Early Treatment.** Philadelphia, WB Saunders, 1983.

6. Dalal SA, Burgess AR, Seigel JH, et al: Pelvic fracture in multiple trauma: Classification by mechanism is key to pattern of organ injury, resuscitative requirements, and outcome. **Journal of Trauma** 1989; 29(7):981–1000.

7. Gustilo RB, Anderson JT: Prevention of infection in the treatment of 1025 open fractures of long bones. **Journal of Bone and Joint Surgery** 1976; 58A:453.

8. Gustilo RB, Mendoza RM, Williams DN: Problems in the management of type III (severe) open fractures: A new classification of type III open fractures. **Journal of Trauma** 1985; 24:742.

9. Hansen ST, Swiontkowski MF: **Orthopedic Trauma Protocols.** New York, Raven Press, 1993.

10. Heppenstall RB, Sapega AA, Scott R, et al: The compartment syndrome: An experimental and clinical study of muscular energy metabolism using phosphorus nuclear magnetic resonance spectroscopy. **Clinical Orthopedics** 1988; 226: 138–155.

11. Hoppenfeld S: **Physical Examination of the Spine and Extremities.** New York, Appleton, 1976.

12. Koury HI, Peschiera JL, Welling RE: Selective use of pelvic roentgenograms in blunt trauma patients. **Journal of Trauma** 1993; 34:236.

13. Maull KI, Capenhart JE, Cardea JA, et al: Limb loss following MAST application. **Journal of Trauma** 1981; 21:60–62.

14. Moore EE, Ducker TB, Edlich RF, et al (eds): **Early Care of the Injured Patient, 4th Edition.** Philadelphia, BC Decker, 1990, chapters 19–24.

15. Ododeh M: The role of reperfusion-induced injury in the pathogenesis of the crush syndrome. **New England Journal of Medicine** 1991; 324: 1417–1421.

16. Rockwood CA, Green DP, Bucholtz R (eds): **Fractures, 3rd Edition.** Philadelphia, JP Lippincott Co, 1991.

17. Trafton PG: Orthopaedic emergencies. In: Ho MT, Saunders CE (eds): **Current Emergency Diagnosis and Treatment, 3rd Edition.** East Norwalk, CT, Appleton & Lange, 1990.

18. Tscherne H, Gotzen L: **Fractures with Soft-Tissue Injuries.** Berlin, Springer Verlag, 1984.

SKILLS STATION

Musculoskeletal Trauma Assessment and Management

■ OBJECTIVES:

Performance at this station will allow the participant to:

1. Perform a rapid assessment of the essential components of the musculoskeletal system.

2. Recognize life- and limb-threatening injuries of the musculoskeletal system, and institute initial management of these problems.

3. Identify the patient at risk for compartment syndrome.

4. Recognize the indications and the value of appropriate splinting of musculoskeletal injuries.

5. Apply standard splints to the extremities, including a traction splint.

6. Recognize the complications associated with the use of splints.

7. Identify pelvic instability associated with pelvic fracture.

8. Recognize the value of the AP pelvic x-ray to identify the potential for massive blood loss and the maneuvers that may be used to reduce pelvic volume and control bleeding.

■ PROCEDURES:

1. Perform a physical examination of the musculoskeletal system.

2. Apply a leg traction splint.

3. Review and discuss a series of x-rays and identify injuries.

INTERACTIVE SKILLS PROCEDURES

Musculoskeletal Trauma Assessment and Management

Note: Standard precautions are required whenever caring for the trauma patient.

Note: A series of x-rays with related scenarios is provided at the conclusion of this section for use during this station in making evaluation and management decisions based on the findings.

Goal of Splinting: To prevent further soft-tissue injury and control bleeding and pain. Consider the immobilization of fractured extremities with the use of splints as "secondary resuscitation devices" that aid in the control of bleeding.

I. PHYSICAL EXAMINATION

A. Look, General Overview

External hemorrhage is identified by obvious external bleeding from an extremity, pooling of blood on the stretcher or floor, blood-soaked dressings, and bleeding that occurs during transport to the hospital. The examiner needs to ask about characteristics of the injury incident and prehospital care.

1. Open wounds may not bleed, but may be indicative of nerve injury or an open fracture.

2. A deformed extremity is indicative of a fracture or joint injury. This type of injury should be splinted before patient transport or as soon as is safely possible.

3. The color of the extremity is important to assess. The presence of bruising indicates muscle injury or significant soft-tissue injury over bones or joints. These changes may be associated with swelling or hematomas. Vascular impairment may be first identified by a pale, distal extremity.

4. Position of the extremity may be helpful in determining certain injury patterns. Certain nerve deficits lead to specific positions of the extremity. For example, injury to the radial nerve results in wrist drop, and injury to the peroneal nerve results in foot drop.

5. Observation of spontaneous activity helps determine the severity of injury. Observing whether the patient spontaneously moves an extremity may suggest to the examiner other obvious or occult injuries. An example is the brain-injured patient who does not follow commands and has no spontaneous lower extremity movement. This patient could have a thoracic or lumbar fracture.

6. Gender and age are important clues to potential injuries. Children may sustain growth plate injuries and fractures that may not manifest themselves (eg, buckle fracture). A woman is less likely to have a urethral injury than a vaginal injury with a pelvic fracture.

7. Drainage from the urinary catheter should be observed. If the urine is bloody or if catheter insertion is difficult, the patient may have a pelvic fracture and a urologic injury.

B. Feel

Life- and limb-threatening injuries are excluded first.

MUSCULOSKELETAL TRAUMA *Musculoskeletal Trauma Assessment and Management*

1. The pelvis is palpated anteriorly and posteriorly to assess for deformity, motion, and/or a gap that indicates a potentially unstable pelvis. The compression-distraction test as well as the push-pull test should be done only once. These tests are dangerous because they may dislodge clots and cause rebleeding.

2. Pulses in all extremities should be palpated and the findings documented. Any perceived abnormality or difference must be explained. Normal capillary refill (<2 seconds) of the pulp space or nail bed provides a good guide to the satisfactory blood flow to the distal parts of the extremity. Loss of or diminished pulses with normal capillary refill indicates a viable extremity; however, surgical consultation is required. **If an extremity has no pulses and no capillary refill, a surgical emergency exists.**

A Doppler device is useful to assess pulses and to determine the ankle/arm systolic pressure ratio. Blood pressure is measured at the ankle and on an uninjured arm. The normal ratio exceeds 0.9. If the ratio is below 0.9, a potential injury exists and surgical consultation is required.

3. The muscle compartments of all the extremities are palpated for compartment syndromes and fractures. This is done by gentle palpation of the muscle and bone. If a fracture is present, the conscious patient complains of pain. If the patient is unconscious, only abnormal motion may be felt. A compartment syndrome is suspected if the muscle compartment is hard, firm, or tender. Compartment syndromes may be associated with fractures.

4. Joint stability is assessed by asking the cooperative patient to move the joint through a range of motion. This should not be done if there is an obvious fracture or deformity, or if the patient cannot cooperate. Each joint is palpated for tenderness, swelling, and intraarticular fluid. Joint stability is assessed by the application of lateral, medial, and anterior-posterior stress. Any deformed or dislocated joint should be splinted and x-rayed before testing for stability.

5. A rapid, thorough neurologic examination of the extremities should be performed and documented. Testing is repeated and recorded as indicated by the patient's clinical condition. Sensation is tested by light touch and pinprick in each of the extremities. Progression of the neurologic findings indicates a potential problem.

   a. C5—Lateral aspect of the upper arm (also axillary nerve)

   b. C6—Palmar aspect of the thumb and index finger (median nerve)

   c. C7—Palmar aspect of the long finger

   d. C8—Palmar aspect of the little finger (ulnar nerve)

   e. T1—Inner aspect of the forearm

   f. L3—Inner aspect of the thigh

   g. L4—Inner aspect of the lower leg, especially over the medial malleolus

   h. L5—Dorsum of the foot between the first and second toes (common peroneal)

   i. S1—Lateral aspect of the foot

6. Motor examination of the extremities also should be performed.

   a. Shoulder abduction—Axillary nerve, C5

   b. Elbow flexion—Musculocutaneous nerve, C5 and C6

   c. Elbow extension—Radial nerve, C6, C7, and C8

   d. Hand and wrist—Power grip tests the dorsiflexion of the wrist (radial nerve, C6) and flexion of the fingers (median and ulnar nerves, C7 and C8).

   e. Finger add/abduction—Ulnar nerve, C8 and T1

   f. Lower extremity—Dorsiflexion of the great toe and ankle tests the deep peroneal nerve, L5, and plantar dorsiflexion tests the posterior tibial nerve, S1.

Musculoskeletal Trauma Assessment and Management **MUSCULOSKELETAL TRAUMA**

g. Muscle power is graded in the standard form. The motor examination is specific to a variety of voluntary movements of each extremity. (See Chapter 7, Spine and Spinal Cord Trauma, Table 1, page 181, Muscle Strength Grading.)

7. The deep tendon reflexes also are assessed.

8. Remember, assess the patient's back!

II. PRINCIPLES OF EXTREMITY IMMOBILIZATION

A. Assess the ABCDEs and treat life-threatening situations first.

B. Remove all clothing and completely expose the patient including the extremities. Remove watches, rings, bracelets, and other potentially constricting devices. Remember, prevent the development of hypothermia.

C. Assess the neurovascular status of the extremity before applying the splint. Assess for pulses, external hemorrhage, which must be controlled, and perform a motor and sensory examination of the extremity.

D. Cover any open wounds with sterile dressings.

E. Select the appropriate size and type of splint for the injured extremity. The device should immobilize the joint above and the joint below the injury site.

F. Apply padding over bony prominences that will be covered by the splint.

G. Splint the extremity in the position in which it is found if distal pulses in the injured extremity are present. If distal pulses are absent, one attempt to realign the extremity should be tried. Gentle traction should be maintained until the splinting device is secured.

H. The extremity is placed in a splint if normally aligned. If malaligned, the extremity needs to be realigned and then splinted.

I. Do not force realignment of a deformed extremity. If it is not easily realigned, splint the extremity in the position in which it is found.

J. Obtain orthopaedic consultation.

K. Document the neurovascular status of the extremity before and after every manipulation or splint application.

L. Administer appropriate tetanus prophylaxis. (See Appendix 4, Tetanus Immunization.)

III. REALIGNING A DEFORMED EXTREMITY

Physical examination determines if the deformity is from a fracture or dislocation. The principle of realigning an extremity fracture is to restore length by applying gentle longitudinal traction to correct the residual angulation and then rotational deformities. While maintaining realignment with manual traction, a splint is applied and secured to the extremity by an assistant.

A. Upper Extremity

1. Humerus

Grasp the elbow and manually apply distal traction. After alignment is obtained, a plaster splint is applied and the arm secured to the chest wall with a sling and swath.

MUSCULOSKELETAL TRAUMA *Musculoskeletal Trauma Assessment and Management*

2. Forearm

Manually apply distal traction through the wrist while holding the elbow and applying countertraction. A splint is then secured to the forearm and the injured extremity is elevated.

B. Lower Extremity

1. Femur

Realign the femur by manually applying traction through the ankle if the tibia and fibula are not fractured. As the muscle spasm is overcome, the leg will straighten and the rotational deformity can be corrected. This maneuver may take several minutes, depending on the size of the patient.

2. Tibia

Manually apply distal traction at the ankle and countertraction just above the knee, provided that the femur is intact.

C. Vascular and Neurologic Deficits

Fractures associated with neurovascular deficit require prompt realignment. Immediate consultation with a surgeon is necessary. If the vascular or neurologic status worsens after realignment and splinting, the splint should be removed and the extremity returned to the position in which blood flow and neurologic status are maximized. The extremity is then immobilized in that position.

IV. APPLICATION OF THE TRACTION SPLINT

A. Application of this device requires 2 people—1 person to handle the injured extremity, the other to apply the splint.

B. Remove all clothing, including footwear, to expose the extremity. Apply sterile dressings to open wounds, and assess the neurovascular status of the extremity.

C. Cleanse any exposed bone and muscle of dirt and debris before applying traction. Document that the exposed bone fragments were reduced into the soft tissues.

D. Determine the length of the splint by measuring the uninjured leg. The upper cushioned ring should be placed under the buttocks and adjacent to the ischial tuberosity. The distal end of the splint should extend beyond the ankle by approximately 6 inches (15 cm). The straps on the splint should be positioned to support the thigh and calf.

E. The femur is aligned by manually applying traction through the ankle. After realignment is achieved, gently elevate the leg to allow the assistant to slide the splint under the extremity so that the padded portion of the splint rests against the ischial tuberosity. Reassess the neurovascular status of the distal injured extremity after applying traction.

F. The ankle hitch is positioned around the patient's ankle and foot while the assistant maintains manual traction on the leg. The bottom strap should be slightly shorter than, or at least the same length as, the 2 upper crossing straps.

G. Attach the ankle hitch to the traction hook while the assistant maintains manual traction and support. Apply traction in increments using the windlass knob until the extremity appears stable, or until pain and muscular spasm are relieved.

H. Reassess the neurovascular status of the injured extremity. If perfusion of the extremity distal to the injury appears worse after applying traction, gradually release the traction.

Musculoskeletal Trauma Assessment and Management **MUSCULOSKELETAL TRAUMA**

I. Secure the remaining straps.

J. Frequently reevaluate the neurovascular status of the extremity. Document the neurovascular status after every manipulation of the extremity.

K. Administer tetanus prophylaxis, as indicated. (See Appendix 4, Tetanus Immunization.)

V. COMPARTMENT SYNDROME—ASSESSMENT AND MANAGEMENT

A. Important Considerations

1. Compartment syndrome may develop insidiously.

2. Compartment syndrome may develop in an extremity from compression or crushing forces and without obvious external injury or fracture.

3. Frequent reevaluation of the injured extremity is essential.

4. The patient who has been hypotensive or is unconscious is at increased risk for developing compartment syndrome.

5. The unconscious or intubated patient cannot communicate the early signs of extremity ischemia.

6. Pain is the earliest symptom that heralds the onset of compartment ischemia, especially pain on passive stretch of the involved muscles of the extremity.

7. Loss of pulses and other classic findings of ischemia occur late, after irreversible damage has occurred.

B. Palpate the muscular compartments of the extremities, comparing the compartment tension in the injured extremity with that in the noninjured extremity.

1. Asymmetry is a significant finding.

2. Frequent examination for tense muscular compartments is essential.

3. Measurement of compartment pressures is helpful.

4. If compartment syndrome is suspected, obtain surgical consultation.

C. Obtain orthopaedic or general surgical consultation early.

VI. IDENTIFICATION AND MANAGEMENT OF PELVIC FRACTURES

A. Identify the mechanism of injury, which can suggest the possibility of a pelvic fracture, eg, ejection from a motor vehicle, crushing injury, pedestrian struck by moving vehicle, or motorcycle collision.

B. Inspect the pelvic area for ecchymosis, perineal or scrotal hematoma, or blood at the urethral meatus.

C. Inspect the legs for differences in length or asymmetry in rotation of the hips.

D. Perform a rectal examination, noting the position and mobility of the prostate gland, any palpable fracture, or the presence of gross or occult blood in the stool.

E. Perform a vaginal examination, noting palpable fractures, the size and consistency of the uterus, or the presence of blood. Remember, females of childbearing age may be pregnant.

MUSCULOSKELETAL TRAUMA *Musculoskeletal Trauma Assessment and Management*

F. If steps B. through E. are abnormal, or if the mechanism of injury suggests a pelvic fracture, obtain an AP x-ray of the patient's pelvis. (Note: The mechanism of injury may suggest the type of fracture.)

G. If steps B. through E. are normal, palpate the bony pelvis to identify painful areas.

H. Determine pelvic stability by gently applying anterior-posterior compression and lateral-to-medial compression over the anterosuperior iliac crests. Testing for axial mobility by gently pushing and pulling on the legs will determine stability in a cranial-caudal direction.

I. Cautiously insert a urinary catheter, if not contraindicated, or perform a retrograde urethrogram if a urethral injury is suspected.

J. Interpret the pelvic x-ray, giving special consideration to those fractures that are frequently associated with significant blood loss, eg, fractures that increase the pelvic volume.

   1. Confirm the patient's identification on the film.

   2. Systematically evaluate the film for:

      a. Width of the symphysis pubis—greater than 1 cm separation signifies significant posterior pelvic injury.

      b. The integrity of the superior and inferior pubic rami bilaterally.

      c. The integrity of the acetabula, as well as femoral heads and necks.

      d. Symmetry of the ilium and width of the sacroiliac joints.

      e. Symmetry of the sacral foramina by evaluating the arcuate lines.

      f. Fracture(s) of the transverse processes of L5.

   3. Remember, the bony pelvis is a ring that rarely sustains an injury in only 1 location. Displacement of ringed structures implies 2 fracture sites.

   4. Remember, fractures that increase the pelvic volume, eg, vertical shear and open-book fractures, are often associated with massive blood loss.

K. Techniques to Reduce Blood Loss from Pelvic Fractures

   1. Avoid excessive and repeated manipulation of the pelvis.

   2. Internally rotate the lower legs to close an open-book type fracture. Pad bony prominences and tie the rotated legs together. This maneuver may reduce a displaced symphysis, decrease the pelvic volume, and be used as a temporary measure until definitive treatment can be provided.

   3. Apply and inflate the PASG. This device also is useful when transporting the patient.

   4. Apply a pelvic external fixation device **(early orthopaedic consultation)**.

   5. Apply skeletal limb traction **(early orthopaedic consultation)**.

   6. Embolize pelvic vessels via angiography.

   7. Obtain early surgical and orthopaedic consultation to determine priorities.

   8. Place sandbags under each buttock if there is no indication of spinal injury and other techniques to close the pelvis are not available.

   9. Apply a pelvic binder.

10. Arrange for transfer to a definitive care facility if local resources are not available to manage this injury.

VII. IDENTIFICATION OF ARTERIAL INJURY

A. Recognize that ischemia is a limb-threatening and potentially life-threatening condition.

B. Palpate peripheral pulses bilaterally (dorsalis pedis, anterior tibial, femoral, radial, and brachial) for quality and symmetry.

C. Document and evaluate any evidence of asymmetry in peripheral pulses.

D. Reevaluate peripheral pulses frequently, especially if asymmetry is identified.

E. Early surgical consultation is required.

VIII. PRINCIPLES OF EXTREMITY EXAMINATION AND IMMOBILIZATION

A. Scenario #1

A 28-year-old man is involved in a head-on motorcycle collision with a car. At the scene, he was combative, his systolic blood pressure was 80 mm Hg, heart rate was 120 beats/minute, and his respiratory rate was 20 breaths/minute. In the emergency department, his vital signs have returned to normal and the patient is complaining of pain in his right upper extremity and both lower extremities. His right thigh and left lower extremity are deformed. Prehospital personnel report a large laceration to the left leg, to which they applied a dressing.

B. Scenario #2

Scenario A: A 20-year-old woman is found trapped in her automobile. Several hours are required to extricate her because her leg was trapped and twisted beneath the dashboard. In the hospital, she is hemodynamically normal and alert. She complains of severe pain in her left leg, which is splinted.

Scenario B: A 34-year-old man is shot in the right leg while cleaning his handgun. He is unable to walk because of knee pain and states his lower extremity is painful, weak, and numb.

C. Scenario #3

A 16-year-old boy is thrown approximately 100 feet (33 meters) from the back of a pickup truck. In the emergency department his skin is cool and he is lethargic and unresponsive. His systolic blood pressure is 75 mm Hg, his heart rate is 145 beats/minute, and his respirations are rapid and shallow. Breath sounds are equal and clear to auscultation. Two large-caliber IVs are initiated, and 2500 mL of warmed crystalloid solution is infused. However, the patient's hemodynamic status does not improve significantly. His blood pressure now is 84/58 mm Hg and his heart rate is 135 beats/minute.

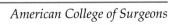

NINE

CHAPTER 9
Injuries Due to Burns and Cold

■ OBJECTIVES:

Upon completion of this topic, the participant will be able to identify methods of assessment and outline measures to stabilize, manage, and transfer patients with burns and cold injuries. Specifically, the participant will be able to:

A. Estimate the burn size and determine the presence of associated injuries.

B. Demonstrate measures of initial assessment and treatment of patients with burns and cold injuries.

C. Identify special problems and methods of treatment of patients with burns and patients with cold injuries.

D. Specify criteria for the transfer of burn patients.

INJURIES DUE TO BURNS AND COLD

I. INTRODUCTION

Burn and cold injuries constitute major causes of morbidity and mortality. Attention to basic principles of initial trauma resuscitation and timely application of simple emergency measures should minimize the morbidity and mortality of these injuries. These principles include a high index of suspicion for the presence of airway compromise in smoke inhalation, and the maintenance of hemodynamic normality with volume resuscitation. The doctor also must have an awareness of measures to be instituted for prevention and treatment of the potential complications of thermal injuries, eg, rhabdomyolysis and cardiac dysrhythmias, sometimes seen in electrical burns. Temperature control and removal from the injury-provoking environment also constitute major principles of thermal injury management.

II. IMMEDIATE LIFESAVING MEASURES FOR BURN INJURIES

A. Airway

Although the larynx protects the subglottic airway from direct thermal injury, the supraglottic airway is extremely susceptible to obstruction as a consequence of exposure to heat. Signs of airway obstruction may not be obvious immediately, although if present, they may warn the examiner of potential airway obstruction. When a patient is admitted to the hospital after sustaining a burn injury, the doctor should be alert to the possibility of airway involvement, identify signs of distress, and initiate supportive measures. Clinical indications of inhalation injury include:

1. Face and/or neck burns

2. Singeing of the eyebrows and nasal vibrissae

3. Carbon deposits and acute inflammatory changes in the oropharynx

4. Carbonaceous sputum

5. Hoarseness

6. History of impaired mentation and/or confinement in a burning environment

7. Explosion with burns to head and torso

8. Carboxyhemoglobin level greater than 10% if patient is involved in a fire

The presence of any of these findings suggests acute inhalation injury. Such injury requires immediate and definitive care, including airway support. **Transfer to a burn center is indicated if there is inhalation injury. If the transport time is prolonged, intubation should be performed prior to transport to protect the airway. The symptom of stridor is an indication for immediate endotracheal intubation. Circumferential burns of the neck may lead to swelling of the tissues around the airway. Therefore, early intubation is indicated in this situation.**

B. Stop the Burning Process

All clothing should be removed to stop the burning process. Synthetic fabrics ignite, burn rapidly at high temperatures, and melt into hot residue that continues to burn the patient. Any clothing with chemical involvement should be removed carefully. Chemical powders (dry) should be brushed from the wound, with the individual caring for the patient avoiding direct contact with the chemical. The involved body surface areas are then rinsed with copious amounts of tap water. The patient then should be covered with warm, clean, and dry linens to prevent hypothermia.

C. Intravenous Lines

Any patient with burns over more than 20% of the body surface area needs circulatory volume support. After establishing airway patency and identifying and treating immediately life-threatening injuries, intravenous access must be established. Large-caliber (at least #16-gauge catheter) intravenous lines must be established immediately in a peripheral vein. If the extent of burn precludes placement of the catheter through unburned skin, overlying burned skin should not deter placement of the catheter in an accessible vein. The upper extremities are preferable to the lower extremities for venous access because of the high incidence of phlebitis and septic phlebitis in the saphenous veins. Begin infusion with Ringer's lactate solution. Guidelines for establishing the flow rate of Ringer's lactate solution are outlined later in this chapter.

III. ASSESSING THE BURN PATIENT

A. History

The injury history often is extremely valuable in the management of the burn patient. Associated injuries may be sustained while the victim attempts to escape the fire. Explosions may throw the patient some distance and may result in internal injuries or fractures, eg, CNS, myocardial, pulmonary, and abdominal injuries. It is essential that the time of the burn injury be established. Burns sustained within an enclosed space should suggest the potential for inhalation injury.

The history, from the patient or relative, should include a brief survey of preexisting illnesses: (1) diabetes; (2) hypertension; (3) cardiac, pulmonary, and/or renal disease; and (4) drug therapy. Allergies and drug sensitivities also are important. The patient's tetanus immunization status also should be ascertained.

B. Body Surface Area (BSA)

The Rule of Nines is a useful and practical guide to determine the extent of the burn. The adult body configuration is divided into anatomic regions that represent 9%, or multiples of 9%, of the total body surface. Body surface area differs considerably for children. The infant's or young child's head represents a larger proportion of the surface area and the lower extremities a lesser proportion, than an adult's. The percentage of total body surface of the infant's head is twice that of the normal adult. (See Figure 1, page 234, Rule of Nines.) **Remember, the palmar surface (including the fingers) of the patient's hand represents approximately 1% of the patient's body surface.** This guideline helps estimate the extent of burns of irregular outline or distribution.

C. Depth of Burn

The depth of burn is important in evaluating the severity of the burn, planning for wound care, and predicting functional and cosmetic results. **First-degree burns** (eg, sunburn) are characterized by erythema, pain, and the absence of blisters. They are not life-threatening, and generally do not require intravenous fluid replacement. This type of burn will not be discussed further in this chapter.

Partial-thickness burns or second-degree burns are characterized by a red or mottled appearance with associated swelling and blister formation. The surface may have a weeping, wet appearance and is painfully hypersensitive, even to air current.

Full-thickness or third-degree burns usually appear dark and leathery. The skin also may appear translucent, mottled, or waxy white. The surface may be red and does not blanch with pressure. The surface is painless and generally dry. (See Figure 2, page 235, Depth of Burn.)

IV. PRIMARY SURVEY AND RESUSCITATION OF THE BURN PATIENT

A. Airway

History of confinement in a burning environment or suggestive signs of early airway injury on arrival in the emergency department necessitate evaluation of the airway and definitive management. Pharyngeal thermal injuries may produce marked upper airway edema, and early maintenance of the airway is important. The clinical manifestations of inhalation injury may be subtle and frequently do not appear in the first 24 hours. If the doctor waits for x-ray evidence of pulmonary injury or change in blood gas determinations, airway edema may preclude intubation, and a surgical airway may be required.

B. Breathing

The initial treatment of injuries is based on the patient's signs and symptoms, which are results of the following possible injuries.

1. Direct thermal injury, producing upper airway edema and/or obstruction

2. Inhalation of products of combustion (carbon particles) and toxic fumes, leading to chemical tracheobronchitis, edema, and pneumonia

3. Carbon monoxide (CO) poisoning

Always assume CO exposure in patients burned in enclosed areas. Diagnosis of CO poisoning is made primarily from a history of exposure. Patients with CO levels of less than 20% usually have no physical symptoms. Higher CO levels may result in (1) headache and nausea (20% to 30%), (2) confusion (30% to 40%), (3) coma (40% to 60%), and (4) death (>60%). Cherry-red skin color is rare. Because of the

INJURIES DUE TO BURNS AND COLD

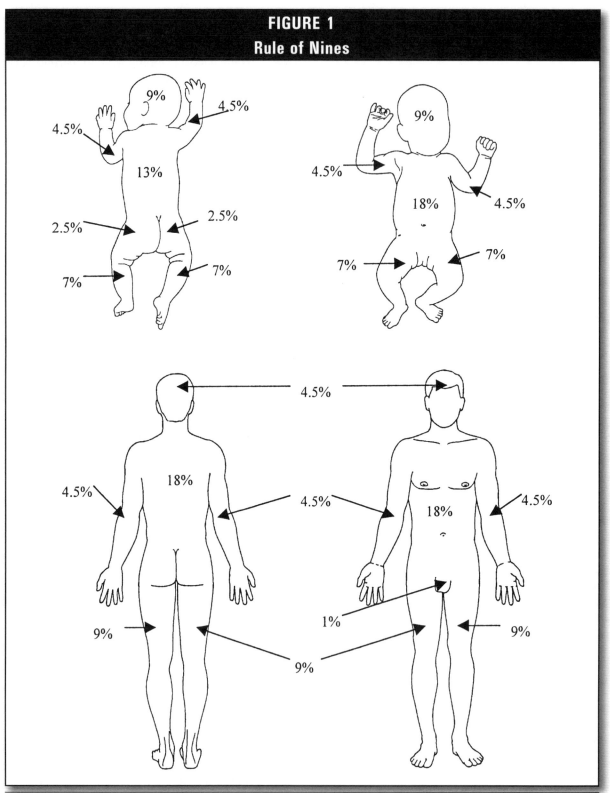

FIGURE 1
Rule of Nines

The Rule of Nines is used in the hospital management of severe burns to determine fluid replacement. It also is useful as a practical guide for the evaluation of severe burns. The adult body is generally divided into surface areas of 9% each and/or fractions or multiples of 9%.

Graphics used with permission from LifeART Collection Images, Copyright ©1989–1997 by TechPool Studios, Cleveland, OH.

FIGURE 2 Depth of Burn		
	DEPTH OF BURN	SIGNS AND SYMPTOMS
Shallow Partial-thickness or Second-degree Burn Injury	• 2° burns are deeper than 1° burns • 2° burns commonly result from contact with hot liquids or flash burns from explosions	• Red or mottled appearance • Blistered and broken epidermis • Considerable swelling • Weeping, wet surfaces • Painful • Sensitive to air
Deep Partial and Full-thickness or Third-degree Burn Injury	• 3° burns cause damage to all skin layers, nerve endings, and even subcutaneous tissues • 3° burns can be caused by fire, prolonged exposure to hot liquids, contact with hot objects, or electricity • Initially, 3° burns may resemble 2° burn injuries	• Pale, white, charred, leathery, mottled, or red appearance • Broken skin with fat exposed • Dry surface • Painless and insensate • Edema

Graphics used with permission from LifeART Collection Images, Copyright ©1989-1997 by TechPool Studios, Cleveland, OH.

increased affinity of CO for hemoglobin (240 times that of oxygen), it displaces oxygen from the hemoglobin molecule and shifts the oxyhemoglobin dissociation curve to the left. CO dissociates very slowly, and its half-life is 250 minutes or 4 hours while the patient is breathing room air, compared with 40 minutes while breathing 100% oxygen. Therefore, patients suspected of exposure to CO should receive high-flow oxygen via a nonrebreathing mask.

Early management of inhalation injury may require endotracheal intubation and mechanical ventilation. Prior to intubation, the patient should be preoxygenated with continuous administration of humidified oxygen. Intubation should be performed early in patients with suspected airway injury. Because there is a high probability of the need for bronchoscopy in burn patients with airway injury, an endotracheal tube of sufficient size should be chosen for a definitive airway. Arterial blood gas determinations

INJURIES DUE TO BURNS AND COLD

should be obtained as a baseline for the evaluation of the patient's pulmonary status. However, measurements of arterial Po_2 do not reliably predict CO poisoning, because a CO partial pressure of only 1 mm Hg results in a carboxyhemoglobin level of 40% or greater. Therefore, baseline carboxyhemoglobin levels should be obtained, and 100% oxygen should be administered.

If the patient's hemodynamic condition permits and spinal injury is excluded, elevation of the head and chest by 20° to 30° is helpful in reducing neck and chest wall edema. If a full-thickness burn of the anterior and lateral chest wall leads to severe restriction of the chest wall motion, even in the absence of a circumferential burn, chest wall escharotomy may be required.

C. Circulating Blood Volume

Evaluation of the circulating blood volume is often difficult in the severely burned patient. In addition, severely burned patients may have accompanying injuries resulting in hypovolemic shock. The shock should be treated according to resuscitation principles as previously outlined. (See Chapter 3, Shock.) Burn resuscitation fluids also should be provided.

Blood pressure may be difficult to obtain and may be unreliable. Monitoring hourly urinary outputs reliably assesses circulating blood volume in the absence of osmotic diuresis (eg, glycosuria). Therefore, an indwelling urinary catheter should be inserted. A good rule to follow is to infuse fluids at a rate sufficient to produce 1.0 mL of urine per kilogram of body weight per hour for children who weigh 30 kilograms or less, and 0.5 mL of urine per kilogram of body weight per hour in the adult.

The burn patient requires 2 to 4 mL of Ringer's lactate solution per kilogram body weight per percent second- and third-degree body surface burns in the first 24 hours to maintain an adequate circulating blood volume and provide adequate renal output. The calculated fluid volume is then proportioned in the following manner: one-half the total fluid is provided in the first 8 hours postburn, and the remaining half is administered in the next 16 hours. **Since third-degree or full-thickness burns and pulmonary burn injury result in increased early fluid requirements, it is better to administer the higher resuscitation volume (4 mL/kg) and assess the patient's response frequently. In children who weigh 30 kg or less, the goal is to maintain an** **average urinary output of 1 mL/kg/hour. In these patients, it is necessary to administer maintenance intravenous fluids containing glucose in addition to the burn formula.**

Any resuscitation formula provides only an estimate of fluid need. Fluid requirement calculations for infusion rates are based on the **time from injury**, not urinary output from the time fluid resuscitation is initiated. The amount of fluid given should be adjusted according to the individual patient's response, ie, urinary output, vital signs, and general condition. Cardiac dysrhythmias may be the first sign of hypoxia and electrolyte or acid-base abnormalities. The ECG should be monitored for cardiac rhythm disturbances.

V. SECONDARY SURVEY AND RELATED ADJUNCTS

A. Physical Examination

The following must be done to plan and direct patient management:

1. Estimate extent and depth of burn

2. Assess for associated injuries

3. Weigh the patient

B. Flow Sheet

A flow sheet, outlining the patient's management, should be initiated when the patient is admitted to the emergency department. This flow sheet should accompany the patient when transferred to the burn unit.

C. Baseline Determinations for the Major Burn Patient

1. Blood

Obtain samples for CBC, type and crossmatch/screen, carboxyhemoglobin, serum glucose, electrolytes, and pregnancy test in all females of childbearing age. Arterial blood samples also should be obtained for blood gas determinations.

2. X-rays

A chest film should be obtained with repeat films as necessary. Other x-rays may be indicated for appraisal of associated injuries.

D. Circumferential Extremity Burns: Maintain Peripheral Circulation

1. Remove all jewelry.

2. Assess the status of distal circulation, checking for cyanosis, impaired capillary refilling, or progressive neurologic signs (ie, paresthesia and deep-tissue pain). Assessment of peripheral pulses in burn patients is best performed with a Doppler ultrasonic flow meter.

3. Circulatory embarrassment in a circumferentially burned limb is best relieved by escharotomy, always with surgical consultation. Escharotomies usually are not needed within the first 6 hours of burn injury.

4. Fasciotomy is seldom required. However, it may be necessary to restore circulation for patients with associated skeletal trauma, crush injury, high-voltage electrical injury, or burns involving tissue beneath the investing fascia.

E. Gastric Tube Insertion

Insert a gastric tube and attach it to suction if the patient experiences nausea, vomiting, abdominal distention, or if burns involve more than 20% of the total BSA. Prior to transfer, it is essential that a gastric tube be inserted and functioning in such patients.

F. Narcotics, Analgesics, and Sedatives

The severely burned patient may be restless and anxious from hypoxemia or hypovolemia rather than pain. Consequently, the patient responds better to oxygen or increased fluid administration rather than to narcotic analgesics or sedatives that may mask the signs of hypoxemia or hypovolemia. Narcotics, analgesics, and sedatives should be administered in small, frequent doses by the intravenous route only.

G. Wound Care

Partial-thickness (second-degree) burns are painful when air currents pass over the burned surface. Gently covering the burn with clean linen relieves the pain and deflects air currents. Do not break blisters or apply an antiseptic agent. Any applied medication must be removed before appropriate antibacterial topical agents can be applied. Application

of cold compresses may cause hypothermia. Do **not** apply cold water to a patient with extensive burns.

H. Antibiotics

Prophylactic antibiotics are not indicated in the early postburn period. Antibiotics should be reserved for the treatment of infection.

I. Tetanus

Determination of the patient's tetanus immunization status is very important. (See Appendix 4, Tetanus Immunization.)

VI. SPECIAL BURN REQUIREMENTS

A. Chemical Burns

Chemical injury can result from exposure to acids, alkalies, or petroleum products. Alkali burns are generally more serious than acid burns, because the alkalies penetrate more deeply. Removal of the chemical and immediate attention to wound care are essential. Chemical burns are influenced by the duration of contact, concentration of the chemical, and amount of the agent. Immediately flush away the chemical with large amounts of water, using a shower or hose if available, for at least 20 to 30 minutes. Alkali burns require longer irrigation. If dry powder is still present on the skin, brush it away **before** irrigation with water. Neutralizing agents have no advantage over water lavage, because reaction with the neutralizing agent may itself produce heat and cause further tissue damage. Alkali burns to the eye require continuous irrigation during the first 8 hours after the burn. A small-caliber cannula can be fixed in the palpebral sulcus for such irrigation.

B. Electrical Burns

Electrical burns result from a source of electrical power making contact with the patient's body. Electrical burns frequently are more serious than they appear on the surface. The body may serve as a volume conductor of electrical energy and the heat generated results in thermal injury of tissue. Different rates of heat loss from superficial and deep tissues account for relatively normal overlying skin coexisting with deep muscle necrosis. Rhabdomyolysis results in myoglobin release, which can cause acute renal failure. The immediate management of a patient with a significant electrical burn includes

INJURIES DUE TO BURNS AND COLD

attention to the airway and breathing, establishment of an intravenous line in an uninvolved extremity, electrocardiographic monitoring, and placement of an indwelling catheter. If the urine is dark, assume that hemochromogens are in the urine. Do not wait for laboratory confirmation before instituting therapy for myoglobinuria. Fluid administration should be increased to ensure a urinary output of at least 100 mL/hour in the adult. If the pigment does not clear with increased fluid administration, 25 g of mannitol should be administered immediately and 12.5 g of mannitol should be added to subsequent liters of fluid to maintain the diuresis. Metabolic acidosis should be corrected by maintaining adequate perfusion and adding sodium bicarbonate to alkalize the urine as necessary and increase the solubility of myoglobin in the urine.

VII. CRITERIA FOR TRANSFER

A. Types of Burn Injuries

The American Burn Association has identified the following types of burn injuries that usually require referral to a burn center:

1. Partial-thickness burns greater than 10% total body BSA

2. Burns that involve the face, hands, feet, genitalia, perineum, or major joints

3. Full-thickness burns in any age group

4. Electrical burns, including lightning injury

5. Chemical burns

6. Inhalation injury

7. Burn injury in patients with preexisting medical disorders that could complicate management, prolong recovery, or affect mortality

8. Any burn-injury patient with concomitant trauma (such as fractures) in which the burn injury poses the greatest risk of morbidity or mortality. In such cases, if the injury poses the greater immediate risk, the patient may be initially stabilized in a trauma center before being transferred to a burn center. The doctor's judgment is necessary in such situations and should be in concert with regional medical control plan and triage protocols.

9. Any burn-injury children who are seen in hospitals without qualified personnel or equipment to manage their care should be transferred to a burn center with these capabilities.

10. Burn injury in patients who will require special social, emotional, or rehabilitative intervention

B. Transfer Procedure

1. Transfer of any patient must be coordinated with the burn center doctor.

2. All pertinent information regarding tests, temperature, pulse, fluids administered, and urinary output should be recorded on the burn/trauma flow sheet and sent with the patient. Any other information deemed important by the referring or receiving doctor also is sent with the patient.

VIII. COLD INJURY: LOCAL TISSUE EFFECT

Severity of cold injury depends on temperature, duration of exposure, environmental conditions, amount of protective clothing, and the patient's general state of health. Lower temperatures, immobilization, prolonged exposure, moisture, the presence of peripheral vascular disease, and open wounds all increase the severity of the injury.

A. Types

Three types of cold injury are seen in the trauma patient:

1. Frostnip is the mildest form of cold injury. It is characterized by initial pain, pallor, and numbness of the affected body part. It is reversible with rewarming and does not result in any tissue loss, unless the injury is repeated over many years, which causes fat pad loss or atrophy.

2. Frostbite is due to freezing of tissue from intracellular ice crystal formations and microvascular occlusion with subsequent tissue anoxia. Some of the tissue damage also may result from a reperfusion injury that occurs on rewarming. Similar to thermal burns, frostbite is classified into first, second, third, and fourth degree according to depth of involvement.

    a. First degree: Hyperemia and edema without skin necrosis

b. Second degree: Large, clear vesicle formation accompanies the hyperemia and edema with partial-thickness skin necrosis

c. Third degree: Full-thickness and subcutaneous tissue necrosis occurs, commonly with hemorrhage vesicle formation

d. Fourth degree: Full-thickness skin necrosis, including muscle and bone with gangrene

While the affected body part is initially nearly always hard, cold, white, and anesthetic, the appearance of the lesion changes frequently during the course of treatment. Additionally, the initial treatment regime is applicable for all degrees of insult and the initial classification is often not prognostically accurate. Hence, some authorities simply classify frostbite as superficial or deep.

3. Nonfreezing injury is due to microvascular endothelial damage, stasis, and vascular occlusion. Trench foot or cold immersion foot (or hand) describes a nonfreezing injury of the hands or feet, typically in soldiers, sailors, or fishermen, resulting from chronic exposure to wet conditions and temperatures just above freezing, ie, 1.6°C to 10°C (35°F to 50°F). Although the entire foot may appear black, deep tissue destruction may not be present. An alternating arterial vasospasm and vasodilatation occurs, with the affected tissue first cold and anesthetic, progressing to hyperemia in 24 to 48 hours. With hyperemia comes an intense painful burning and dysesthesia, as well as tissue damage characterized by edema, blistering, redness, ecchymosis, and ulcerations. Complications of local infection, cellulitis, lymphangitis, or gangrene can occur. Proper attention to foot hygiene can prevent the occurrence of most such injuries.

Chilblain, or pernio, is primarily a dermatologic manifestation of chronic repetitive damp cold exposure as might occur in fisherman, or chronic dry cold exposure as might occur in mountain climbers. It typically occurs on the face, anterior tibial surface, or dorsum of the hands and feet, areas poorly protected or chronically exposed to the environment. It is characterized by pruritic, red-purple skin lesions (papules, macules, plaques, or nodules). With continued exposure, ulcerative or hemorrhagic lesions appear and progress to scarring, fibrosis, or atrophy with itching replaced by tenderness and pain. It is more annoying and chronic than destructive. Careful protection from further exposure and the use of antiadrenergics or calcium channel blockers are often helpful.

B. Management of Frostbite and Nonfreezing Cold Injuries

Treatment should be immediate to decrease duration of tissue freezing, although rewarming should not be undertaken if there is the risk of refreezing. Constricting, damp clothing should be replaced by warm blankets and the patient should be given hot fluids by mouth, if able to drink.

Place the injured part in circulating water at a constant 40°C (104°F) until the pink color and perfusion return (usually within 20 to 30 minutes). This is best accomplished in an inpatient setting in a large tank, such as a whirlpool tank. Avoid dry heat and do not rub or massage the area. Rewarming can be extremely painful, and adequate analgesics (IV narcotics) are essential. Cardiac monitoring during rewarming is advised.

C. Local Wound Care of Frostbite

The goal of wound care for frostbite is to preserve damaged tissue by preventing infection, avoiding opening uninfected vesicles, and elevating the injured area, which is left open to air. The affected tissue should be protected by a tent or cradle and pressure spots should be avoided.

Only rarely is fluid loss massive enough to require resuscitation with intravenous fluids, although patients may be dehydrated. Tetanus prophylaxis depends on the patient's tetanus immunization status. Systemic antibiotics are reserved for identified infections. The wounds should be kept clean and uninfected blebs left intact for 7 to 10 days to provide a sterile biologic dressing to protect underlying epithelialization. Tobacco nicotine and other vasoconstrictive agents must be withheld. Weight bearing is prohibited until edema is resolved.

Numerous adjuvants have been tried in an effort to restore blood supply to cold-injured tissue. Unfortunately, most are ineffective. Sympathetic blockade (sympathectomy, drugs) and vasodilating agents have generally not helped in altering the natural history of the acute cold injury. Heparin, thrombolytic agents, and hyperbaric oxygen also have failed to demonstrate substantial treatment benefit. Low-molecular-weight dextran has shown some benefit during the rewarming phase in animal models.

With all cold injuries, estimations of depth of injury and extent of tissue damage are not usually accurate until demarcation is evident. This often requires

INJURIES DUE TO BURNS AND COLD

several weeks or months of observation. Earlier surgical debridement or amputation is seldom warranted unless infection with sepsis intervenes.

IX. COLD INJURY: SYSTEMIC HYPOTHERMIA

Hypothermia is defined as a core body temperature below 35°C (95°F). In the absence of concomitant traumatic injury, hypothermia may be classified as mild (35°C to 32°C or 95°F to 89.6°F), moderate (32°C to 30°C or 89.6°F to 86°F), or severe (below 30°C or 86°F). This drop in core temperature may be rapid, as in immersion in near-freezing water, or slow, as in exposure to more temperate environments. The elderly are particularly susceptible to this condition because of their impaired ability to increase heat production and decrease heat loss by vasoconstriction. Children also are more susceptible because of relative increased BSA and limited energy sources. Because determination of the core temperature, preferably esophageal, is essential for the diagnosis, special thermometers capable of registering low temperatures are required. Trauma patients also are susceptible to hypothermia, and **any** degree of hypothermia in the trauma patient may be detrimental. In these patients hypothermia should be considered to be any core temperature below 36°C (96.8°F), and severe hypothermia is any core temperature below 32°C (89.6°F). Hypothermia is common in the severely injured, but further loss of core temperature can be limited with the administration of **only** warmed intravenous fluids and blood, judicious exposure of the patient, and maintenance of a warm environment.

A. Signs of Hypothermia

In addition to a decrease in core temperature, a depressed level of consciousness is the most common feature of hypothermia. The patient is cold to touch and appears gray and cyanotic. Vital signs, including pulse rate, respiratory rate, and blood pressure, are all variable, and the absence of respiratory or cardiac activity is not uncommon in patients who eventually recover. Because of severe depression of the respiratory rate and heart rate, signs of respiratory and cardiac activity are easily missed unless careful assessment is conducted.

B. Management of Hypothermia

Immediate attention is devoted to the ABCDEs, including the initiation of cardiopulmonary resus-

citation (CPR) and the establishment of intravenous access if the patient is in cardiopulmonary arrest. Care must be taken to identify the presence of an organized cardiac rhythm; if one exists, sufficient circulation in patients with markedly reduced metabolism is probably present, and vigorous chest compressions may convert this rhythm to fibrillation. In the absence of an organized rhythm, CPR should be instituted and continued until the patient is rewarmed or there are other indications to discontinue CPR. However, the exact role of CPR as an adjunct to rewarming remains controversial.

Prevent heat loss by removing the patient from the cold environment and replacing wet, cold clothing with warm blankets. Administer oxygen via a bag-reservoir device. The patient should be managed in a critical care setting whenever possible. Cardiac monitoring is required. A careful search for associated disorders, such as diabetes, sepsis, and drug or alcohol ingestion, or occult injuries should be conducted. These disorders should be treated promptly. Blood should be drawn for CBC, electrolytes, blood glucose, alcohol, toxins screen, creatinine, amylase, and blood cultures. Abnormalities should be treated accordingly. For example, hypoglycemia would require intravenous glucose administration.

Determination of death can be very difficult in the hypothermic patient. Patients who appear to have suffered a cardiac arrest or death as a result of hypothermia should not be pronounced dead until they are rewarmed. **Remember the axiom: you are not dead until you are warm and dead!** An exception to this axiom is the hypothermic patient who has sustained an anoxic event while still normothermic, is without pulse or respiration, and has a serum potassium level greater than 10 mmol/L.

The rewarming technique depends on the patient's temperature and his or her response to simpler measures, as well as the presence or absence of concomitant injuries. For example, treat mild and moderate exposure hypothermia by **passive external rewarming** in a warm room using warm blankets, clothing, and warmed intravenous fluids. Severe hypothermia may require **active core rewarming methods** that may include invasive surgical rewarming techniques, eg, peritoneal lavage, thoracic/pleural lavage, A-V rewarming, or cardiopulmonary bypass, all of which are better done in a critical care setting.

Cardiac output falls proportional to the degree of hypothermia, and cardiac irritability begins at about 33°C (91.4°F). Ventricular fibrillation becomes increasingly common as the temperature falls below 28°C (82.4°F), and at temperatures below 25°C (77°F) asystole may occur. Cardiac drugs and defibrillation are not usually effective in the presence of acidosis, hypoxia, and hypothermia. In general, these treatment modalities should be reserved until the patient is warmed to at least 28°C (82.4°F). Bretylium tosylate is the only dysrhythmic agent known to be effective; lidocaine is reportedly ineffective in the hypothermic patient with ventricular fibrillation. Dopamine is the single inotropic agent that has some degree of action in the hypothermic patient. Administer 100% oxygen while the patient is being rewarmed. Arterial blood gases are probably best interpreted "uncorrected," ie, the blood warmed to 37°C (98.6°F), and those values used as guides to administering sodium bicarbonate and adjusting ventilation parameters during rewarming and resuscitation. Attempts to actively rewarm the patient should not delay transfer to a critical care setting.

X. SUMMARY

A. Burn Injury: Thermal, Chemical, Electrical

Immediate lifesaving measures for the burn patient include the **recognition of inhalation injury** and subsequent endotracheal intubation, and the rapid institution of intravenous fluid therapy. **All clothing should be removed rapidly.** Early stabilization and management of the burn patient include:

1. Identifying the extent and depth of the burn

2. Establishing fluid guidelines according to the patient's weight

3. Initiating a patient-care flow sheet

4. Obtaining baseline laboratory and x-ray studies

5. Maintaining peripheral circulation in circumferential burns by performing an escharotomy if necessary

6. Identifying which burn patients require transfer to a burn unit or center

B. Cold Injuries

Diagnose the cause and severity of cold injury by obtaining an adequate history and noting the physical findings as well as measuring the core tempera-

ture using a low-temperature range thermometer (esophageal temperature probe preferred). The patient should be removed from the cold environment immediately, and vital signs should be monitored and supported continuously. Rewarming techniques should be applied as soon as possible. The patient with hypothermia should not be considered dead until rewarming has occurred.

Early management of cold-injured patients includes:

1. Adhering to the ABCDEs of resuscitation

2. Identifying the type and extent of cold injury

3. Measuring the patient's core temperature

4. Initiating a patient-care flow sheet

5. Initiating rapid rewarming techniques

6. Determining the patient's life or death status after rewarming

■ BIBLIOGRAPHY

1. Amy BW, McManus WF, Goodwin CW Jr, et al: Lightning injury with survival in five patients. **Journal of the American Medical Association** 1985; 253:243–245.

2. Britt LD, Dascombe WH, Rodriguez A: New horizons in management of hypothermia and frostbite injury. **Surgical Clinics of North America** 1991; 71(2):345–370.

3. Cioffi WG, Graves TA, McManus WF, et al: High frequency percussive ventilation in patients with inhalation injury. **Journal of Trauma** 1989; 29:350–354.

4. Danzl D, Pozos R, Auerbach P, et al: Multicenter hypothermia survey. **Annals of Emergency Medicine** 1987; 16:1042–1055.

5. Demling HR: Burn care in the immediate resuscitation period. Section III, Thermal injury. In: Wilmor DW (ed): **Scientific American Surgery.** Scientific American Inc., New York, 1998.

6. Edlich R, Change D, Birk K, et al: Cold injuries. **Comprehensive Therapy** 1989; 15(9):13–21.

7. Gentilello LM, Cobean RA, Offner PJ, et al: Continuous arteriovenous rewarming: Rapid reversal of hypothermia in critically ill patients. **Journal of Trauma** 1992; 32(3):316–327.

INJURIES DUE TO BURNS AND COLD

8. Gentilello LM, Jurkovich GJ, Moujaes S: Hypothermia and injury: Thermodynamic principles of prevention and treatment. In: Levine B (ed): **Perspectives in Surgery.** St. Louis, Quality Medical Publishers, 1991.

9. Graves TA, Cioffi WG, McManus WF, et al: Fluid resuscitation of infants and children with massive thermal injury. **Journal of Trauma** 1988; 28(12):1656–1659.

10. Gunning K (ed): **Burns Trauma Handbook, 5th Edition.** The Liverpool Hospital Department of Trauma Services, July 1994.

11. Halebian P, Robinson N, Barie P, et al: Whole body oxygen utilization during carbon monoxide poisoning and isocapneic nitrogen hypoxia. **Journal of Trauma** 1986; 26:110–117.

12. Haponik EF, Munster AM (eds): **Respiratory Injury: Smoke Inhalation and Burns.** New York, McGraw-Hill, 1990.

13. Jacob J, Weisman M, Rosenblatt S, et al: Chronic pernio. A historical perspective of cold-induced vascular disease. **Archives of Internal Medicine** 1986; 146:1589–1592.

14. Jurkovich GJ: Hypothermia in the trauma patient. In: Maull KI, Cleveland HC, Strauch GO, et al (eds): **Advances in Trauma.** Chicago, Yearbook Medical Publishers, 1989, volume 4, pp 11–140.

15. Jurkovich GJ, Greiser W, Luterman A, et al: Hypothermia in trauma victims: An ominous predictor of survival. **Journal of Trauma** 1987; 27:1019–1024.

16. Lund T, Goodwin CW, McManus WF, et al: Upper airway sequelae in burn patients requiring endotracheal intubation or tracheostomy. **Annals of Surgery** 1985; 201:374–382.

17. McManus WF, Pruitt BA: Thermal injuries. In: Mattox RH, Moore EE, Feliciano CV (eds): **Trauma, 2nd Edition.** East Norwalk, CT, Appleton & Lange, 1991, pp 751–764.

18. Millard LG, Rowell NR: Chilblain lupus erythematosus (Hutchinson): A clinical and laboratory study of 17 patients. **British Journal of Dermatology** 1978; 98(5):497–506.

19. Mills WJ Jr: Summary of treatment of the cold injured patient: Frostbite [1983 classic article]. **Alaska Medicine** 1993; 35(1):61–66.

20. Moss J: Accidental severe hypothermia. **Surgery, Gynecology and Obstetrics** 1986; 162: 501–513.

21. Mozingo DW, Smith AA, McManus WF, et al: Chemical burns. **Journal of Trauma** 1988; 28: 642–647.

22. O'Malley J, Mills W, Kappes B, et al: Frostbite: General and specific treatment, the Alaskan method. **Alaska Medicine** 1993; 27(1):pullout.

23. Perry RJ, Moore CA, et al: Determining the approximate area of burn: An inconsistency investigated and reevaluated. **British Medical Journal** 1996; 312(7042):1338.

24. Pruitt BA Jr: The burn patient: I. Initial care. **Current Problems in Surgery** 1979; 16(4):1–55.

25. Pruitt BA Jr: The burn patient: II. Later care and complications of thermal injury. **Current Problems in Surgery** 1979; 16(5):1–95.

26. Reed R, Bracey A, Hudson J, et al: Hypothermia and blood coagulation: Dissociation between enzyme activity and clotting factor levels. **Circulatory Shock** 1990; 32:141–152.

27. Rustin M, Newton J, Smith N, et al: The treatment of chilblains with nifedipine: The results of a pilot study, a double-blind placebo-controlled randomized study and a long-term open trial. **British Journal of Dermatology** 1989; 120: 267–275.

28. Saffle JR, Crandall A, Warden GD: Cataracts: A long-term complication of electrical injury. **Journal of Trauma** 1985; 25:17–21.

29. Schaller M, Fischer A, Perret C: Hyperkalemia: A prognostic factor during acute severe hypothermia. **Journal of the American Medical Association** 1990; 264(14):1842–1845.

30. Sheehy TW, Navari RM: Hypothermia. **Alaskan Journal of Medical Science** 1984; 21(4):374–381.

31. Stratta RJ, Saffle JR, Kravitz M, et al: Management of tar and asphalt injuries. **American Journal of Surgery** 1983; 146:766–769.

CHAPTER 10

Extremes of Age:
A. Pediatric Trauma

■ OBJECTIVES:

Upon completion of this topic, the participant will be able to demonstrate an ability to apply the principles of trauma care for managing the acutely injured pediatric patient. Specifically, the participant will be able to:

A. Identify the unique characteristics of the child as a trauma patient.

1. Types of injury

2. Patterns of injury

3. Anatomic and physiologic differences in children as compared with adults

4. Long-term effects of injury

B. Discuss the primary management of the following critical injuries in children based on the anatomic and physiologic differences as compared with adults.

1. Airway management

2. Shock and maintenance of body heat

3. Fluid and electrolyte management

4. Medications and dosages

5. Central nervous system and cervical spine injuries

6. Psychologic support

C. Identify the injury patterns associated with the abused child and the elements that lead to the suspicion of child abuse.

EXTREMES OF AGE: A. PEDIATRIC TRAUMA

I. INTRODUCTION

Injury continues to be the most common cause of death and disability in childhood. Over 10 million children require emergency department care each year in the United States for treatment of injuries, representing nearly 1 out of every 6 children. More than 10,000 children die each year in the United States from serious injury. (See Table 1, Top Five Injury Mechanisms and Related Mortality.) Injury morbidity and mortality surpass all major diseases in children and young adults, making injury the most serious public health and health care problem in this population. Motor vehicle-associated injuries are the most common cause of deaths in children of all ages, whether the child is an occupant, a pedestrian, or a cyclist. Deaths due to drowning, house fires, homicides, and falls follow in descending order. Child battering accounts for the majority of homicides in infants. Firearm injuries account for the majority of homicides in children and adolescents. Falls account for the majority of all pediatric injuries, but infrequently result in death. Blunt mechanisms of injury and the child's body habitus result in multisystem injury being the rule rather than the exception. (See Table 2, page 245, Common Mechanisms of Injury and Associated Patterns of Injury.) Therefore, it must be presumed that all organ systems are injured until proven otherwise. Penetrating injuries have increased in childhood and adolescence in many large cities. **Children with multisystem injuries can deteriorate rapidly and develop serious complications. Therefore, such patients should be transferred early to a facility capable of managing the child with multisystem injuries.**

The priorities of assessment and management of the injured child are the same as in the adult. However, the unique anatomic and physiologic characteristics of the pediatric patient combine with the different mechanisms of injury to produce distinct patterns of injury. (See Table 2, page 245, Common Mechanisms of Injury and Associated Patterns of Injury.) For example, most serious pediatric trauma is blunt trauma that involves the brain. As a result, apnea, hypoventilation, and hypoxia occur five (5) times more commonly than hypovolemia with hypotension in seriously injured children. Therefore, management protocols for the pediatric trauma patient include greater emphasis on aggressive management of the airway and breathing.

A. Size and Shape

Because of the smaller body mass of children, the energy imparted from fenders, bumpers, and falls results in a greater force applied per unit body area. This more intense energy is transmitted to a body with less fat, less connective tissue, and close proximity of multiple organs. This results in the high frequency of multiple organ injuries seen in the pediatric population. Additionally, the head is

Table 1—Top Five Injury Mechanisms and Related Mortality

	0–5 YEARS	6–10 YEARS	>10 YEARS
Proportion	35%	27%	37%
Mortality	3.1%	2.2%	3.3%
Mechanism	Fall (0.8%) MV (5.3%) Peds (5.3%) Struck (1.9%) Stab (1%)	Fall (0.1%) Peds (4.7%) Bike (1.5%) MV (4.6%) Sport (0.7%)	MV (3.9%) Fall (0.5%) Bike (2.2%) GSW (9.6%) Sport (0.2%)
Proportion of all injuries	82%	83%	69%

Abbreviations: MV = motor vehicular; peds = pedestrian; stab = stabbing; struck = inadvertently struck by object; GSW = gunshot wound; sport = sports-related. Mortality for each mechanism listed is identified in parentheses beside abbreviation.

Table 2—Common Mechanisms of Injury and Associated Patterns of Injury

MECHANISM OF INJURY	COMMON PATTERNS OF INJURY
Motor vehicle crash (child is passenger)	• Unrestrained: Multiple trauma, head and neck injuries, scalp and facial lacerations • Restrained: Chest and abdomen injuries, lower spine fractures
Motor vehicle crash (child is pedestrian)	• Low speed: Lower extremity fractures • High speed: Multiple trauma, head and neck injuries, lower extremity fractures
Fall from a height	• Low: Upper extremity fractures • Medium: Head and neck injuries, upper and lower extremity fractures • High: Multiple trauma, head and neck injuries, upper and lower extremity fractures
Fall from a bicycle	• Without helmet: Head and neck lacerations, scalp and facial lacerations, upper extremity fractures • With helmet: Upper extremity fractures • Striking handlebar: Internal abdominal injuries

proportionately larger in young children, resulting in a higher frequency of blunt brain injuries in this age group.

B. Skeleton

The child's skeleton is incompletely calcified, contains multiple active growth centers, and is more pliable. For these reasons, internal organ damage is often noted without overlying bony fracture. For example, rib fractures in the child are uncommon, but pulmonary contusion is frequent. Other soft tissues of the thorax, the heart, and mediastinal structures also may sustain significant damage without evidence of bony injury. The identification of rib fractures in a child suggests the transfer of a massive amount of energy, and multiple, serious organ injuries should be suspected.

C. Surface Area

The ratio of a child's body surface area to body volume is highest at birth and diminishes as the child matures. As a result, thermal energy loss is a significant stress factor in the child. Hypothermia may

develop quickly and complicate the management of the hypotensive pediatric patient.

D. Psychologic Status

Psychologic ramifications of caring for an injured child can present significant challenges. In the very young, emotional instability frequently leads to a regressive psychologic behavior when stress, pain, or other perceived threats intervene in the child's environment. The child's ability to interact with unfamiliar individuals in strange and difficult situations is limited, making history taking and cooperative manipulation, especially if it is painful, extremely difficult. The doctor who understands these characteristics and is willing to cajole and soothe an injured child is more likely to establish a good rapport. This facilitates comprehensive assessment of the child's psychologic as well as physical injuries.

E. Long-term Effects

A major consideration in dealing with injured children is the effect that injury may have on subsequent growth and development. Unlike the adult, the child must not only recover from the effects of the traumatic event, but also must continue the normal process of growth and development. The physiologic and psychologic effects of injury on this process should not be underestimated, particularly in those cases involving long-term function, growth deformity, or subsequent abnormal development. Children sustaining even a minor injury may have prolonged disability in either cerebral function, psychologic adjustment, or organ system disability. Recent evidence suggests that as many as 60% of children who sustain severe multisystem trauma have residual personality changes at 1 year following hospital discharge, and 50% show cognitive and physical handicaps. Social, affective, and learning disabilities are present in half of seriously injured children. Additionally, childhood injuries have a significant impact on the family structure, with personality and emotional disturbances found in two-thirds of uninjured siblings. Frequently, a child's injuries impose a strain on the parents' marital relationship, including financial and sometimes employment hardships.

Trauma may affect not only the child's survival, but also perhaps just as importantly, the quality of the child's life for years to come. Bony and solid visceral injuries are cases in point. Injuries through growth centers may result in growth abnormalities of the injured bone. If the injured bone is a femur, a leg length discrepancy may result in lifelong disability with running and walking. If the fracture is through the growth center of a thoracic vertebra(e), the result may be scoliosis, kyphosis, or even gibbus. Massive disruption of a child's spleen may require a splenectomy. The loss of the spleen predisposes the child to a lifelong risk of overwhelming postsplenectomy sepsis and death.

F. Equipment

Immediately available equipment of the appropriate size is essential for successful initial management of the injured child. (See Table 6, page 262, Pediatric Equipment.) Broselow™ Pediatric Emergency Tape is an ideal adjunct for rapid determination of weight based on length for appropriate drug doses and equipment size. (See Skills Station IV, page 87, Shock Assessment and Management.)

II. AIRWAY: EVALUATION AND MANAGEMENT

The "A" of the ABCDEs of initial assessment is the same in the child as it is in the adult. Establishing a patent airway to provide adequate tissue oxygenation is the first objective. The inability to establish and/or maintain a patent airway with lack of oxygenation and ventilation is the most common cause of cardiac arrest in the child. Therefore, the child's airway is the first priority.

A. Anatomy

The smaller the child, the greater is the disproportion between the size of the cranium and the midface. This produces a greater propensity for the posterior pharyngeal area to buckle as the relatively larger occiput forces passive flexion of the cervical spine. Avoiding passive flexion of the cervical spine requires that the plane of the midface be kept parallel to the spine board in the "sniffing position." (See Figure 1, page 247, Improper Positioning of the Child to Maintain a Patent Airway.) Careful attention to maintaining this position while providing maximum protection to the cervical spine is especially important in the obtunded child. Because of the larger occiput, placement of a layer of padding is required beneath the infant's or toddler's entire torso to preserve neutral alignment of the spinal column. (See Figure 2, page 248, Proper Positioning of the Child to Maintain a Patient Airway.) Soft tissues in the infant's oropharynx (ie, tongue, tonsils) are relatively large compared with the oral cavity, which may make visualization of the larynx difficult.

A child's larynx is funnel-shaped, allowing secretions to accumulate in the retropharyngeal area. It is also more cephalad and anterior in the neck and the vocal cords have a slightly more anterocaudal angle. The vocal cords are frequently more difficult to visualize during intubation when the child's head is in the normal supine anatomical position. The infant's trachea is approximately 5 cm long and grows to 7 cm by about 18 months. Failure to appreciate this short length may result in intubation of the right mainstem bronchus, inadequate ventilation, accidental tube dislodgment and/or mechanical barotrauma.

B. Management

In a spontaneously breathing child with a partially obstructed airway, the airway should be optimized by placing the child's head in the sniffing position while maintaining neutral alignment of the cervical spine. (See Figure 2, page 248, Proper Positioning of the Child to Maintain a Patent Airway.) The airway also may be opened by the chin lift or jaw thrust maneuver combined with bimanual inline spinal immobilization. After the mouth and oropharynx are cleared of secretions or debris, supplemental oxygen should be administered. If the patient is unconscious, mechanical methods of maintaining the airway may be necessary. **Before attempts are made to mechanically establish an airway, the child should be oxygenated.**

1. Oral airway

The oral airway should only be inserted when a child is unconscious. If placed when the child's gag reflex is maintained, vomiting is likely. The practice of inserting the airway backwards and rotating it 180° is not recommended for the pediatric patient. Trauma with resultant hemorrhage into soft-tissue structures of the oropharynx may occur. The oral airway should be gently inserted directly into the oropharynx. The use of a tongue blade to depress the tongue may be helpful.

2. Orotracheal intubation

Endotracheal intubation is indicated for the injured child in a variety of situations, eg, the child with severe brain injury requiring controlled ventilation, the child who cannot maintain an airway, the child exhibiting signs of ventilatory failure, or the child suffering significant hypovolemia who requires operative intervention.

Orotracheal intubation is the most reliable means of establishing an airway and ventilating the child. Uncuffed tubes of appropriate size should be used to avoid subglottic edema, ulceration, and disruption of the infant's fragile airway. The smallest area of the child's airway is at the cricoid ring, which forms a natural seal with the endotracheal tube. Therefore, cuffed endotracheal tubes are rarely needed in children under the age of 9 years. A simple technique to gauge the size of the endotracheal tube is to approximate the diameter of the child's external nares or the child's little finger to the tube diameter. The Broselow™ Pedi-

FIGURE 1
Improper Positioning of the Child to Maintain a Patent Airway

Plane of face is **not** parallel to spine board

When placed on a spine board without padding, a young child's relatively large head forces the neck into a kyphotic position and buckles the airway, causing partial obstruction.

(Adapted with permission from Herzenberg JE, Hensinger RN, Dedrick DK, et al: Emergency transport and positioning of young children who have an injury of the cervical spine. The standard backboard may be hazardous. *Journal of Bone and Joint Surgery* 1989; 71-A:15-22.

EXTREMES OF AGE: A. PEDIATRIC TRAUMA

FIGURE 2
Proper Positioning of the Child to Maintain a Patent Airway

Plane of face is parallel to spine board

When placed on a spine board with a layer of padding, a young child's chest is raised, allowing for safe cervical spine positioning and maintenance of the airway in a sniffing position.

(Adapted with permission from Herzenberg JE, Hensinger RN, Dedrick DK, et al: Emergency transport and positioning of young children who have an injury of the cervical spine. The standard backboard may be hazardous. *Journal of Bone and Joint Surgery* 1989; 71-A:15-22.

atric Emergency Tape also lists appropriate tube sizes for endotracheal intubation.

Most trauma centers utilize a protocol for emergency intubation, referred to as rapid sequence intubation (RSI). Careful attention must be paid to the child's weight, vital signs (pulse and blood pressure), and level of consciousness to determine which branch of the algorithm is to be utilized. (See Algorithm 1, page 249, Rapid Sequence Intubation [RSI] for the Pediatric Patient.)

The child who requires an endotracheal tube for airway control should first be preoxygenated. Infants and children have a more pronounced vagal response to endotracheal intubation than adults do. Such responses may be caused by hypoxia, vagal stimulation during laryngoscopy or pharmacologic agents. They can be minimized by atropine pretreatment. Atropine also dries oral secretions, permitting easier visualization of landmarks for intubation. The dose of atropine is 0.02 mg/kg with a minimal dose of 0.1 mg and maximal initial dose of 1.0 mg given at least 1 to 2 minutes before intubation. The child should then be sedated. The normovolemic child can be se-

dated with etomidate (0.3 mg/kg) or midazolam (0.3 mg/kg). However, the hypotensive child should be sedated with etomidate (0.3 mg/kg) or midazolam (0.1 mg/kg). The specific antidote for midazolam is flumazenil, which should be immediately available. After sedation, cricoid pressure is maintained to help avoid aspiration of gastric contents. This is followed by paralysis with 1 of 2 agents. Ideally, short-acting paralysis agents should be used, eg, succinylcholine. Succinylcholine has a rapid onset, its action is of short duration, and it may be a safer drug of choice. If a longer period of paralysis is needed, eg, the child who needs a CT scan for further evaluation, vecuronium may be indicated. After the endotracheal tube is inserted, its position must be assessed and, if correct, the cricoid pressure then can be released. If it is not possible to place the endotracheal tube after the child is paralyzed, the child must be ventilated with a bag-valve-mask device until a definitive airway is secured.

Orotracheal intubation under direct vision with adequate immobilization and protection of the cervical spine is the preferred method of obtaining initial airway control. Nasotracheal

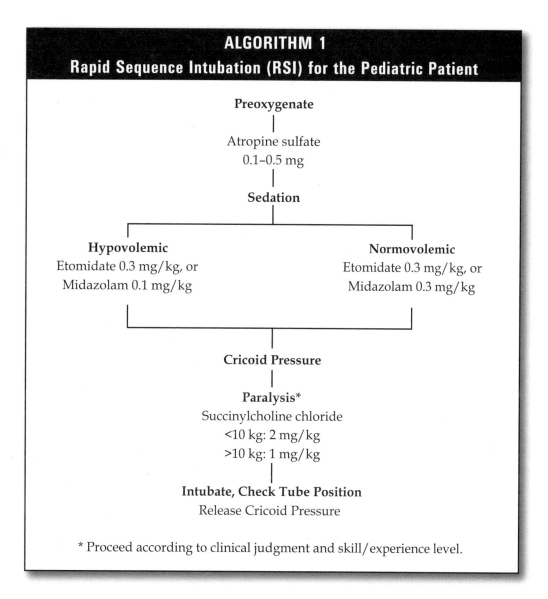

ALGORITHM 1
Rapid Sequence Intubation (RSI) for the Pediatric Patient

Preoxygenate

Atropine sulfate
0.1–0.5 mg

Sedation

Hypovolemic	**Normovolemic**
Etomidate 0.3 mg/kg, or	Etomidate 0.3 mg/kg, or
Midazolam 0.1 mg/kg	Midazolam 0.3 mg/kg

Cricoid Pressure

Paralysis*
Succinylcholine chloride
<10 kg: 2 mg/kg
>10 kg: 1 mg/kg

Intubate, Check Tube Position
Release Cricoid Pressure

* Proceed according to clinical judgment and skill/experience level.

intubation should not be performed in children under the age of 9 years. Nasotracheal intubation requires blind passage around a relatively acute angle in the nasopharynx toward the anterosuperiorly located glottis, making intubation by this route difficult. The potential for penetrating the child's cranial vault or damaging the more prominent nasopharyngeal (ie, adenoidal) soft tissues resulting in hemorrhage also makes the nasotracheal route for airway control ill-advised.

Once past the glottic opening, the endotracheal tube should be positioned 2 to 3 cm below the level of the vocal cords and carefully secured in place. Auscultation of both hemithoraces in the axillae should be performed to ensure that right mainstem bronchial intubation has not occurred, and that both sides of the chest are being adequately ventilated. A chest x-ray may be obtained to accurately identify the position of the endotracheal tube. Any movement of the head may result in displacement of the endotracheal tube. Breath sounds should be evaluated periodically to ensure that the tube remains in the appropriate position and to identify the possibility of evolving ventilatory dysfunction.

3. Cricothyroidotomy

When airway access and control cannot be accomplished by bag-valve-mask or orotracheal intubation, needle cricothyroidotomy is the

EXTREMES OF AGE: A. PEDIATRIC TRAUMA

preferred method. Needle jet insufflation via the cricothyroid membrane is an appropriate, temporizing technique for oxygenation, but it does not provide adequate ventilation, and progressive hypercarbia may occur. (See Chapter 2, Airway and Ventilatory Management.)

Surgical cricothyroidotomy is rarely indicated for the infant or small child. Surgical cricothyroidotomy can be performed in the older child in whom the cricothyroid membrane is easily palpable (usually by the age of 12 years).

III. BREATHING: EVALUATION AND MANAGEMENT

A. Breathing and Ventilation

The respiratory rate in the child decreases with age. An infant requires 40 to 60 breaths/minute, whereas the older child breathes 20 times/minute. Normal spontaneous tidal volumes vary from 6 to 8 mL/kg for infants and children, although slightly larger tidal volumes of 7 to 10 mL/kg may be required during assisted ventilation. Although most bag-valve-mask devices used with pediatric patients are designed to limit the amount of pressure that can be exerted manually on the child's airway, the doctor must remember the fragile nature of the immature tracheobronchial tree and alveoli to minimize the potential for iatrogenic bronchoalveolar injury.

Hypoxia is the most common cause of cardiac arrest in the child. However, before cardiac arrest occurs, hypoventilation causes a respiratory acidosis, which is the most common acid-base abnormality encountered during resuscitation of the injured child. With adequate ventilation and perfusion the child should be able to maintain a relatively normal pH. **Caution: In the absence of adequate ventilation and perfusion, attempting to correct an acidosis with sodium bicarbonate results in further hypercarbia and worsened acidosis.**

B. Tube Thoracostomy

Injuries that disrupt pleural apposition, eg, hemothorax, pneumothorax, or hemopneumothorax occur in children as in adults with similar physiologic consequences. These injuries are managed with pleural decompression. Chest tubes are of smaller size (see Table 6, page 262, Pediatric Equipment) and are placed into the thoracic cavity by tunnel-ing the tube over the rib above the skin incision site and directing it superiorly and posteriorly along the inside of the chest wall. The site of chest tube insertion is the same in the child as in the adult, the 5th intercostal space, just anterior to the anterior midaxillary line.

IV. CIRCULATION AND SHOCK: EVALUATION AND MANAGEMENT

A. Recognition

Injury in childhood may result in significant blood loss. The increased physiologic reserve of the child allows maintenance of most vital signs in the normal range, even in the presence of shock. This may be misleading to those not familiar with the subtle physiologic changes manifested by the child in hypovolemic shock. Tachycardia and poor skin perfusion often are the only keys to early recognition of hypovolemia and the early initiation of appropriate crystalloid fluid resuscitation. **Early assessment of the child by a surgeon is essential to the appropriate management of the injured child.** A 30% diminution in circulating blood volume is required to manifest a change in the child's vital signs.

The primary response to hypovolemia in the child is tachycardia. However, caution must be exercised when monitoring only the child's heart rate because tachycardia also may be caused by pain, fear, and psychological stress. Other more subtle signs of blood loss in the child include loss of peripheral pulses, a narrowing of pulse pressure to less than 20 mm Hg, skin mottling, cool extremities compared with torso skin, and a decrease in level of consciousness with a dulled response to pain. A decrease in blood pressure and other indices of inadequate organ perfusion, eg, urinary output, should be monitored closely but generally develop later than tachycardia, skin mottling, and decreased pulse pressure during blood loss. All of the aforementioned findings are considered to be hemodynamic abnormalities. Changes in vital organ function are outlined in Table 3, page 251, Systemic Responses to Blood Loss in the Pediatric Patient.

The lower limit of normal systolic blood pressure in the child is 70 mm Hg plus twice the age in years, and the diastolic pressure should be two-thirds of the systolic blood pressure. Hypotension in the child represents a state of uncompensated shock and indicates severe blood loss of greater than 45% of his or

Table 3—Systemic Responses to Blood Loss in the Pediatric Patient

SYSTEM	MILD BLOOD VOLUME LOSS (<30%)	MODERATE BLOOD VOLUME LOSS (30%–45%)	SEVERE BLOOD VOLUME LOSS (>45%)
Cardiovascular	↑ Heart rate; weak, thready peripheral pulses	Low normal blood pressure, narrowed pulse pressure, markedly ↑ heart rate; absent peripheral pulses with weak, thready central pulses	Hypotension; tachycardia then bradycardia
Central Nervous System	Anxious, irritable, confused	Lethargic, dulled response to pain[1]	Comatose
Skin	Cool, mottled; prolonged capillary refill	Cyanotic; markedly prolonged capillary refill	Pale, cold
Urinary Output	Minimal ↓	Minimal	None

[1]The child's dulled response to pain with this degree of blood loss (30%-45%) is often indicated by the decreased response noted when an IV catheter is inserted.

her circulating blood volume. Tachycardia changing to bradycardia often accompanies this hypotension. This change may occur suddenly in infants. These physiologic changes must be treated by a rapid infusion of both crystalloid and blood. (See Table 4, page 252, Vital Functions.)

B. Fluid Resuscitation

The goal in fluid resuscitation in the child is to rapidly replace the circulating volume. A child's blood volume can be estimated at 80 mL/kg. When shock is suspected, a fluid bolus, using warmed fluids, of 20 mL/kg of crystalloid solution is required. This initial 20 mL/kg bolus, if it were to remain in the vascular space, would represent 25% of the child's blood volume. Because the goal is to replace the lost intravascular volume, it may be necessary to give 3 boluses of 20 mL/kg or a total of 60 mL/kg to achieve a replacement of the lost 25%. The 3-for-1 rule applies to the pediatric patient as well as the adult patient. (See Chapter 3, Shock.) When starting the third 20 mL/kg bolus, consideration should be given to the use of packed red blood cells (PRBCs). PRBCs are administered as a bolus of 10 mL/kg. (See Algorithm 2, page 253, Resuscitation Flow Diagram for the Pediatric Patient with Normal and Abnormal Hemodynamics.)

Fluid resuscitation in the child is based on the child's weight. It is often very difficult for emergency department personnel to estimate the weight of a child, particularly if these personnel do not treat many children. The easiest and quickest method of determining the child's weight to accurately calculate fluid volumes and drug dosages is with the Broselow™ Pediatric Emergency Tape. This tool rapidly provides the child's approximate weight, respiratory rate, fluid resuscitation volume, and a variety of drug dosages.

The injured child should be monitored carefully for response to fluid resuscitation and to the adequacy of organ perfusion. A return toward hemodynamic normality is indicated by:

- Slowing of the heart rate (<130 beats/minute with improvement of other physiologic signs) (age dependent)
- Clearing of the sensorium
- Return of peripheral pulses
- Return of normal skin color
- Increased warmth of extremities
- Increased systolic blood pressure (approximately 90 mm Hg plus twice the age in years)
- Increased pulse pressure (>20 mm Hg)

EXTREMES OF AGE: A. PEDIATRIC TRAUMA

Table 4—Vital Functions

AGE GROUP (in years)	WEIGHT RANGE (in kg)	HEART RATE (beats/min)	BLOOD PRESSURE (mm Hg)	RESPIRATORY RATE (breaths/min)	URINARY OUTPUT (mL/kg/hr)
Infant 0–1	0–10	<160	>60	<60	2.0
Toddler 1–3	10–14	<150	>70	<40	1.5
Preschool 3–5	14–18	<140	>75	<35	1.0
School age 6–12	18–36	<120	>80	<30	1.0
Adolescent >12	36–70	<100	>90	<30	0.5

- Urinary output of 1 to 2 mL/kg/hour (age dependent)

Children generally have 1 of 3 responses to fluid resuscitation. Most children will be stabilized by the use of crystalloid fluid only and do not require blood (responders). Some children respond to crystalloid and blood resuscitation (responders). Some children initially respond to crystalloid fluid and blood then deteriorate (transient responders). Other children do not respond at all to crystalloid fluid and blood infusion (nonresponders). These children (transient and nonresponders) are candidates for prompt infusion of additional blood and consideration for operation.

The resuscitation flow diagram is a useful aid in the initial management of the injured child. (See Algorithm 2, page 253, Resuscitation Flow Diagram for the Pediatric Patient with Normal and Abnormal Hemodynamics.)

C. Blood Replacement

Failure to improve hemodynamic abnormalities following the first bolus of resuscitation fluid raises the suspicion of continuing hemorrhage, prompts the need for administration of a second and perhaps a third 20 mL/kg bolus of crystalloid fluid, and requires the prompt involvement of a surgeon. When starting the third bolus of crystalloid fluid or if the child's condition deteriorates, consideration must be given to the use of 10 mL/kg of type-specific or O-negative warmed PRBCs.

D. Venous Access

Severe hypovolemic shock usually occurs as the result of disruption of intrathoracic or intraabdominal organ systems or blood vessels. Venous access should preferably be established by a peripheral percutaneous route. If percutaneous access is unsuccessful after 2 attempts, consideration should be given to intraosseous infusion or direct venous cutdown. In special situations, a doctor with skill and expertise can safely insert a femoral venous line.

The preferred sites for venous access in children are:

- Percutaneous peripheral (2 attempts)
- Intraosseous
- Percutaneous placement—Femoral vein
- Venous cutdown—Saphenous vein at the ankle
- Percutaneous placement—External jugular vein (do not use if airway compromise or cervical collar applied)

Intravenous access in the hypovolemic child younger than 6 years of age is a perplexing and challenging problem, even in the most experienced hands. Intraosseous infusion, cannulating the marrow cavity of a long bone in an uninjured extremity, is an emergent-access procedure for the critically ill or injured child. The intraosseous route is safe, efficacious, and requires less time than does venous cutdown. However, intraosseous infusion should

American College of Surgeons

EXTREMES OF AGE: A. PEDIATRIC TRAUMA

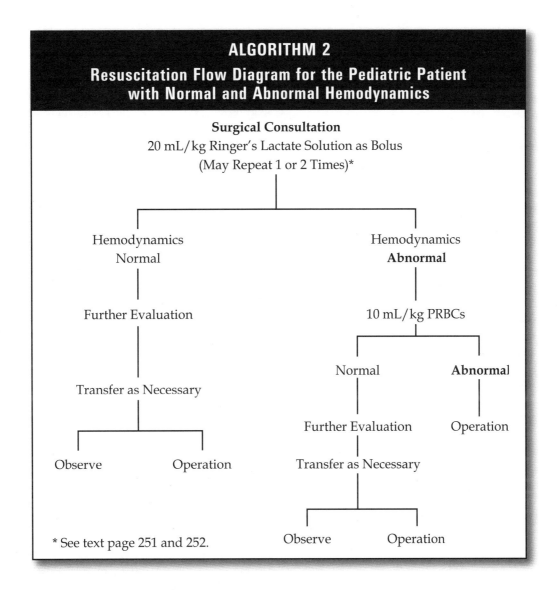

ALGORITHM 2

Resuscitation Flow Diagram for the Pediatric Patient with Normal and Abnormal Hemodynamics

Surgical Consultation

20 mL/kg Ringer's Lactate Solution as Bolus

(May Repeat 1 or 2 Times)*

Hemodynamics Normal

Further Evaluation

Transfer as Necessary

Observe   Operation

Hemodynamics **Abnormal**

10 mL/kg PRBCs

Normal   **Abnormal**

Further Evaluation   Operation

Transfer as Necessary

Observe   Operation

* See text page 251 and 252.

be discontinued when suitable peripheral venous access has been established.

Indications for intraosseous infusion are limited to children for whom venous access is impossible due to circulatory collapse or for whom percutaneous peripheral venous cannulation has failed on 2 attempts. Complications of this procedure include cellulitis rarely, osteomyelitis, compartment syndrome, and iatrogenic fracture. The preferred site for intraosseous cannulation is the proximal tibia, below the level of the tibial tuberosity. If the tibia is fractured, the needle may be inserted into the distal femur. Intraosseous cannulation should not be performed distal to a fracture site. (See Skills Station IV, Shock Assessment and Management.)

E. Urinary Output

Urinary output varies with age, as does the blood volume. Urinary output for the newborn and infant, up to 1 year, is 2 mL/kg/hour. The toddler has a urinary output of 1.5 mL/kg/hour, and the older child has a urinary output of 1 mL/kg/hour through adolescence. Not until the child has stopped growing does the lower limit of urinary output achieve the normal adult value of 0.5 mL/kg/hour. (See Table 4, page 252, Vital Functions.)

Urinary output combined with urinary specific gravity is an excellent method of determining the adequacy of volume resuscitation. Once the circulating blood volume has been restored, the urinary

EXTREMES OF AGE: A. PEDIATRIC TRAUMA

output can be expected to return to normal. A urinary catheter should be inserted to accurately measure the child's urinary output. A straight catheter, rather than a catheter with an inflatable retaining device, may be used in children weighing less than 15 kg.

F. Thermoregulation

The high ratio of BSA to body mass in children increases heat exchange with the environment and directly affects the child's ability to regulate core temperature. Thin skin and the lack of substantial subcutaneous tissue contribute to increased evaporative heat loss and caloric expenditure. Hypothermia may render the injured child refractory to treatment, prolong coagulation times, and adversely affect CNS function. While the child is exposed during the initial survey and resuscitation phase, overhead heat lamps or heaters or thermal blankets may be necessary to maintain body temperature to preserve body heat, warm the room as well as the intravenous fluids, blood products, and inhaled gases.

V. CHEST TRAUMA

Eight percent of all injuries in children involve the chest. Chest injury also is a marker for other organ system injury, since more than two-thirds of children with chest injury have been shown to have other organ system injuries. Certain types of chest injury, specifically rib fractures, represent an additional marker for the severity of the injuring force. The mechanism of injury and the anatomy of the child's chest are directly responsible for the spectrum of injuries seen.

The vast majority of chest injuries in childhood are due to blunt mechanisms, caused principally by the motor vehicle. The pliability and softness of the child's chest wall results in transmission of forces within the thoracic skeleton to the lung resulting in injury to the pulmonary parenchyma. Rib fractures in childhood are not common. However, when they do occur, the force required to break the ribs is significantly greater than it is in adults, and thus is an indication of the severity of the injuring force. The compliant chest wall causes the high frequency of pulmonary contusion seen in the child. The specific injuries caused by thoracic trauma in the child are identical to those encountered in the adult, although the frequencies of occurrence of those injuries are

somewhat different. Thoracotomy is not generally needed in the child.

Mobility of mediastinal structures makes the child more sensitive to tension pneumothorax and flail segments. The pliable chest wall increases the frequency of pulmonary contusions and direct intrapulmonary hemorrhage, usually without overlying rib fractures. Diaphragmatic rupture, aortic transection, major tracheobronchial tears, flail chest, and cardiac contusions are rarely encountered in childhood. When identified, treatment is the same as in the adult. Significant injuries rarely occur alone and are frequently a component of major multisystem injury.

The incidence of penetrating thoracic injury increases after 10 years of age. Penetrating trauma to the chest is managed in the same manner as in the adult.

VI. ABDOMINAL TRAUMA

Most pediatric abdominal injuries occur as the result of blunt trauma, primarily involving motor vehicles and falls. Penetrating abdominal injuries dictate prompt involvement by the surgeon. The hypotensive child who sustains penetrating abdominal trauma requires prompt operative intervention.

A. Assessment

The conscious infant and young child are generally frightened by the events preceding admission to the emergency department, and this may influence the examination of the abdomen. While talking quietly and calmly to the child, ask questions about the presence of abdominal pain and gently assess the tone of the abdominal musculature. Deep painful palpation of the abdomen should be avoided at the onset of the examination to prevent voluntary guarding that may confuse the abdominal findings. Almost all infants and young children who are stressed and crying will swallow large amounts of air. Decompression of the stomach by inserting a gastric tube should be a part of the resuscitation phase. Orogastric tube decompression is preferred in infants. Tenseness of the abdominal wall often decreases as gastric distention is relieved, allowing for more careful and reliable evaluation. Abdominal examination in the unconscious patient does not vary greatly with age. Decompression of the urinary bladder also facilitates abdominal evaluation.

EXTREMES OF AGE: A. PEDIATRIC TRAUMA

B. Diagnostic Adjuncts

1. Computed tomography (CT)

The advent of helical CT scanning allows for extremely rapid and precise identification of injuries. CT scanning is often used to evaluate the abdomen of children who have sustained blunt trauma and who are hemodynamically normal. It must be immediately available, performed early, and when employed **not delay further treatment.** The identification of intraabdominal injuries by CT scan in hemodynamically normal pediatric patients may allow nonoperative management by the surgeon.

The injured child who requires a CT scan as an adjunctive study often requires sedation to prevent movement during the scanning process. CT may be performed with contrast as appropriate.

2. Diagnostic peritoneal lavage (DPL)

DPL is used to detect intraabdominal bleeding in the hypotensive child, when ultrasonography is not readily available.

As in the adult, warmed Ringer's lactate solution in volumes of 10 mL/kg (up to 1000 mL) is used. **Remember,** the child's abdominal wall is relatively thin compared with that of the adult. Uncontrolled penetration of the peritoneal cavity can produce iatrogenic injury to the abdominal contents, even with an open technique. DPL has utility in diagnosing injuries to intraabdominal viscera only. Retroperitoneal organs cannot be evaluated reliably by this technique. The interpretation of a positive lavage is the same in both children and adults. Aspiration of blood on catheter insertion or greater than 100,000 RBCs/mm³ in the lavage is considered a positive finding. Although the definition of a positive peritoneal lavage is the same for children and adults, the presence of blood in the peritoneum does not in and of itself mandate celiotomy in a child who responds to resuscitation. The presence of leukocytosis, feces, vegetable fibers, and/or bile in the lavage mandates celiotomy. (See C., Nonoperative Management.)

Only the surgeon who will care for the child should perform the diagnostic peritoneal lavage.

3. Focused Assessment Sonography in Trauma (FAST)

Few studies on the efficacy of ultrasound in the child with abdominal injury have been reported. Therefore, the role of abdominal ultrasound in children in the emergency department remains to be defined. In children, FAST performed in the emergency department may identify intraabdominal blood.

C. Nonoperative Management

Selective, nonoperative management of children with blunt abdominal injuries is performed in many trauma centers. The presence of intraperitoneal blood on CT, DPL, or FAST does not necessarily mandate a celiotomy. It has been well demonstrated that bleeding from an injured spleen, liver, and kidney generally is self-limited. Therefore, a FAST or DPL that is positive for fluid or blood alone does not mandate a celiotomy in a child with initial abnormal hemodynamics that are readily normalized by fluid resuscitation. **If the child cannot be normalized hemodynamically and if the diagnostic procedure performed is positive for blood, a prompt celiotomy to control hemorrhage is indicated.**

When nonoperative management is selected as the treatment modality, these children **must** be managed in a facility offering pediatric intensive care capabilities and under the supervision of a qualified surgeon with special interest in and commitment to the care for the injured child. Intensive care must include continuous nursing staff coverage, continuous monitoring of vital signs, and **immediate** availability of surgical personnel and operating room resources. Frequent, repeated examinations by the surgeon are necessary to adequately assess the evolving status of the child.

Nonoperative management of confirmed abdominal visceral injuries is a surgical decision made by surgeons, just as is the decision to operate. Therefore, the surgeon must provide the management of the pediatric trauma patient.

D. Specific Visceral Injuries

A number of abdominal visceral injuries are more common in children than in adults. Duodenal hematoma results from a combination of undeveloped abdominal muscular tone and a bicycle handlebar or an elbow striking the child in the right upper quad-

EXTREMES OF AGE: A. PEDIATRIC TRAUMA

rant, but also may be caused by child abuse. This injury is most often treated nonoperatively with nasogastric suction and parenteral nutrition. Similarly, blunt pancreatic injuries often occur from like mechanisms. Small bowel perforations at or near the ligament of Treitz are more common in children than in adults, as are mesenteric, small bowel avulsion injuries. These particular injuries are often diagnosed late due to the vague early symptoms and the potential for late perforation. Bladder rupture is more common than in adults due to the shallowness of the child's pelvis. Penetrating injuries of the perineum or straddle injuries occur when a child falls on a fence, and often result in intraperitoneal injuries due to the nearness of the peritoneum to the perineum. **Rupture of a hollow viscus requires early operative intervention.**

Children who are restrained by a lap belt are at particular risk for enteric disruption, especially if they sustain a flexion disruption (Chance) fracture of the lumbar spine. Any patient with this mechanism of injury and these findings should be considered as potentially having a disrupted gastrointestinal tract until proven otherwise.

The child's spleen, liver, and kidneys are frequently disrupted from blunt force. It is uncommon for these injuries to require operative repair. It is common for a hemodynamically abnormal child to present to the emergency department and receive rapid crystalloid fluid resuscitation, with return to hemodynamic normality. When an injury to the liver, spleen, or kidney is diagnosed, the child should undergo a CT scan. The child should be placed in the intensive care unit for continuous monitoring. Delayed hemorrhage from splenic rupture usually does not occur.

VII. HEAD TRAUMA

Information provided in Chapter 6, Head Trauma, also applies to pediatric patients. This section emphasizes additional points peculiar to children.

Most head injuries in the pediatric population are the result of motor vehicle crashes, bicycle accidents, and falls. Data from the National Pediatric Trauma Registry indicate that an understanding of the interaction between the CNS and extracranial injuries is imperative, as hypotension and hypoxia from associated injuries have an adverse effect on the outcome from intracranial injury. Lack of attention to the ABCDEs and associated injuries significantly increases mortality from head injury. As in the adult,

hypotension is rarely, if ever, caused by head injury alone, and other explanations for this finding should be investigated aggressively.

The brain of the child is anatomically different from that of the adult. The brain doubles in size in the first 6 months of life and achieves 80% of the adult brain size by 2 years of age. There is increased water content of the brain up to 2 years of age. Neuronal plasticity occurs after birth and includes incomplete neuronal synapse formation and arborization, incomplete myelinization, and a vast number of neurochemical changes. The subarachnoid space is relatively smaller and hence offers less protection to the brain due to less buoyancy. Thus, head momentum is more likely to impart parenchyma structural damage. Normal cerebral blood flow increases proportionately to nearly twice that of adult levels by the age of 5 years, and then decreases. This accounts in part for the child's severe susceptibility to cerebral hypoxia.

A. Assessment

Children and adults may differ in their response to head trauma, which may influence the evaluation of the injured child. The principal differences include:

1. Outcome in children suffering severe brain injury is better than in adults. However, the outcome in children less than 3 years of age is worse than a similar injury in the older child. Children are particularly susceptible to the effects of the secondary brain injury that may be produced by hypovolemia with reduced cerebral perfusion, hypoxia, seizures, or hyperthermia. The combination of hypovolemia and hypoxia on the injured brain is devastating, but hypotension from hypovolemia is the worst single risk factor. **Adequate and rapid restoration of an appropriate circulating blood volume is mandatory and hypoxia must be avoided.**

2. Although an infrequent occurrence, infants may become hypotensive from blood loss into either the subgaleal or epidural space. This hypovolemia, due to intracranial injury, occurs because of open cranial sutures and fontanelle in infants. Treatment is directed toward appropriate volume restoration as it is with blood loss from other body regions.

3. The young child with an open fontanelle and mobile cranial sutures is more tolerant of an expanding intracranial mass lesion. Signs of an expanding mass may be hidden until rapid decompensation occurs. Therefore, an infant who is not in coma but who has bulging fontanelles or suture diastases **should be treated as having a more severe injury.** Early neurosurgical consultation is essential.

4. Vomiting and even amnesia are common after brain injury in children and do not necessarily imply increased intracranial pressure. However, persistent vomiting or vomiting that becomes more frequent is of concern and demands CT of the head. Gastric decompression is essential, because of the risk of aspiration.

5. Impact seizures, ie, seizures occurring shortly after brain injury, are more common in children and are usually self-limited. Recurrent seizure activity requires investigation by CT scanning.

6. Children tend to have fewer focal mass lesions than do adults, but elevated intracranial pressure due to brain swelling is more common. Rapid restoration of normal circulating blood volume is necessary. Some practitioners fear that restoration of a child's circulating blood volume places the child at greater risk of making the existing head injury worse. The opposite is true. If hypovolemia is not corrected promptly, the outcome from head injury is made worse due to secondary brain injury. Emergency CT is vital to identify those children who require emergency surgery.

7. The GCS is useful when applied to the pediatric age-group. However, the verbal score component must be modified for children younger than 4 years. (See Table 5, Pediatric Verbal Score, and Appendix 5, Trauma Scores—Revised and Pediatric.)

8. Because of the frequency of developing increased intracranial pressure in children, neurosurgical consultation to consider intracranial pressure monitoring should be obtained **early** in the course of resuscitation for children with:

a. A GCS Score of 8 or less, or motor scores of 1 or 2.

b. Multiple injuries associated with brain injury that require major volume resuscitation, immediate lifesaving thoracic or abdominal surgery, or for which stabilization and assessment is prolonged.

c. An abnormal CT scan of the brain.

9. Medication dosages must be adjusted as dictated by the child's size, and in consultation with a neurosurgeon. Drugs often used in children with head injuries include:

a. Phenobarbital 10 to 20 mg/kg/dose.

b. Diazepam 0.1 to 0.2 mg/kg/dose, slow IV bolus.

c. Phenytoin or fosphenytoin 15 to 20 mg/kg, administered at 0.5 to 1.5 mL/kg/minute as a loading dose, then 4 to 7 mg/kg/day for maintenance.

d. Mannitol 0.5 to 1.0 g/kg (rarely required). Diuresis with the use of mannitol or furosemide may worsen hypovolemia and should be withheld early in the resuscitation of the child with a head injury unless there are incontrovertible signs of transtentorial herniation.

Table 5—Pediatric Verbal Score

VERBAL RESPONSE	V-SCORE
Appropriate words or social smile, fixes and follows	5
Cries, but consolable	4
Persistently irritable	3
Restless, agitated	2
None	1

EXTREMES OF AGE: A. PEDIATRIC TRAUMA

B. Management

Management of traumatic brain injury in children currently involves:

1. Rapid, early assessment and management of the child's ABCDEs.

2. Appropriate neurosurgical involvement from the beginning of treatment.

3. Appropriate sequential assessment and management of the brain injury with attention directed toward the prevention of secondary brain injury, ie, hypoxia and hypoperfusion. Early endotracheal intubation with adequate oxygenation and ventilation are indicated to avoid progressive CNS damage. Attempts to orally intubate the trachea in the uncooperative, brain-injured child may be difficult and actually increase intracranial pressure. In the hands of the doctors who have considered the risks and benefits of intubating such children, pharmacologic sedation and paralysis may be used to facilitate intubation.

4. Continuous reassessment of all parameters.

VIII. SPINAL CORD INJURY

Information provided in Chapter 7, Spine and Spinal Cord Trauma, also applies to pediatric patients. This section emphasizes the differences of pediatric spinal injury.

Spinal cord injury in children is fortunately uncommon, as only 5% of all spinal cord injuries occur in the pediatric age-group. For children younger than 10 years, motor vehicle crashes most commonly produce these injuries. For children aged 10 to 14 years, motor vehicles and sporting activities account for an equal number of spinal injuries.

A. Anatomic Differences

1. Interspinous ligaments and joint capsules are more flexible.

2. Vertebral bodies are wedged anteriorly and tend to slide forward with flexion.

3. The facet joints are flat.

4. The child has a relatively large head compared with the neck. Therefore, the angular forces applied to the upper neck are relatively greater than in the adult.

B. Radiologic Considerations

Pseudosubluxation frequently complicates the radiographic evaluation of the child's cervical spine. About 40% of children younger than 7 years show anterior displacement of C2 on C3, and 20% of children up to 16 years exhibit this phenomenon. This radiographic finding is seen less commonly at C3 to C4. More than 3 mm of movement can be seen when these joints are studied by flexion and extension maneuvers.

When subluxation is seen on a lateral c-spine x-ray, it must be ascertained whether this is a pseudosubluxation or a c-spine injury. Pseudosubluxation of the cervical vertebrae is made more pronounced by the flexion of the c-spine that occurs when a child lies supine on a hard surface. To correct this radiographic anomaly, place the child's head in a neutral position by bringing the head forward into the sniffing position and repeat the x-ray. (See Figure 2, page 248, Proper Positioning of the Child to Maintain a Patent Airway.) The presence of a c-spine injury usually can be identified from neurologic examination findings and, on careful palpation of the posterior c-spine, an area of soft tissue swelling or a step-off deformity.

Increased distance between the dens and the anterior arch of C1 occurs in about 20% of young children. Gaps exceeding the upper limit of normal for the adult population are seen frequently.

Skeletal growth centers can resemble fractures. Basilar odontoid synchondrosis appears as a radiolucent area at the base of the dens, especially in children younger than 5 years. Apical odontoid epiphyses appear as separations on the odontoid x-ray and are usually seen between the ages of 5 and 11 years. The growth center of the spinous process may resemble fractures of the tip of the spinous process.

Children may sustain spinal cord injury without radiographic abnormalities (SCIWORA) more commonly than do adults. A normal spine series can be found in up to two-thirds of children suffering spinal cord injury. Therefore, if spinal cord injury is suspected, based on history or results of the neurologic examination, normal spine x-rays do not exclude significant spinal cord injury. **When in doubt about the integrity of the cervical spine, assume that an unstable injury exists, maintain immobilization of the child's head and neck, and obtain appropriate consultation.**

Spinal cord injury in childhood is treated in the same way as spinal cord injuries occurring in adults. Methylprednisolone may be used for nonpenetrating spinal cord injuries in the same dosages as those recommended for adults. (See Chapter 7, Spine and Spinal Cord Trauma.) Consultation with a neurosurgeon should be obtained early.

IX. MUSCULOSKELETAL TRAUMA

The initial priorities in the management of skeletal trauma in the child are similar to those for the adult, with the additional concerns about potential injury to the growth plate.

A. History

History is of vital importance. In the younger child, x-ray diagnosis of fractures and dislocations is difficult because of the lack of mineralization around the epiphysis and the presence of a physis (growth plate). Information about the magnitude, mechanism, and time of the injury facilitates better correlation of the physical findings and x-rays. Radiographic evidence of fractures of differing ages should alert the doctor to possible child abuse.

B. Blood Loss

Blood loss associated with long-bone and pelvic fractures is proportionately less in the child than in the adult. Blood loss associated with an isolated closed femur fracture and treated appropriately is associated with an average fall in hematocrit of 4 points, which is not enough to cause shock. Hemodynamic instability in the presence of an isolated femur fracture should prompt evaluation for other sources of blood loss.

C Special Considerations of the Immature Skeleton

Bones lengthen as new bone is laid down by the physis near the articular surfaces. Injuries to, or adjacent to, this area before the physis has closed can potentially retard the normal growth or alter the development of the bone in an abnormal way. Crush injuries to the physis, which are often difficult to recognize radiographically, have the worst prognosis.

The immature, pliable nature of bones in children may lead to a so-called greenstick fracture. Such fractures are incomplete, with angulation maintained by cortical splinters on the concave surface. The torus or "buckle" fracture, seen in small children, involves angulation due to cortical impaction with a radiolucent fracture line. Supracondylar fractures at the elbow or knee have a high propensity for vascular injury as well as injury to the growth plate.

D. Principles of Immobilization

Simple splinting of fractured extremities in children usually is sufficient until definitive orthopaedic evaluation can be performed. Injured extremities with evidence of vascular compromise require emergent evaluation to prevent the adverse sequelae of ischemia. A single attempt at reduction of the fracture to restore blood flow is appropriate followed by simple splinting or traction splinting of the femur.

X. THE BATTERED, ABUSED CHILD

The battered, abused child syndrome refers to any child who sustains an intentional injury as the result of acts by parents, guardians, or acquaintances. Children who die within the first year of life from injury usually do so as the result of child abuse. Therefore, a history and careful evaluation of the child suspected of being abused is critically important to prevent eventual death, especially in children who are younger than 1 year. A doctor should suspect abuse if:

1. A discrepancy exists between the history and the degree of physical injury.

2. A prolonged interval has passed between the time of the injury and the seeking of medical advice.

3. The history includes repeated trauma, treated in different emergency departments.

4. Parents respond inappropriately or do not comply with medical advice, eg, leaving a child in the emergency facility.

5. The history of injury changes or differs between parents or guardians.

These findings, on careful physical examination, should suggest child abuse and indicate more intensive investigation:

1. Multiple subdural hematomas, especially without a fresh skull fracture

2. Retinal hemorrhage

3. Perioral injuries

4. Ruptured internal viscera without antecedent major blunt trauma

EXTREMES OF AGE: A. PEDIATRIC TRAUMA

5. Trauma to the genital or perianal area

6. Evidence of frequent injuries typified by old scars or healed fractures on x-ray

7. Fractures of long bones in children younger than 3 years of age

8. Bizarre injuries such as bites, cigarette burns, or rope marks

9. Sharply demarcated second- and third-degree burns in unusual areas

In the United States, doctors are bound by law to report incidences of child abuse to governmental authorities, even cases where abuse is only suspected. Abused children are at increased risk for fatal injuries, and no one is served by failing to report. The system protects doctors from legal liability for identifying confirmed or even suspicious cases of abuse. Although the reporting procedures may vary from state to state, it is most commonly handled through local social service agencies or the state's health and human services department. The process of reporting child abuse assumes greater importance when one realizes that 50% of abused children who return to the hospital dead were victims of previous episodes of abuse that went unreported or were not taken seriously.

XI. PITFALLS IN CHILDHOOD INJURY

The unique anatomic and physiologic characteristics of children occasionally produce pitfalls in the management of these patients. The small size of the endotracheal tube promotes obstruction from inspissated secretions. Additionally, uncuffed tubes can be dislodged, especially during patient movement or transportation. The necessity of frequent reassessment cannot be overemphasized. The same prudent attention to all tubes and catheters used for resuscitation and stabilization is essential.

The child's ability to compensate in the early phases of blood loss can create an illusion of hemodynamic normality, resulting in inadequate fluid resuscitation and rapid deterioration, which is often precipitous. Delays in the recognition of abdominal hollow viscus injury are possible, especially when the decision to manage solid organ injury nonoperatively is made. Such an approach to the management of these injuries in children must be accompanied by an attitude of anticipation, frequent reevaluation, and preparation for immediate surgical intervention. These children should all be managed by a surgeon

in a facility equipped to handle any contingencies in an expeditious manner.

Many orthopaedic injuries in children produce only subtle symptoms, and positive findings on physical examination are difficult to detect. Any evidence of unusual behavior, eg, the child who refuses to use an arm or bear weight on an extremity, must be carefully evaluated for an occult bony or soft-tissue injury. The parents are often the ones who note behavior that is out of the ordinary for their child. Additionally, the doctor must remember the potential for child abuse. The history of the injury event should be viewed suspiciously when the findings do not corroborate the parent's story.

XII. SUMMARY

The recognition and management of pediatric injuries require the same astute skills as those required for adults. However, unwary doctors can make serious errors unless they are fully cognizant of the unique features of the pediatric trauma patient. These unique characteristics include airway anatomy and management, fluid requirements, recognition of CNS as well as thoracic and abdominal injuries, diagnosis of extremity fractures, and the recognition of the battered, abused child. It is vitally important that the child with multiple injuries, including head injury, be rapidly and appropriately resuscitated to avoid the untoward effects of hypovolemia and secondary brain injury.

Early involvement of the general surgeon or the pediatric surgeon is imperative in the management of the injured child. Nonoperative management of abdominal visceral injuries should be performed only by surgeons in facilities equipped to handle any contingency in an expeditious manner.

■ BIBLIOGRAPHY

1. **Injury Facts.** Itasca, IL, National Safety Council, 1999.

2. Barlow B, Niemirska M, et al: Response to injury in children with closed femur fractures. **Journal of Trauma** 1987; 27:429–430.

3. Chesnut RM, Marshall LF, et al: The role of secondary brain injury in determining outcome from severe head injury. **Journal of Trauma** 1993; 43:216–222.

4. Cooper A, Barlow B, DiScala C: Vital signs and trauma mortality: The pediatric perspective. **Pediatric Emergency Care** 2000; 16:66.

5. Cooper A, Barlow B, DiScala C, et al: Mortality and truncal injury: The pediatric perspective. **Journal of Pediatric Surgery** 1994; 29:33.

6. DiScala C, Sage R, Li G, et al: Child abuse and unintentional injuries. **Archives of Pediatric and Adolescent Medicine** 2000; 154(1):16–22.

7. Garcia VF, Gotshall CS, et al: Rib fractures in children: A marker of severe trauma. **Journal of Trauma** 1990; 30:695–700.

8. Gerardi MJ, Sacchett AD, Cantor RM, et al: Rapid-sequence intubation of the pediatric patient. **Annals of Emergency Medicine** July 1996; 28:55–74.

9. Hannan E, Meaker P, Fawell L, et al: Predicting inpatient mortality for pediatric blunt trauma patients: A better alternative. **Journal of Pediatric Surgery** 2000; 35(2):155–159.

10. Harris BH, Schwaitzberg SD, Seman TM, et al: The hidden morbidity of pediatric trauma. **Journal of Pediatric Surgery** 1989; 24:103–106.

11. Herzenberg JE, Hensinger RN, Dedrick DE, et al: Emergency transport and positioning of young children who have an injury of the cervical spine. **Journal of Bone and Joint Surgery** 1989; 71-A:15–22.

12. Keller MS, Vane DW: Management of blunt splenic injury: Comparison of pediatric and adult. **Journal of Pediatric Surgery** 1987; 153:462–468.

13. Luersson TG, Klauber MR, Marshall LF: Outcome from head injury related to a patient's age: A longitudinal prospective study of adult and pediatric injury. **Journal of Neurosurgery** 1988; 68:409–416.

14. Luna GK, Dellinger EP: Nonoperative observation therapy for splenic injuries: A safe therapeutic option. **American Journal of Surgery** 1987; 153:462–468.

15. Mutabagani KH, Coley BD, Zumberge N, et al: Preliminary experience with focused abdominal sonography for trauma (FAST) in children: Is it useful? **Journal of Pediatric Surgery** 1999; 34:48–54.

16. Nakayama DK, Ramenofsky ML, Rowe MI: Chest injuries in children. **Annals of Surgery** 1989; 210:770–775.

17. O'Neill JA, Meacham WF, Griffen PO, et al: Patterns of injury in the battered children syndrome. **Journal of Trauma** 1973; 13:332.

18. Pang D, Wilberger JE: Spinal cord injury without radiographic abnormalities in children. **Journal of Neurosurgery** 1982; 57:114–129.

19. Patel JC, Tepas JJ: The efficacy of focused abdominal sonography for trauma (FAST) as a screening tool in the assessment of injured children. **Journal of Pediatric Surgery** 1999; 34:44–47.

20. Peclet MH, Newman KD, et al: Thoracic trauma in children: An indicator of increased mortality. **Journal of Pediatric Surgery** 1990; 25:961–966.

21. Pugula FA, Wald SL, Shackford SR, et al: The effect of hypotension and hypoxia on children with severe head injuries. **Journal of Pediatric Surgery** 1993; 28(3):310–316.

22. Schwaitzberg SD, Bergman KS, Harris BW: A pediatric trauma model of continuous hemorrhage. **Journal of Pediatric Surgery** 1988; 23:605–609.

23. Swischuk LE, Swischuk PN, John SD: Wedging of C-3 in infants and children: Usually a normal finding and not a fracture. **Radiology** 1993; 188:523–526.

24. Tepas JJ, DiScala C, Ramenofsky ML, et al: Mortality and head injury: The pediatric perspective. **Journal of Pediatric Surgery** 1990; 25:92–96.

25. Tepas JJ, Ramenofsky ML, et al: The Pediatric Trauma Score as a predictor of injury severity: An objective assessment. **Journal of Trauma** 1988; 28:425–429.

EXTREMES OF AGE: A. PEDIATRIC TRAUMA

Table 6—Pediatric Equipment

AGE AND WEIGHT	AIRWAY AND BREATHING						CIRCULATION		SUPPLEMENTAL EQUIPMENT				
	O₂ Mask	Oral Airway	Bag-valve	Laryngo-scope	ET tube	Stylet	Suction	BP Cuff	IV Catheter	NG Tube	Chest Tube	Urinary Catheter	Cervical Collar
Premie 3 kg	Premie, newborn	Infant	Infant	0 straight	2.5–3.0 no cuff	6 Fr	6–8 Fr	Premie, newborn	22 ga	12 Fr	10–14 Fr	5 Fr feeding	–
0–6 mos 3.5 kg	Newborn	Infant, small	Infant	1 straight	3.0–3.5 no cuff	6 Fr	8 Fr	Newborn, infant	22 ga	12 Fr	12–18 Fr	5–8 Fr feeding	–
6–12 mos 7 kg	Pediatric	Small	Pediatric	1 straight	3.5–4.0 no cuff	6 Fr	8–10 Fr	Infant, child	22 ga	12 Fr	14–20 Fr	8 Fr	Small
1–3 yr 10–12 kg	Pediatric	Small	Pediatric	1 straight	4.0–4.5 no cuff	6 Fr	10 Fr	Child	20–22 ga	12 Fr	14–24 Fr	10 Fr	Small
4–7 yr 16–18 kg	Pediatric	Medium	Pediatric	2 straight or curved	5.0–5.5 no cuff	14 Fr	14 Fr	Child	20 ga	12 Fr	20–32 Fr	10–12 Fr	Small
8–10 yr 24–30 kg	Adult	Medium, large	Pediatric, adult	2–3 straight or curved	5.5–6.5 cuffed	14 Fr	14 Fr	Child, adult	18–20 ga	12 Fr	28–38 Fr	12 Fr	Medium

CHAPTER

Extremes of Age:
B. Trauma in the Elderly

■ OBJECTIVES:

Upon completion of this topic, the participant will be able to demonstrate an ability to apply the principles of trauma care for managing the acutely injured geriatric patient. Specifically, the participant will be able to:

A. Identify the unique characteristics of the elderly trauma patient.

   1. Types of injury

   2. Patterns of injury

   3. Anatomic and physiologic differences in the elderly

B. Discuss the primary management of the following critical injuries in geriatric patients based on their anatomic and physiologic differences.

   1. Airway management

   2. Breathing and ventilation

   3. Shock, fluid, and electrolyte management

   4. Central nervous system and cervical spine injuries

C. Identify the elements that lead to suspicion of abuse of the elderly.

EXTREMES OF AGE: B. TRAUMA IN THE ELDERLY

I. INTRODUCTION

People aged 65 and older represent the fastest-growing segment of the American population. The elderly currently comprise 15% of the United States' population and it is projected that they will represent 25% of the population by the year 2025. The senior population's rapid growth has already made a significant economic impact because of its unique medical requirements as well as the fact that seniors consume more than one-third of the health care resources. Currently, trauma is the seventh leading cause of death in the elderly, surpassed only by heart disease, cancer, chronic obstructive pulmonary disease, stroke, diabetes, and pneumonia.

Even though patients aged 65 or older are less likely than younger individuals to be injured, they are more likely to have a fatal outcome from injuries that do occur. However, over 80% of the injured can return to their preexisting level of independent living after aggressive resuscitation and follow-up care. Despite this, in the United States in 1997 over 36,000 elderly died due to injury, accounting for 25% of all injury fatalities. This excess mortality probably reflects the decreased physical reserves of the elderly due to the physiologic changes of aging, the comorbidities they develop, and a lack of understanding of their needs by many health care providers. (See Table 1, pages 265–266, Comorbid Conditions and Impact on Management of the Injured Patient, and Figure 1, page 267, Effects of Aging on Organ Systems.)

II. BIOMECHANICS OF INJURY

The 3 leading causes of death due to injury among the elderly in the United States are falls, motor vehicle crashes, and burns. Falls, the most common cause of unintentional injury and death among the elderly, account for 40% of the deaths in this age-group. Both the incidence of falls and the severity of complications rise with age. However, the majority of the elderly persons who fall do not die, and large numbers of emergency department visits and subsequent hospital admissions occur as a result. The accumulated effects of the aging process and environmental hazards most frequently cause falls. Due to changes in both the central nervous and musculoskeletal systems, older people are stiffer, less coordinated, and may have an unsteady gait. Visual, hearing, and memory impairments place them at high risk in the environment for hazards that can cause

falls. Falls from dizziness or vertigo are extremely common. Finally drugs—including alcohol—are a cause of or a contributing factor to many falls.

Over 4000 elderly people are killed annually in motor vehicle crashes, either as drivers or passengers. Additionally, 2000 elderly people are killed as pedestrians when struck by a motor vehicle. The effects of the aging process are a major influence on the incidence of injury and death. Often, the elderly have lessened visual and auditory acuity. Daylight acuity, glare resistance, and night vision decrease markedly with age. Medical conditions and their treatment may alter attention and consciousness. Because of the onset of senile changes in the brain, judgment may be altered. Finally, there often is decreased ability to implement appropriate actions because of impairment from medical conditions, including severe arthritis, osteoporosis, emphysema, heart disease, and decreased muscle mass.

Thermal injury is the third leading cause, accounting for almost 2000 deaths annually. One-third of these individuals are fatally injured while under the influence of alcohol, while smoking in bed, and/or caught in a building fire with exposure to heat and toxic products of combustion. Of the remainder, the majority sustain injury and death by ignition of clothing or prolonged contact with hot substances. As with falls, factors associated with degenerative disease and physical impairment appear to contribute substantially to the overrepresentation of the elderly. Elderly persons who come into contact with hot surfaces or liquids or are exposed to fire often are not able to remove themselves until extensive injury occurs. Finally, preexisting cardiovascular, respiratory, and renal diseases often make it impossible for the injured person to overcome serious but potentially survivable burns.

III. AIRWAY

The "A" of the ABCDE mnemonic of the primary survey is the same in the elderly as for any other trauma patient in all other patient populations. Establishing and maintaining a patent airway to provide adequate tissue oxygenation is the first objective. Supplemental oxygen should be administered as soon as possible, even in the presence of chronic pulmonary disease. Because of the elderly patient's likely limitation in cardiopulmonary reserve, early intubation of the injured elder should be considered for those presenting in shock. Early intubation also

EXTREMES OF AGE: B. TRAUMA IN THE ELDERLY

Table 1—Comorbid Conditions and Impact on Management of the Injured Patient

PRIMARY SURVEY	CONDITION	CLINICAL SEQUELAE	MANAGEMENT
Airway and c-spine control	• Rheumatoid disease	• Difficulty in opening mouth—cord injury	Consider • Nasopharyngeal intubation, or • Surgical airway
Breathing	• Asthma	• Hypoxia • Hypercarbia • Pneumothorax • Hypotension	• Bronchodilator • Steroids • Chest drain • IV fluids
	• Chronic obstructive pulmonary disease	• Hypoxia • Hypercarbia • V̇/Q̇ shunts	• Early ventilation
Circulation with hemorrhage control	• Ischemic heart disease	• Pain • Infarction • Dysrhythmia	• Titrated analgesia • IV fluids • Antidysrhythmic drugs • Cardioversion
	• Hypertension	• Exclude ↑ICP • Pain	• IV vasodilator • Invasive monitoring
	• Left ventricular failure	• Hypoxia • Bronchospasm • Hypotension	• Bronchodilator • Vasodilator • Inotropes • Invasive monitoring
	• Right ventricular failure	• Hypoxia • Hypotension	• Fluid challenge • Invasive monitoring
Disability	• Drugs	• Airway compromise • Hypoxia • Hypercarbia • Tachycardia • Neurostimulation • Neuroinhibition	• Specific antagonists • Thiamine
	• Psychoses • Stroke	• Spectrum of neurologic signs according to vascular territory affected	• Exclude hypoglycemia and intracranial trauma • Dextrose • Glucagon
	• Diabetes mellitus	• Sweating • Tachycardia • Confusion • Coma	• Exclude intracranial trauma • Nasopharyngeal airway • Benzodiazepines
	• Epilepsy	• Airway compromise • Hypoxia • Hypercarbia • Confusion • Coma • Transient or permanent memory loss (according to cause)	• Anticonvulsants • Consult with intensivist or neurologist • Paralyze, sedate, ventilate

EXTREMES OF AGE: B. TRAUMA IN THE ELDERLY

Table 1—Comorbid Conditions and Impact on Management of the Injured Patient (continued)

PRIMARY SURVEY	CONDITION	CLINICAL SEQUELAE	MANAGEMENT
Other	• Cancer	• Diagnosis often • Site dictates signs, eg, pleural effusion	• Treat according to ATLS guidelines
	• Acid/pepsin disorder	• Anemia • Abdominal pain • Headaches • Hematemesis	• Exclude acute GI trauma and/or intraabdominal pathology
	• Irritable bowel disease	• Anemia • Rectal bleeding • Abdominal pain • Hypoxia • Metabolic acidosis	• Exclude acute GI trauma and intraabdominal pathology • Steroids may mask intraabdominal pathology
	• Chronic renal failure	• Fluid overload • Hypertension	• Invasive monitoring • Careful fluid balance • Consult with nephrologist
	• Chronic liver failure	• Hypoxia • Hypovolemia • Hypoglycemia • Malnutrition	
	• Anemia	• Chronic, often asymptomatic	• Transfuse according to hemodynamic indices
	• Anticoagulation	• Increased bleeding	• Reverse with FFP

should be considered for those with chest wall injury or alteration in their level of consciousness.

Particular concerns of airway maintenance in the elderly include dentition, nasopharyngeal fragility, macroglossia and microstomia, and cervical arthritis. Edentulousness may interfere with achieving a proper seal on a face mask. Consequently, while broken dentures should be removed, intact well-fitted dentures are often best noted and left in place until after airway control is achieved. Care must be taken when placing nasogastric or nasotracheal tubes because of nasopharyngeal tissue friability, especially around the turbinates. Profuse bleeding may ensue, complicating an already dangerous situation. The oral cavity may be compromised by either macroglossia, associated with amyloidosis or acromegaly, or microstomia such as the constricted small bird-like mouth of progressive systemic sclerosis. Finally, arthritis may affect the temporo-

mandibular joints and cervical spine, making endotracheal intubation more difficult. Degenerative changes and calcification in laryngeal cartilage place the elderly population at increased risk of injury from minor blows to the neck.

The principles of airway management remain the same, with endotracheal intubation as the preferred method for definitive airway control. If acute airway obstruction exists or the vocal cords cannot be visualized, surgical cricothyroidotomy should be performed. (See Chapter 2, Airway and Ventilatory Management.)

IV. BREATHING AND VENTILATION

Many of the changes that occur in the airway and lungs in elderly patients are difficult to ascribe purely to the process of senescence and may be the result of chronic exposure to toxic agents such as tobacco

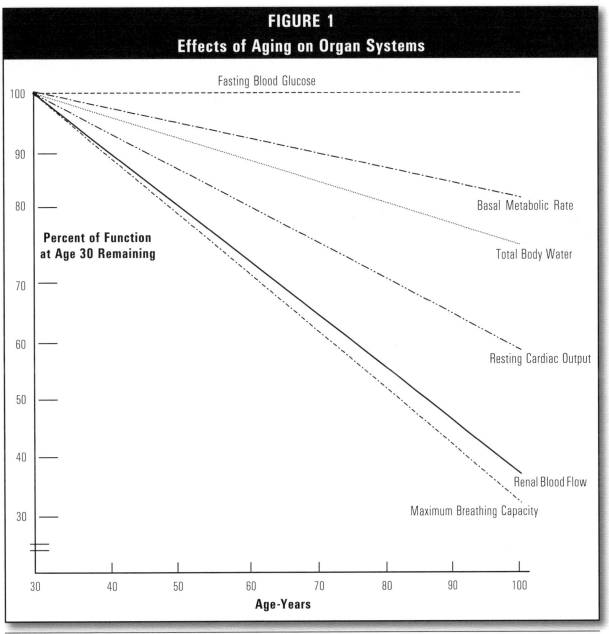

FIGURE 1
Effects of Aging on Organ Systems

Steady decline in function in organ systems is noted during aging. Data are expressed as percentages of the volume observed at 30 years of age. (Reprinted with permission from Shock NW, The physiology of aging. In: Powers JH (ed): *Surgery of the Aged and Debilitated Patient.* Philadelphia, WB Saunders, 1968, Figure 1-16.)

smoke and other environmental toxins throughout life. The loss of respiratory reserve, due to the effects of aging and chronic diseases (eg, chronic bronchitis and emphysema), makes careful monitoring of the geriatric patient's respiratory system imperative. Administration of supplemental oxygen is mandatory. Caution should be exercised with the use of supplemental oxygen because some elderly patients with chronic pulmonary disease may retain carbon dioxide. Such patients lose the normal respiratory drive produced by an elevated $Paco_2$ and have a hypoxemic respiratory drive. These patients must not be allowed to remain hypoxic. High-flow oxygen should be administered by nonrebreathing face mask. If somnolence results from a rising $Paco_2$, intubation is necessary.

EXTREMES OF AGE: B. TRAUMA IN THE ELDERLY

Chest injuries occur in elderly and nonelderly patients with similar frequency, but the mortality rate for elderly patients is higher. Chest wall injury with rib fractures or pulmonary contusions are common and not well tolerated. Simple pneumothorax and hemothorax also are poorly tolerated. The likelihood of respiratory failure may not be adequately appreciated in these patients because of failure to recognize the increased work of breathing and excess of energy expenditure. Adequate pain control and vigorous pulmonary toilet are essential for a satisfactory outcome. Pulmonary complications, predominately atelectasis, pneumonia, and pulmonary edema, occur in the elderly with great frequency. Marginal cardiopulmonary reserve coupled with overzealous crystalloid fluid infusion increases the potential for pulmonary edema or worsening of pulmonary contusions. Admission to the hospital usually is necessary even with apparently minor injuries.

V. CIRCULATION

As the heart ages there is progressive loss of function. By the age of 65 years, nearly 50% of the population has coronary artery stenosis. Cardiac index falls off linearly with age. Maximal heart rate also begins to decrease from about 40 years of age. The formula for maximal heart rate is 220 minus the individual's age in years. Although resting heart rate varies little, the maximum tachycardic response decreases with age.

The cause of this diminution of function is multifaceted. Total blood volume decreases and circulation time increases. There is increasing myocardial stiffness, slowed electrophysiologic conduction, and loss of myocardial cell mass. The response to endogenous catecholamine release with stress is also different, which is likely related to a reduction in responsiveness of the cellular membrane receptor. These changes predispose the aged heart to reentry dysrhythmias. Additionally, diastolic dysfunction makes the heart more dependent on atrial filling to increase cardiac output.

The kidney loses mass rapidly after the age of 50 years. This loss involves entire nephron units, and is accompanied by a decrement in glomerular filtration rate and renal blood flow. Serum creatinine usually remains within normal limits, presumably due to a reduction in muscle creatinine production. The aged kidney is less able to reabsorb sodium or excrete potassium or hydrogen ions. Maximum concentration ability of the kidney of an octogenarian is only 850 mOsm/kg, 70% of the ability of the 30-year-old kidney. A decrease in the production of, and responsiveness of the kidney to, renin and angiotensin is seen. As a result, creatinine clearance in the elderly is markedly reduced and the aged kidney is more susceptible to injury from hypovolemia, medications, and other nephrotoxins.

A. Evaluation and Management

A common pitfall in the evaluation of older patients after sustaining injury is the mistaken impression that "normal" blood pressure and heart rate indicate normovolemia. **Early monitoring of the cardiovascular system must be instituted.** Blood pressure generally increases with age. Thus, a systolic blood pressure of 120 mm Hg may represent hypotension in an elderly patient whose normal preinjury blood pressure was 170 to 180 mm Hg. Significant blood volume loss may be masked by the absence of early tachycardia. The onset of hypotension also may be delayed. Additionally, the chronic high afterload state induced by elevated peripheral vascular resistance may limit cardiac output and ultimately cerebral, renal, coronary, and peripheral oxygen delivery.

Geriatric patients have a limited physiologic reserve and may have difficulty generating an adequate response to injury. Severely injured hypotensive elderly patients with metabolic acidosis almost always die, especially if they have sustained brain injury. Fluid requirements, once corrected for the lesser lean body mass, are similar to those of younger patients. The elderly hypertensive patient on chronic diuretic therapy may have a chronically contracted vascular volume and a serum potassium deficit. Careful monitoring of the administration of crystalloid solutions is important to prevent electrolyte disorders.

Isotonic electrolyte solutions are used for initial resuscitation. Ringer's lactate solution is the initial fluid of choice. Initially, 1 or 2 liters are administered rapidly while observing the patient's physiologic response. Further decisions with respect to fluid resuscitation are predicated on this observed response. (See Chapter 3, Shock.)

The optimal hemoglobin level for the injured elderly patient is controversial. Current consensus suggests that in people over the age of 65 years, hemoglobin concentrations of over 10 gm should be maintained to maximize oxygen-carrying capacity and delivery. However, indiscriminate blood transfusion is condemned because of the attendant risk of blood-borne infections as well as its known impairment of immune host response and resulting complications.

Because elderly patients may have such a limited cardiac reserve, a rapid and complete assessment for all sources of blood loss is necessary. The FAST examination is a rapid means of determining the presence of abnormal intraabdominal fluid collections. DPL may also be of use. There is at present little role for nonoperative management of blunt abdominal solid viscus injuries in elderly patients. The risk of nonoperative management may be greater than the risk of an early operation.

The retroperitoneum is an often-unrecognized source of blood loss. Elderly patients may develop exsanguinating retroperitoneal hemorrhage after relatively minor pelvic or hip fractures. A patient with pelvic, hip, or lumbar vertebral fractures who demonstrates continuing blood loss without a specific source, especially after a negative DPL or FAST examination, should have prompt angiography and attempted control with transcatheter embolization.

The process of aging along with superimposed disease states make close monitoring mandatory, especially in cases of injury with acute intravascular volume loss and shock. Patients who on initial assessment appear to have only minor injuries or be uninjured may have a significant mortality (up to 44%). About 33% of those elderly patients who do not die directly from the consequences of injury, die from "inexplicable" sequential organ failure which may reflect early, unsuspected states of hypoperfusion. Failure to recognize inadequate oxygen delivery creates an oxygen deficit from which the geriatric patient is not able to recover. Because of associated coronary artery disease, hypotension from hypovolemia frequently results in impaired cardiac performance from myocardial ischemia. Thus, hypovolemic and cardiogenic shock may coexist. Early and aggressive invasive monitoring, perhaps with a pulmonary artery catheter, may be beneficial. Hemodynamic resuscitation may require the use of inotropes after volume restoration in these patients. Prompt transfer to a trauma center may be lifesaving.

VI. DISABILITY: BRAIN AND SPINAL CORD INJURIES

A. Changes with Aging

Brain weight decreases about 10% by 70 years of age with progressive loss of neurons, resulting in cerebral atrophy. This loss is replaced by cerebrospinal fluid. Concomitantly, the dura becomes tightly adherent to the skull. While the increased space created around the brain may serve to protect the brain from contusion, it also causes stretching of the parasagittal bridging veins, making them more prone to rupture on impact. This brain volume loss also allows for more brain movement in response to angular acceleration/deceleration. Surprising amounts of blood can collect around the brain of an elderly individual before overt symptoms become apparent.

As the brain shrinks, abnormal proteins tangle inside the neuron while plaque from dendritic degeneration accumulates. Cerebral blood flow is reduced by 20% by the age of 70 years. This is further reduced if atheromatous debris occludes conducting arteries. Peripheral conduction velocity slows due to demyelination. Reduced acquisition or retention of information may cause clinically subtle changes in mental status. Visual and auditory acuity declines, vibratory and position sensation is impaired, and reaction time increases. In addition to complicating the evaluation process of the injured elderly patient, these changes place the elderly individual at greater risk for injury. Finally, preexisting medical conditions or their treatment may be a cause of confusion in the elderly.

In the spine, the most dramatic changes occur in the intervertebral disc. Loss of water and proteins affect the shape and compressibility of the disc. These changes shift the loads on the vertebral column to the facets, ligaments, and paraspinal muscles and contribute to degeneration of the facet joints and development of spinal stenosis. Progressively, these alterations place the spine and spinal cord at increased risk for injury. This risk is increased in the presence of osteoporosis, whether apparent radiographically or not. Finally, osteoarthritis can cause diffuse canal stenosis, segmental immobility, and kyphotic deformity which are most severe in the cervical region.

EXTREMES OF AGE: B. TRAUMA IN THE ELDERLY

B. Evaluation and Management

Elderly patients with brain injury have fewer severe cerebral contusions than do younger patients. However, the elderly have a higher incidence of subdural and intraparenchymal hematoma. Subdural hematomas are nearly 3 times as frequent in the elderly as in younger patients. This may be in part because elderly individuals are more likely to be taking anticoagulant medications for cardiac or cerebral disease. A subdural hematoma may produce a rather gradual onset of neurologic decline, especially in the elderly patient. In fact, chronic subdural hematomas resulting from an earlier fall may be the cause of the fall for which the doctor is currently examining the patient. CT scans of the head provide rapid, accurate, and detailed information on structural damage to the brain, skull, and supporting elements. Liberal use of this modality is encouraged in elderly patients with brain injury. (See Chapter 6, Head Trauma.)

Cervical spine injuries appear to be more common in the elderly trauma patient. They may be more occult and be particularly difficult to diagnose if osteoporosis and osteoarthritis are present. Severe osteophytic disease makes diagnosis of fracture challenging. Degeneration of intervertebral ligaments can increase the degree of intervertebral subluxation that is physiologic. Preexisting canal stenosis due to anterior osteophytes and posterior ligamentous hypertrophy increase the risk for central and anterior cord syndromes. These injuries often result from relatively mild extension injuries after falls or rear-end motor vehicle crashes. Magnetic resonant imaging (MRI) is particularly useful for diagnosing these injuries. (See Chapter 7, Spine and Spinal Cord Trauma.)

VII. EXPOSURE AND ENVIRONMENT

The skin and connective tissues of elderly individuals undergo extensive changes, including cell number decrease, loss of strength, and impaired function. The epidermal keratinocytes lose a significant proportion of their proliferate ability with aging. The dermis loses as much as 20% of its thickness, undergoes a significant loss of vascularity, and has a marked decrease in mast cell number. These changes result in loss of thermal regulatory ability, decreased barrier function against bacterial invasion, and significant impairment to wound healing.

The injured elderly patient must be protected from hypothermia. Hypothermia not attributable to shock or exposure should alert the physician to the possibility of occult disease, in particular sepsis, pancreatitis, hypothyroidism, and phenothiazine overdose.

The potential for invasive bacterial infection through injured skin must be recognized. Appropriate care, including assessing tetanus immunization status to prevent infection, must be instituted early. (See Appendix 4, Tetanus Immunization.)

VIII. OTHER ORGAN SYSTEMS

A. Musculoskeletal System

Disorders of the musculoskeletal system are the most common complaint of the middle-aged and elderly population. They are the most likely cause of restrictions in an individual's daily life and are the key components to loss of independence. Aging results in stiffening of ligaments, cartilage, intervertebral discs, joint capsules, etc. Deterioration of tendons, ligaments, and joint capsules leads to increased risk of injury, spontaneous rupture, and less joint stability. The risk of injury increases not only to the musculoskeletal system, but also to adjacent soft tissues.

Aging causes a general decline in responsiveness to many anabolic hormones and an absolute reduction in the levels of growth hormones. After the age of 25 years, muscle mass decreases by 4% every 10 years. After the age of 50 years, the rate is 10% per decade unless the levels of growth factors are low, and then the rate of decrease approaches 35%. This is manifested by a reduction in size and total number of muscle cells. The decrease in muscle mass is directly correlated to the decrease in strength seen with the aging process.

Osteoporosis results in a decrease of histologic normal bone with a consequent loss of strength and resistance to fractures. This disorder is endemic in the elderly population, clinically affecting almost 50%. The causes of osteoporosis include loss of estrogen hormones, loss of body mass, decreasing levels of physical activity, and inadequate consumption and inefficient use of calcium.

The consequences of these changes on the musculoskeletal system are frequently disabling and at times devastating. Injuries to ligaments and tendons affect joints and adjacent soft tissues. Osteoporosis contributes to the occurrence of spontaneous vertebral

EXTREMES OF AGE: B. TRAUMA IN THE ELDERLY

compression fractures and to the high incidence of hip fractures in the elderly. This incidence approaches 1% per year for men and 2% for women over the age of 85 years. The ease with which fractures occur in the elderly patient magnifies the degree of trauma that the elderly patient might otherwise survive.

Elderly individuals are particularly susceptible to long-bone fractures with attendant disability and associated pulmonary morbidity and mortality. Early stabilization of long-bone fractures may decrease this risk, provided the patient is in an optimal hemodynamic state. Resuscitation should be targeted at normalizing tissue perfusion as early as possible and before fracture fixation is performed.

The most common locations of fractures in the elderly patient are the proximal femur, hip, humerus, and wrist. Patients complain of pain in the area of the greater trochanter or anterior pelvis. In general, these individuals are unable to walk. Isolated hip fractures do not usually cause Class III or IV shock. Neurovascular integrity should be assessed and compared with the opposite extremity.

Fractures of the humerus usually result from falls on an outstretched extremity. The resulting injury is a fracture of the surgical neck of the humerus. Usually, there is pain and tenderness in the shoulder or upper humerus area. Of major importance in the evaluation of these patients is the determination of whether the fracture is impacted or nonimpacted. Impacted fractures demonstrate no false motion of the humerus when the shoulder is rotated gently from a flexed elbow. Patients with nonimpacted fractures generally experience pain on movement of the arm. These latter fractures require hospitalization for orthopaedic consultation and often operation.

Colles' fracture results from a fall on the outstretched, dorsiflexed hand causing a metaphyseal fracture of the distal radius. The classic finding of a fracture at the base of the ulna styloid process occurs in 69% of the cases. Evaluation should include careful testing of the median nerve and motor function of the finger flexors. The wrist should be examined radiographically and all the carpal bones should be visualized to exclude a more complex injury.

The aim of treatment for musculoskeletal injuries should be to undertake the least invasive, most definitive procedure that will permit early mobilization. Prolonged inactivity and disease often lim- its the ultimate functional outcome and impacts survival.

B. Nutrition and Metabolism

The caloric needs of men and women decline with age as lean body mass and metabolic rate gradually decrease. Protein requirements actually may increase as a result of inefficient utilization. There is a widespread occurrence of chronically inadequate nutrition among the elderly. Poor nutritional status contributes to a significantly increased complication rate. Early and adequate nutritional support of injured elderly patients is a cornerstone of successful trauma care.

C. The Immune System and Infections

Mortality from most diseases increases with age. Why this is true is uncertain, but the loss of competence of the immune system with age certainly plays a role. Thymic tissue is less than 15% of its maximum by 50 years of age. Liver and spleen size also decrease. With aging, cell-mediated and humoral immune response to foreign antigens is decreased, while the response to autologous antigens is increased. It is not clear if aging alters granulocyte function, but chronic diseases of the elderly, eg, diabetes mellitus, may do so. As a consequence of this, elderly persons have an impaired ability to respond to bacteria and viruses, a reduced ability to respond to vaccination, and a lack of reliable response to skin antigen testing. Clinically, elderly individuals are less able to tolerate infection and are more prone to develop multiple organ system failure. The absence of fever, leukocytosis, and other manifestations of the inflammatory response may be caused by poor immune function.

IX. SPECIAL CIRCUMSTANCES

A. Medications

Concomitant disease may require the use of medications and elderly patients are often taking many pharmacologic agents. Drug interactions are frequently encountered and side effects are much more common due to the very narrow therapeutic range in the elderly. Adverse reactions to some medications may even contribute to the injury-producing event. Beta-adrenergic blocking agents may limit chronotropic activity. Calcium channel blockers may prevent peripheral vasoconstriction and con-

EXTREMES OF AGE: B. TRAUMA IN THE ELDERLY

tribute to hypotension. Nonsteroidal antiinflammatory agents may contribute to blood loss due to their adverse effects on platelet function. Steroids and other drugs may further reduce the inflammatory response. Chronic anticoagulant use may increase blood loss. Chronic diuretic use may render the elderly patient dehydrated and with total body deficits of potassium and sodium. Hypoglycemic agents not only may contribute to the injury event itself but also may make control of serum glucose difficult if their use is unrecognized. Psychotropic medications, commonly prescribed for elderly patients, may mask injuries or become problematic if discontinued abruptly. Changes in CNS function as a result of these medications also may contribute to the injury. Finally, elderly individuals frequently neglect to keep their tetanus immunization current.

Pain relief in injured elderly trauma patients should not be neglected after resuscitation. Morphine is safe and effective and should be given in small-titrated (0.5 to 1.0 mg) intravenous doses. Antiemetics should be given with caution to avoid extrapyramidal effects. Finally, nephrotoxic drugs (antibiotics, radiographic dyes, etc) must be given in appropriate doses reflecting the elderly patient's decreased renal functions, contracted intravascular volume, and other comorbid conditions.

B. Abuse of the Geriatric Patient

When evaluating an injured elderly patient, consider that the injury may be intentionally inflicted. Abuse of elderly individuals may be as common as child abuse. Abuse is defined as any willful infliction of injury, unreasonable confinement, intimidation, or cruel punishment resulting in physical harm, pain, mental anguish, or other willful deprivation by a caretaker of goods or services that are necessary to avoid physical harm, mental anguish, or mental illness. Multifaceted in etiology, elder abuse often is not recognized and is underreported. Many cases of abused elderly persons involve only subtle signs, eg, poor hygiene or dehydration, and have great potential to go undetected. Although every state in the United States has reporting requirements, it is estimated that only 1 in 6 cases of geriatric abuse is brought to the attention of the proper authorities. A multidisciplinary approach to the patient is required.

C. Decisions at the End of Life

Many elderly patients return to their preinjury level of function and independence after recovery from injury. Age significantly increases mortality from injury, but more aggressive care, especially early in the evaluation and resuscitation of the elderly trauma patient, has been shown to improve survival. Attempts to identify which elderly trauma patients are at greatest risk for mortality have not found much utility in clinical practice.

Certainly there are circumstances in which the doctor and patient, or family member(s), may choose to forego lifesaving measures and provide only supportive care. This decision is particularly clear in the elderly patient who has sustained extensive burns and where survival is unprecedented. In other circumstances, it is sometimes more difficult to be certain about patient outcome, or be dogmatic about therapy. In many situations, the doctor confronts poorly defined probabilities. The trauma team should always seek the existence of a living will, advance directives, or similar legal documents. While no absolute ethical guidelines can be given, the following observations may be helpful: (1) the patient's right to self-determination is paramount; (2) medical intervention is only appropriate when it is in the patient's best interests; and (3) medical therapy is only appropriate when its likely benefits outweigh its likely adverse consequences. The ethical issue of appropriateness of care in an environment of declining hospital resources and restrictions on finances is more challenging.

X. SUMMARY

The number of elderly persons is increasing in the population of the United States and other industrialized nations. Although less likely to be injured than younger populations, the mortality rate for the elderly population is higher. Many elderly-aged trauma patients can be returned to their preinjury medical status and independence. A knowledge of the changes that occur with aging, an appreciation of the injury patterns seen in the elderly, and an understanding of the need for aggressive resuscitation and monitoring of the injured geriatric patient are necessary for improved outcome.

■ BIBLIOGRAPHY

1. Alexander BH, Rivara FP, Wolf ME: The cost and frequency of hospitalization for fall-related injuries in older adults. **American Journal of Public Health** 1992; 82(7):1020–1023.

2. Allen JE, Schwab CW: Blunt chest trauma in the elderly. **American Surgery** 1985; 51(12):697–700.

3. Bouchard JA, Barei D, Cayer D, et al: Outcome of femoral shaft fractures in the elderly. **Clinical Orthopedics** 1996 Nov; (332):105–109.

4. Burdge JJ, Katz B, Edwards R, et al: Surgical treatment of burns in elderly patients. **Journal of Trauma** 1988; 28(2):214–217.

5. Clayton MC, Solem LB, Ahrenholtz DH: Pulmonary failure in geriatric patients with burns: The need for diagnostic-related group modifier. **Journal of Burn Care and Rehabilitation** 1995; 16(4):451–454.

6. Council Report: Decisions near the end of life. **Journal of the American Medical Association** 1992; 267:2229–2233.

7. Curreri PW, Luterman A, Braun DW Jr, et al: Brain injury: Analysis of survival and hospitalization time for 937 patients. **Annals of Surgery** 1980; 192(4):472–478.

8. Demarest GB, Osler TM, Clevenger FW: Injuries in the elderly: Evaluation and initial response. **Geriatrics** 1990; 45(8):36–38, 41–42 [review].

9. DeMaria EJ, Kenney PR, Merriam MA, et al: Aggressive trauma care benefits the elderly. **Journal of Trauma** 1987; 27(11):1200–1206.

10. DeMaria EJ, Merriam MA, Casanova LA, et al: Do DRG payments adequately reimburse the costs of trauma care in geriatric patients? **Journal of Trauma** 1989; 28(8):1244–1249.

11. Fairman R, Rombear JL: Physiologic problems in the elderly surgical patient. In: Miller A (ed), Rowlands J (contrib ed): **Physiologic Basis of Modern Surgical Care.** Washington, DC, Mosby, 1988, p 1108.

12. Finelli FC, Jonsson J, Champion HR, et al: A case control study for major trauma in geriatric patients. **Journal of Trauma** 1989; 29(5):541–548.

13. Gakuu LN, Kabetu CE: An overview on management of the traumatised elderly patient. **East African Medicine Journal** 1997; 74(10):618–621.

14. Gubler KD, Maier RV, Davis R, et al: Trauma recidivism in the elderly. **Journal of Trauma** 1996; 41(6):952–956.

15. Horan MA, Clague JE: Injury in the aging: Recovery and rehabilitation. **British Medical Bulletin** 1999; 55(4):895–909.

16. Horst HM, Obeid FJ, Sorensen VJ, et al: Factors influencing survival of elderly trauma patients. **Critical Care Medicine** 1986; 14(8):681–684.

17. Kanis JA: The incidence of hip fracture in Europe. **Osteoporosis International** 1993; 3 Supplement 1:10–15.

18. Kauder DR, Schwab CW: Comorbidity in geriatric patients. In: Maull K, Cleveland H, Strauch G, et al (eds): **Advances in Trauma.** St. Louis, Mosby, 1990, pp 215–230.

19. Koepsell TD, Wolf ME, McCloskey L, et al: Medical conditions and motor vehicle collisions in older adults. **Journal of American Geriatrics Society** 1994; 42(7):695–700.

20. Lachs MS, Pillemer K: Abuse and neglect of elderly persons. **New England Journal of Medicine** 1995; 332(7):437–443.

21. Mackenzie EJ, Morris JA, Edelstein SL: Effect of pre-existing disease on length of stay in trauma patients. **Journal of Trauma** 1989; 29(6):757–764.

22. Mackenzie EJ, Morris JA, Smith GS, et al: Acute hospital costs of trauma in the United States: Implications for regionalized systems of care. **Journal of Trauma** 1990; 30(9);1096–1101.

23. Manton DK, Vaupel JW: Survival after the age of 80 in the United States, Sweden, France, England, and Japan. **New England Journal of Medicine** 1995; 333(18):1232–1235.

24. McMahon DJ, Schwab CW, Kauder DR: Comorbidity and the elderly trauma patient. **World Journal of Surgery** 1996; 20(8):1113–1119.

25. Milzman DP, Boulanger BR, Rodriguez A, et al: Pre-existing disease in trauma patients: A predictor of fate independent of age and injury severity score. **Journal of Trauma** 1992; 31(2):236–244.

26. Morris JA, Auerbach PS, Marshall GA, et al: The Trauma Score as a triage tool in the prehospital setting. **Journal of the American Medical Association** 1986; 256:1319–1325.

27. Morris JA, Mackenzie EJ, Edelstein SL: The effect of pre-existing conditions on mortality in trauma patients. **Journal of the American Medical Association** 1990; 263(14):1942–1946.

28. Oreskovich MR, Howard JD, Copass MK, et al: Geriatric trauma: Injury patterns and outcome. **Journal of Trauma** 1984; 24(7):565–572.

29. Osler T, Hales K, Baack B, et al: Trauma in the elderly. **American Journal of Surgery** 1988; 156(6):537–543.

30. Pennings JL, Bachulis BL, Simons CT, et al: Survival after severe brain injury in the aged. **Archives of Surgery** 1993; 128(7):787–794.

31. Phillips S, Rond PC, Kelly SM, et al: The failure of triage criteria to identify geriatric patients with trauma: Results from the Florida trauma triage study. **Journal of Trauma** 1996; 40(2): 278–283.

32. Riggs JE: Mortality from accidental falls among the elderly in the United States, 1962–1988: Demonstrating the impact of improved trauma management. **Journal of Trauma** 1993; 35(2): 212–219.

33. Rowe JW: Health care myths at the end of life. **Bulletin of the American College of Surgeons** 1996; 81(6):11–18.

34. Scalea TM, Simon HM, Duncan AO, et al: Geriatric blunt multiple trauma: Improved survival with early invasive monitoring. **Journal of Trauma** 1990; 30(2):129–134.

35. Schwab CW, Kauder DR: Trauma in the geriatric patient. **Archives of Surgery** 1992; 127(6): 701–706.

36. Shabot MM, Johnson CL: Outcome from critical care in the "oldest old" trauma patients. **Journal of Trauma** 1995; 39(2):254–259.

37. Smith DP, Enderson BL, Maull KI: Trauma in the elderly: Determinants of outcomes. **Southern Medical Journal** 1990; 83(2):171–177.

38. Timberlake GA: Elder abuse. In: Kaufman HH (ed): **The Physician's Perspective on Medical Law.** Neurosurgical Topics; American Association of Neurological Surgeons, Park Ridge, IL, 1997.

39. van Aalst JA, Morris JA, Yates HK, et al: Severely injured geriatric patients return to independent living: A study of factors influencing function and independence. **Journal of Trauma** 1991; 31(8):1096–1101; discussion 1101–1102.

40. van der Sluis CK, Klasen HJ, Eisma WH, et al: Major trauma in young and old: What is the difference? **Journal of Trauma** 1996; 40(1):78–82.

41. Wardle TD: Co-morbid factors in trauma patients. **British Medical Bulletin** 1999; 55(4): 744–756.

42. Zietlow SP, Capizzi PJ, Bannon MP, et al: Multisystem geriatric trauma. **Journal of Trauma** 1994; 37(6):985–988.

ELEVEN

Trauma in Women

OBJECTIVES:

Upon completion of this topic, the participant will be able to initially assess and manage the pregnant trauma patient and her fetus, and special problems in women. Specifically, the student will be able to:

A. Identify the alterations of pregnancy and discuss effects on patient management.

B. Identify and discuss the mechanisms of injury to the pregnant patient and fetus.

C. Outline the priorities and assessment methods for both patients (mother and fetus).

D. Outline indications for operative intervention unique to the injured pregnant patient.

E. Recognize the potential for isoimmunization.

F. Identify patterns of domestic violence.

TRAUMA IN WOMEN

I. INTRODUCTION

The potential for pregnancy must be considered in any girl or woman between the ages of 10 and 50 years. Pregnancy causes major physiologic changes and altered anatomic relationships involving nearly every organ system of the body. These changes of structure and function may influence the evaluation of the injured pregnant patient by altering the signs and symptoms of injury, the approach and responses to resuscitation, as well as the results of diagnostic tests. Pregnancy also may affect the patterns of injury or severity of injury. The doctor attending a pregnant trauma patient must remember that there are 2 patients. Nevertheless, **initial treatment** priorities for an injured pregnant patient remain the same as for the nonpregnant patient. A thorough understanding of the physiologic relationship between a pregnant patient and her fetus is essential if the best interests of both are to be served. The best initial treatment for the fetus is the provision of optimum resuscitation of the mother and the early assessment of the fetus. Monitoring and evaluation techniques should allow not only assessment of the mother but also of the fetus. The use of x-rays, if indicated during critical management, should not be withheld because of the pregnancy. **A qualified surgeon and obstetrician should be consulted early in the evaluation of the pregnant trauma patient.**

II. ANATOMIC AND PHYSIOLOGIC ALTERATIONS OF PREGNANCY

A. Anatomic

The uterus remains an intrapelvic organ until approximately the 12th week of gestation, when it begins to rise out of the pelvis. By 20 weeks, the uterus is at the umbilicus. At 34 to 36 weeks, it reaches the costal margin. During the last 2 weeks of gestation, the fundus frequently descends as the fetal head engages the pelvis. As the uterus enlarges, the bowel is pushed cephalad, so that the bowel lies mostly in the upper abdomen. As a result, the bowel is somewhat protected in blunt abdominal trauma, whereas the uterus and its contents (fetus and placenta) become more vulnerable. However, penetrating trauma to the upper abdomen during late gestation can result in complex intestinal injury due to this cephalad displacement.

During the first trimester, the uterus is a thick-walled structure of limited size, confined within the bony pelvis. During the second trimester, the uterus enlarges beyond its protected intrapelvic location, but the small fetus remains mobile and cushioned by a relatively generous amount of amniotic fluid. The amniotic fluid itself could be a source of amniotic fluid embolism and disseminated intravascular coagulation following trauma if the fluid gains access to the intravascular space. By the third trimester, the uterus is large and thin walled. In the vertex presentation, the fetal head is usually within the pelvis, with the remainder of the fetus exposed above the pelvic brim. Pelvic fracture(s) in late gestation may result in skull fracture or serious intracranial injury to the fetus. Unlike the elastic myometrium, the placenta has little elasticity. This lack of placental elastic tissue predisposes to shear forces at the uteroplacental interface, which may lead to abruptio placentae. The placental vasculature is maximally dilated throughout gestation, yet it is exquisitely sensitive to catecholamine stimulation. Likewise, an abrupt decrease in maternal intravascular volume may result in a profound increase in uterine vascular resistance, reducing fetal oxygenation despite reasonably normal maternal vital signs.

B. Blood Volume and Composition

1. Volume

Plasma volume increases steadily throughout pregnancy and plateaus at 34 weeks' gestation. A smaller increase in red blood cell (RBC) volume occurs, resulting in a decreased hematocrit (physiologic anemia of pregnancy). In late pregnancy, a hematocrit of 31% to 35% is normal. With hemorrhage, otherwise healthy pregnant patients may lose 1200 to 1500 mL of their blood volume before exhibiting signs and symptoms of hypovolemia. However, this amount of hemorrhage may be reflected by fetal distress evidenced by an abnormal fetal heart rate.

2. Composition

The white blood cell (WBC) count increases during pregnancy. It is not unusual to see WBC counts of 15,000/mm³ during pregnancy or as high as 25,000/mm³ during labor. Levels of serum fibrinogen and other clotting factors are mildly elevated. Prothrombin and partial thromboplastin times may be shortened but bleeding and clotting times are unchanged. The serum albumin level falls to 2.2 to 2.8 g/dL during pregnancy, causing a drop in serum protein levels by approximately

1.0 g/dL. Serum osmolarity remains at about 280 mOsm/L throughout pregnancy.

C. Hemodynamics

1. Cardiac output

After the 10th week of pregnancy, cardiac output can be increased by 1.0 to 1.5 L/minute due to the increase in plasma volume and decrease in vascular resistance of the uterus and placenta, which during the third trimester of pregnancy receive 20% of the patient's cardiac output. This increased output can be greatly influenced by the maternal position in the second half of pregnancy. In the supine position, vena cava compression may decrease cardiac output by 30% due to decreased venous return from the lower extremities.

2. Heart rate

Heart rate increases gradually by 10 to 15 beats/minute throughout pregnancy, reaching a maximum rate by the third trimester. This change in heart rate must be considered in interpreting the tachycardic response to hypovolemia.

3. Blood pressure

Pregnancy results in a 5- to 15-mm Hg fall in systolic and diastolic pressures during the second trimester. Blood pressure returns to near-normal levels at term. Some women may exhibit hypotension (supine hypotensive syndrome) when placed in the supine position due to compression of the inferior vena cava. This hypotension is corrected by relieving uterine pressure on the inferior vena cava as described in V., Assessment and Management in this chapter. The normal changes in blood pressure, pulse, hemoglobin, and hematocrit during pregnancy must be interpreted carefully in the pregnant trauma patient.

4. Venous pressure

The resting central venous pressure (CVP) is variable with pregnancy, but the response to volume is the same as in the nonpregnant state. Venous hypertension in the lower extremities is present during the third trimester.

5. Electrocardiographic changes

The axis may shift leftward by approximately 15°. Flattened or inverted T waves in leads III, AVF,

and the precordial leads may be normal. Ectopic beats are increased during pregnancy.

D. Respiratory

Minute ventilation increases primarily as a result of an increase in tidal volume due to increased levels of progesterone during pregnancy. Hypocapnea ($Paco_2$ of 30 mm Hg) is therefore common in late pregnancy. A $Paco_2$ of 35 to 40 mm Hg may indicate impending respiratory failure during pregnancy. Although the forced vital capacity fluctuates slightly during pregnancy, it is largely maintained throughout pregnancy due to equal and opposite changes in inspiratory capacity (which increases) and residual volume (which decreases). Anatomic alterations in the thoracic cavity appear to account for the decreased residual volume that is associated with diaphragmatic elevation with increased lung markings and prominence of the pulmonary vessels seen on chest x-ray.

Oxygen consumption is increased during pregnancy. Therefore, it is important to maintain and ensure adequate arterial oxygenation during the resuscitation of the injured pregnant patient.

E. Gastrointestinal

Gastric emptying time is prolonged during pregnancy, and the doctor should always assume that the stomach of a pregnant patient is full. Therefore, early gastric tube decompression is particularly important to avoid aspiration of gastric contents. The intestines are relocated to the upper part of the abdomen and may be shielded by the uterus. Position of the patient's spleen and liver are essentially unchanged by pregnancy.

F. Urinary

The glomerular filtration rate and the renal plasma blood flow increase during pregnancy. Levels of creatinine and serum urea nitrogen fall to approximately one-half of normal prepregnancy levels. Glycosuria is common during pregnancy. There is a physiologic dilatation of the renal calyces, pelves, and ureters outside of the pelvis, which may persist for several weeks following pregnancy. Because of frequent dextrorotation of the uterus, the right renal collection system is often more dilated than the left.

G. Endocrine

The pituitary gland increases in size and weight by 30% to 50% during pregnancy. Shock may cause necrosis of the anterior pituitary gland, resulting in pituitary insufficiency.

H. Musculoskeletal

The symphysis pubis widens to 4 to 8 mm and the sacroiliac-joint spaces increase by the 7th month of gestation. These factors must be considered in interpreting x-rays of the pelvis.

I. Neurologic

Eclampsia is a complication of late pregnancy that may mimic head injury. Eclampsia should be considered if seizures occur with associated hypertension, hyperreflexia, proteinuria, and peripheral edema. Expert neurologic and obstetric consultation frequently is helpful in differentiating between eclampsia and other causes of seizures.

III. MECHANISMS OF INJURY

Most mechanisms of injury are similar to those in the nonpregnant patient. However, certain differences must be recognized in the pregnant patient.

A. Blunt Injury

The abdominal wall, uterine myometrium, and amniotic fluid act as buffers to direct fetal injury from blunt trauma. Nonetheless, fetal injuries may occur when the abdominal wall strikes an object such as the dashboard or steering wheel, or if the pregnant patient is struck by a blunt instrument. Indirect injury to the fetus may occur from rapid compression, deceleration, contrecoup effect, or a shearing force resulting in abruptio placentae.

Seat belts decrease maternal injury and death by preventing ejection. However, the type of restraint system affects the frequency of uterine rupture and fetal death. The use of a lap belt alone allows forward flexion and uterine compression with possible uterine rupture or abruptio placentae. A lap belt worn too high over the uterus could produce uterine rupture because of direct force transmission to the uterus on impact. The use of shoulder restraints in conjunction with the lap belt reduces the likelihood of direct or indirect fetal injury, presumably because of the greater surface area over which the deceleration force is dissipated as well as the prevention of forward flexion of the mother over the gravid uterus. Therefore, determination of the type of restraint device worn by the pregnant patient, if any, is important in the overall assessment.

B. Penetrating Injury

As the gravid uterus increases in size, the remainder of the viscera is relatively protected from penetrating injury, while the likelihood of uterine injury increases. The dense uterine musculature in early pregnancy can absorb a great amount of energy from penetrating missiles, which decreases missile velocity and lessens the likelihood of injury to other viscera. The amniotic fluid and conceptus also absorb energy and contribute to slowing of the penetrating missile. The resulting low incidence of associated maternal visceral injuries accounts for the generally excellent maternal outcome in the penetrating wounds of the gravid uterus. However, the fetus generally fares poorly when there is a penetrating injury to the uterus.

IV. SEVERITY OF INJURIES

Severity of maternal injuries determines maternal and fetal outcome. Therefore, treatment methods also depend on the severity of maternal injuries. All pregnant patients with major injuries require admission to a facility with trauma and obstetric capabilities, since there is an increased maternal and fetal mortality rate in this group of patients. Eighty percent of pregnant females who survive hemorrhagic shock will experience fetal death. Even the pregnant patient with minor injuries should be carefully observed, since occasionally even minor injuries may be associated with abruptio placentae and fetal loss. Direct fetal injuries usually occur in late pregnancy and are typically associated with serious maternal trauma.

V. ASSESSMENT AND MANAGEMENT

For optimal outcome of mother and fetus, it is recommended to assess and resuscitate the mother first, and then to assess the fetus before conducting a secondary survey of the mother.

A. Primary Survey and Resuscitation

1. Maternal

Assure a patent airway, adequate ventilation and

oxygenation, and effective circulatory volume. If ventilatory support is required, intubation as described in Chapter 2, Airway and Ventilatory Management, is appropriate for the pregnant patient and consideration should be given to hyperventilating her.

Uterine compression of the vena cava may reduce venous return to the heart, thereby decreasing cardiac output and aggravating the shock state. Therefore, **unless a spinal injury is suspected,** the pregnant patient should be transported and evaluated on her left side. If the patient is in a supine position, the patient can be logrolled **4 to 6 inches to her left and supported** with a bolstering device. The uterus should be displaced manually to the left side to relieve pressure on the inferior vena cava. **Because of the increased intravascular volume, the pregnant patient can lose a significant amount of blood before tachycardia, hypotension, and other signs of hypovolemia occur. Thus, the fetus may be in distress and the placenta deprived of vital perfusion while the mother's condition and vital signs appear stable.** Crystalloid fluid resuscitation and early type-specific blood administration are indicated to support the physiologic hypervolemia of pregnancy. Avoid administering vasopressors to restore maternal blood pressure, because these agents further reduce uterine blood flow, resulting in fetal hypoxia. As intravenous lines are started, blood samples are drawn for appropriate laboratory analyses, including type and crossmatch, toxicology studies, and fibrinogen levels.

2. Fetus

The abdominal examination during pregnancy is critically important, as rapid identification of serious maternal injuries and fetal well-being are dependent on a thorough evaluation. Uterine rupture is suggested by findings of abdominal tenderness, guarding, rigidity, or rebound tenderness, especially if there is profound shock. Frequently, peritoneal signs are difficult to appreciate in advanced gestation due to expansion and attenuation of the abdominal wall musculature. Other abnormal findings suggestive of uterine rupture include abdominal fetal lie (eg, oblique or transverse lie), easy palpation of fetal parts due to extrauterine location, and inability to readily palpate the uterine fundus when there is fundal rupture). X-ray evidence of rupture includes extended fetal extremities, abnormal fetal position,

or free intraperitoneal air. Diagnosis of uterine rupture mandates operative exploration.

Abruptio placentae may be suggested by vaginal bleeding (70% of the cases), uterine tenderness, frequent uterine contractions, uterine tetany, or uterine irritability (uterus contracts when touched). Thirty percent of abruptions following trauma may not exhibit vaginal bleeding. Uterine ultrasonography may demonstrate the lesion, but the test is not definitive. Late in pregnancy, abruption can occur following relatively minor injuries.

In most cases of uterine rupture or abruptio placentae, the patient will complain of abdominal pain or cramping. Signs of hypovolemia can accompany either of these injuries.

Initial fetal heart tones can be auscultated with a Doppler (≥10 weeks' gestation). Continuous fetal monitoring should be performed beyond 20 to 24 weeks' gestation. (See B., Adjuncts to Primary Survey and Resuscitation in this section.)

B. Adjuncts to Primary Survey and Resuscitation

1. Maternal

If possible, the patient should be monitored on her left side after physical examination. Monitoring of the CVP response to fluid challenge may be valuable in maintaining the relative hypervolemia required in pregnancy. Monitoring should include pulse oximetry and arterial blood gas determinations. Remember, maternal bicarbonate is normally low during pregnancy.

2. Fetus

Obstetric consultation should be obtained since fetal distress can occur at any time and without warning. Fetal heart rate is a sensitive indicator of both maternal blood volume status, as well as fetal well-being. Fetal heart tones should be monitored in every injured pregnant woman. Intermittent and repeated Doppler examination can be used to detect fetal heart tones after 10 weeks' gestation. Continuous fetal monitoring with a cardiotocodynamometer is useful after 20 to 24 weeks' gestation. The normal range for fetal heart rate is between 120 to 160 beats/minute. An abnormal fetal heart rate, repetitive decelerations, absence of accelerations or beat-to-beat variabil-

TRAUMA IN WOMEN

ity, or frequent uterine activity may be a sign of impending maternal and/or fetal decompensation (eg, hypoxia and/or acidosis) and should prompt immediate obstetric consultation, if not already obtained.

Indicated radiographic studies should be performed, because the benefits certainly outweigh potential risk to the fetus. However, unnecessary duplication of films should be avoided.

C. Secondary Assessment

The maternal secondary survey should follow the same pattern as in the nonpregnant patient. Indications for abdominal CT, FAST, or DPL are the same. However, if DPL is performed, the catheter should be placed above the umbilicus using the open technique. Pay careful attention to the presence of uterine contractions suggesting early labor or tetanic contractions suggesting premature separation of the placenta. Evaluation of the perineum should include a formal pelvic examination, ideally performed by a doctor skilled in obstetric care. The presence of amniotic fluid in the vagina, evidenced by a pH of 7 to 7.5, suggests ruptured chorioamniotic membranes. Cervical effacement and dilatation, fetal presentation, and the relationship of the fetal presenting part to the ischial spines should be noted. Because vaginal bleeding in the third trimester may indicate disruption of the placenta and impending death of the fetus, a vaginal examination is vital. Repeated vaginal examinations should be avoided. The decision regarding an emergency cesarean section should be made in conjunction with an obstetrician.

Admission to the hospital is mandatory in the presence of vaginal bleeding, uterine irritability, abdominal tenderness, pain or cramping, evidence of hypovolemia, changes in or absence of fetal heart tones, or leakage of amniotic fluid. Care should be provided at a facility with appropriate fetal and maternal monitoring and treatment capabilities. **The fetus may be in jeopardy even with apparently minor maternal injury.**

D. Definitive Care

Obstetric consultation should be obtained whenever specific uterine problems exist or are suspected.

With extensive placental separation or with amniotic fluid embolization, widespread intravascular clotting may develop, causing depletion of fibrino-gen (<250 mg/dL), other clotting factors, and platelets. This consumptive coagulopathy may emerge rapidly. In the presence of life-threatening amniotic fluid embolism and/or disseminated intravascular coagulation, uterine evacuation should be accomplished on an urgent basis along with replacement of platelets, fibrinogen, and other clotting factors if necessary.

Consequences of fetomaternal hemorrhage include not only fetal anemia and death, but also isoimmunization if the mother is Rh-negative. Because as little as 0.01 mL of Rh-positive blood will sensitize 70% of Rh-negative patients, the presence of fetomaternal hemorrhage in an Rh-negative mother should warrant Rh immunoglobulin therapy. Although a positive Kleihauer-Betke test (a maternal blood smear allowing detection of fetal RBCs in the maternal circulation) indicates fetomaternal hemorrhage, a negative test does not exclude minor degrees of fetomaternal hemorrhage that are capable of sensitizing the Rh-negative mother. **Therefore, all pregnant Rh-negative trauma patients should be considered for Rh immunoglobulin therapy unless the injury is remote from the uterus** (eg, isolated distal extremity injury). Immunoglobulin therapy should be instituted within 72 hours of injury.

The large, engorged pelvic vessels that surround the gravid uterus can contribute to massive retroperitoneal bleeding after blunt trauma with associated pelvic fractures.

Initial management is directed at resuscitation and stabilization of the pregnant patient because the fetal life at this point is totally dependent on the mother's condition. Fetal monitoring should be maintained after satisfactory resuscitation and stabilization of the mother. The presence of 2 patients (mother and fetus) and the potential for multiple injuries emphasize the importance of a surgeon working in concert with an obstetric consultant.

VI. PERIMORTEM CESAREAN SECTION (c-section)

There are few data to support perimortem c-section in pregnant trauma patients suffering from hypovolemic cardiac arrest. Fetal distress can be present when the mother is hemodynamically normal. Progressive maternal instability compromises fetal survival. At the time of maternal hypovolemic cardiac arrest, the fetus already has suffered prolonged hypoxia. For other causes of maternal cardiac arrest, perimortem c-section occasionally may be successful if performed within 4 to 5 minutes of the arrest.

VII. DOMESTIC VIOLENCE

Domestic violence is a major cause of injury to women during cohabitation, marriage, and pregnancy regardless of ethnic background, cultural influences, or socioeconomic status. Seventeen percent of injured pregnant patients experience trauma as the result of another person, and 60% of these patients have repeated episodes of domestic violence. According to estimates from the United States Department of Justice (1994), 2 to 4 million per year and almost half of all women over their lifetimes are abused in some manner. As with child abuse, this information must be identified and documented. These attacks can result in death and disability. They also represent an increasing number of emergency department visitations.

Indicators that may **suggest** the presence of domestic violence include:

1. Injuries inconsistent with stated history
2. Diminished self-image, depression, suicide attempts
3. Self-abuse
4. Frequent emergency department or doctor's office visits
5. Symptoms suggestive of substance abuse
6. Self-blame for injuries

7. Partner insists on being present for interview and examination and monopolizes discussion

These indicators only raise the suspicion of the potential for domestic violence and should serve to initiate further investigation. Three questions, when asked in a nonjudgmental manner and without the patient's partner being present, detect 65% to 70% of domestic violence victims. (See Table 1, Partner Violence Screen.) Suspected cases of domestic violence should be handled through local social service agencies or the state health and human services department.

VIII. SUMMARY

Important and predictable anatomic and physiologic changes occur during pregnancy that may influence the evaluation and treatment of the injured pregnant patient. Vigorous fluid and blood replacement should be given to correct and prevent maternal as well as fetal hypovolemic shock. A search should be made for conditions unique to the injured pregnant patient, such as blunt or penetrating uterine trauma, abruptio placentae, amniotic fluid embolism, isoimmunization, and premature rupture of membranes. Attention also must be directed toward the fetus, the second patient of this unique duo, after its environment is stabilized. A qualified surgeon and obstetrician should be consulted early in the evaluation of the pregnant trauma patient.

Table 1—Partner Violence Screen

1. Have you been kicked, hit, punched, or otherwise hurt by someone within the past year? If so, by whom?

2. Do you feel safe in your current relationship?

3. Is there a partner from a previous relationship who is making you feel unsafe now?

Reprinted with permission, Feldhaus KM, Koziol-McLain J, Amsbury HL, et al: Accuracy of 3 brief screening questions for detecting partner violence in the emergency department. *Journal of the American Medical Association* 1997; 277: 1357-1361.

TRAUMA IN WOMEN

BIBLIOGRAPHY

1. Berry MJ, McMurray RG, Katz VL: Pulmonary and ventilatory responses to pregnancy, immersion, and exercise. **Journal of Applied Physiology** 1989; 66(2):857–862.

2. Buchsbaum HG, Staples PP Jr: Self-inflicted gunshot wound to the pregnant uterus: Report of two cases. **Obstetrics and Gynecology** 1985; 65(3):32S–35S.

3. Eisenstat SA, Sancroft L: Domestic violence. **New England Journal of Medicine**; 1999; 341: 886–892.

4. Esposito TJ: Trauma during pregnancy. **Emergency Medicine Clinics of North America** 1994; 12:167–199.

5. Feldhaus KM, Koziol-McLain J, Amsbury HL, et al: Accuracy of 3 brief screening questions for detecting partner violence in the emergency department. **Journal of the American Medical Association** 1997; 277:1357–1361.

6. Grisso JA, Schwarz DF, Hirschinger N, et al: Violent injuries among women in an urban area. **New England Journal of Medicine** 1999; 341: 1899–1905.

7. Hamburger KL, Saunders DG, Hovey M: Prevalence of domestic violence in community practice and rate of physician inquiry. **Family Medicine** 1992; 24:283–287.

8. Higgins SD, Garite TJ: Late abruptio placenta in trauma patients: Implications for monitoring. **Obstetrics and Gynecology** 1984; 63(3): 10S–12S.

9. Kissinger DP, Rozycki GS, Morris JA, et al: Trauma in pregnancy — Predicting pregnancy outcome. **Archives of Surgery** 1991; 125:1079–1086.

10. Knudson MM, Rozycki GS, Strear CM: Reproductive system trauma. In: Mattox KL, Feliciano DV, Moore EE (eds): **Trauma.** New York, McGraw-Hill, 2000, pp 879–906.

11. Kyriacou DN, Anglin D, Taliaferro E, et al: Risk factors for injury to women from domestic violence. **New England Journal of Medicine** 1999; 341:1892–1898.

12. Minow M: Violence against women—A challenge to the supreme court. **New England Journal of Medicine** 1999; 341:1927–1929 [editorial].

13. Mollison PL: Clinical aspects of Rh immunization. **American Journal of Clinical Pathology** 1973; 60:287.

14. Nicholson BE (ed): Family violence. **The Journal of the South Carolina Medical Association** 1995; 91(10):409–446.

15. Pearlman MD, Tintinalli JE, Lorenz RP: Blunt trauma during pregnancy. **New England Journal of Medicine** 1991; 323:1606–1613.

16. Rose PG, Strohm PL, Zuspan FP: Fetomaternal hemorrhage following trauma. **American Journal of Obstetrics and Gynecology** 1985; 153: 844–847.

17. Schoenfeld A, Ziv E, Stein L, et al: Seat belts in pregnancy and the obstetrician. **Obstetrical and Gynecological Survey** 1987; 42(5):275–282.

18. Sisley A, Jacobs LM, Poole G, et al: Violence in America: A public health crisis—Domestic violence. **Journal of Trauma** 1999; 46:1105–1113.

19. Timberlake GA, McSwain NE: Trauma in pregnancy, a ten-year perspective. **The American Surgeon** 1989; 55:151–153.

20. Towery RA, English TP, Wisner DW: Evaluation of pregnant women after blunt injury. **Journal of Trauma** 1992; 35:731–736.

21. Statement on Domestic Violence. **Bulletin of the American College of Surgeons**, 2000; 85:26.

RESOURCE

National Coalition Against Domestic Violence, PO Box 18749, Denver, CO 80218-0749, 303/839-1852, 303/831-9251 (Fax).

TWELVE

Transfer to Definitive Care

12

■ OBJECTIVES:

Upon completion of this topic, the participant will be able to define and apply general principles for the **safe** transfer of an injured patient to definitive care. Specifically, the doctor will be able to:

A. Identify those injured patients who may require transfer from a primary care institution to a facility capable of providing the necessary level of trauma care.

B. Initiate procedures to **optimally** prepare the trauma patient for safe transfer to a higher-level trauma care facility via the appropriate mode of transportation.

TRANSFER TO DEFINITIVE CARE

I. INTRODUCTION

This course is designed to train students to be more proficient in their ability to assess, stabilize, and prepare the patient for definitive care. Definitive care, whether it be support and monitoring in an intensive care unit (ICU) or operative intervention, requires the presence and active involvement of a surgeon and the trauma team. If definitive care cannot be rendered at the local hospital, the patient requires transfer to a hospital that has the resources and capabilities to care for the patient. Ideally, this facility should be a verified trauma center, the level of which depends on the patient's needs. The decision to transfer the patient to another facility depends on the patient's injuries and the local resources. Decisions as to which patients should be transferred, and when, are matters of medical judgment. Recent evidence supports the view that trauma outcome is enhanced if critically injured patients are cared for in trauma centers. **The trauma patient should be transferred to the closest appropriate hospital, preferably a verified trauma center.** (Reference: ACS Committee on Trauma, *Resources for Optimal Care of the Injured Patient*; guidelines for trauma system development and trauma center verification processes and standards may be obtained from the ACS, c/o Customer Service/Publications, 633 N. Saint Clair St., Chicago, IL 60611; or order online at www.facs.org.)

The major principle of trauma management is to **do no further harm**. Indeed, care of the trauma patient should consistently improve with each step, from the scene of the incident to the facility that can provide the patient with the necessary, proper treatment. All those who care for trauma patients must ensure that the level of care never declines from one step to another.

II. DETERMINING THE NEED FOR PATIENT TRANSFER

The vast majority of patients receive their total care in the local hospital, and movement beyond that point is not necessary. **It is essential that doctors assess their own capabilities and limitations, as well as those of their institution. This allows for early recognition of patients who may be safely cared for in the local hospital and those who require transfer for definitive care.** Once the need for transfer is recognized, arrangements should be expedited and not delayed for diagnostic procedures (eg, DPL,

CT scan) that do not change the immediate plan of care.

Patient outcome is directly related to time from injury to properly delivered definitive care. In those institutions in which there is no full-time, in-house emergency department coverage, the timeliness of transfer is partly dependent on the response of the doctor to the emergency department. Consequently, it is recommended that appropriate communication with the prehospital system be developed such that those patients can be identified who require the presence of a doctor in the emergency department at the time of arrival. Subsequently, the attending doctor should be committed to respond to the emergency department prior to the arrival of critically injured patients. Identification of those patients requiring prompt attention can be based on physiologic measurements, specific identifiable injuries, and mechanism of injury.

The timing of interhospital transfer varies based on the distance of transfer, the available skill levels for transfer, circumstances of the local institution, and intervention that is necessary before the patient can be transferred safely. If the resources are available and if the necessary procedures can be performed expeditiously, life-threatening injuries should be treated before patient transport. (See Table 1, page 286, Interhospital Transfer Criteria.) This treatment may require operative intervention to ensure that the patient is in the best possible condition for transfer. **Intervention prior to transfer is a surgical decision.**

To help the doctor determine which patients might need care at a higher-level facility, the ACS Committee on Trauma recommends using certain physiologic indices, injury mechanisms and patterns, and historical information. These factors also help the doctor decide which stable patients might benefit from transfer.

Certain clinical measurements of physiologic status are useful in determining the need for transfer to an institution that provides a higher level of care. Patients who exhibit evidence of shock, significant physiologic deterioration, or progressive deterioration in neurologic status require the highest level of care and should benefit from timely transfer.

Stable patients with blunt abdominal trauma and documented liver or spleen injuries may be candidates for nonoperative management. Implicit in such practice is the immediate availability of an operating room and a qualified surgical team. A general or trauma surgeon should supervise nonoperative management, regardless of the patient's age. Such patients should not be treated expectantly at facilities that are not prepared for urgent operative intervention. They should be transferred to a trauma center.

Patients with certain specific injuries, combinations of injuries (particularly those involving the brain), or who have historical findings indicating high-energy transfer may be at risk for death and are candidates for early transfer to a trauma center. High-risk criteria suggesting the necessity for early transfer are outlined in Table 1, page 286, Interhospital Transfer Criteria.

Management of the combative or uncooperative patient with an altered level of consciousness is difficult and fraught with hazards. The patient is often in a supine position, immobilized, and has wrist/leg restraints applied. If sedation is required, the patient should be intubated. Therefore, before administering any sedation, the treating doctor must:

1. Assure that the patient's ABCDEs are appropriately managed.
2. Relieve the patient's pain if possible, eg, apply splint fractures, administer small, intravenous doses of narcotics.
3. Attempt to calm and reassure the patient.

Remember, benzodiazepines, fentanyl, propofol, and ketamine are all hazardous in the hypovolemic, intoxicated, or head-injured patient. **When in doubt, pain management, sedation, and intubation should be accomplished by the individual most skilled in these procedures.** (See Chapter 2, Airway and Ventilatory Management.)

Abuse of alcohol and/or other drugs is common to all forms of trauma and is particularly important to identify. Doctors should recognize that alcohol and drugs can alter pain perception and mask significant physical findings. Alterations in the patient's responsiveness may be related to alcohol and/or drugs, but absence of cerebral injury should never be assumed in the presence of alcohol or drugs. If the examining doctor is unsure, transfer to a higher-level facility may be appropriate. Death of another individual involved in the incident suggests the possibility of severe, occult injury in survivors. **A thor-**

ough and careful evaluation of the patient, even in the absence of obvious signs of severe injury, is mandatory.

III. TRANSFER RESPONSIBILITIES

A. Referring Doctor

The referring doctor is responsible for the initiation of transfer of the patient to the receiving institution and for the selection of an appropriate mode of transportation and level of care required for optimal management of the patient en route. The referring doctor should consult with the receiving doctor and should be thoroughly familiar with the transporting agencies, their capabilities, and the arrangements for patient management during transport.

The referring doctor is responsible for stabilizing the patient's condition, within the capabilities of the initial institution, before the patient is actually transferred to another facility. Initiation of the transfer process should begin while resuscitative efforts are in progress.

Transfer agreements must be established to provide for the consistent and efficient movement of patients between institutions. These agreements allow for feedback to the referring hospital and enhance the efficiency and quality of the patient's management during transfer.

B. Receiving Doctor

The receiving doctor must be consulted with regard to the transfer of a trauma patient. The receiving doctor must assure that the proposed receiving institution is qualified, able, and willing to accept the patient, and is in agreement with the intent to transfer. The receiving doctor should assist the referring doctor in making arrangements for the appropriate mode and level of care during transport. If the proposed receiving doctor and facility are unable to accept the patient, they should assist in finding an alternative placement for the patient.

The quality of care rendered en route also is of vital importance to the patient's outcome. Only by direct communication between the referring and receiving doctors can the details of patient transfer be clearly delineated. If adequately trained ambulance personnel are not available, a nurse or doctor should accompany the patient. All monitoring and management rendered en route should be documented.

TRANSFER TO DEFINITIVE CARE

Table 1—Interhospital Transfer Criteria
When the Patient's Needs Exceed Available Resources

CLINICAL CIRCUMSTANCES

Central Nervous System
• Head Injury
  • Pentrating injury or depressed skull fracture
  • Open injury with or without CSF leak
  • GCS Score <15 or neurologically abnormal
  • Lateralizing signs
• Spinal Cord Injury or Major Vertebral Injury

Chest
  • Widened mediastinum or signs suggesting great vessel injury
  • Major chest wall injury or pulmonary contusion
  • Cardiac injury
  • Patients who may require prolonged ventilation

Pelvis/Abdomen
  • Unstable pelvic-ring disruption
  • Pelvic-ring disruption with shock and evidence of continuing hemorrhage
  • Open pelvic injury
  • Solid organ injury

Extremity
  • Severe open fractures
  • Traumatic amputation with potential for replantation
  • Complex articular fractures
  • Major crush injury
  • Ischemia

Multisystem Injury
  • Head injury with face, chest, abdominal, or pelvic injury
  • Injury to more than 2 body regions
  • Major burns or burns with associated injuries
  • Multiple, proximal long-bone fractures

Comorbid Factors
  • Age >55 years
  • Children ≤5 years of age
  • Cardiac or respiratory disease
  • Insulin-dependent diabetics, morbid obesity
  • Pregnancy
  • Immunosuppression

Secondary Deterioration (Late Sequelae)
  • Mechanical ventilation required
  • Sepsis
  • Single or multiple organ system failure (deterioration in central nervous, cardiac, pulmonary, hepatic, renal, or coagulation systems)
  • Major tissue necrosis

Adapted with permission, ACS Committee on Trauma: *Resources for Optimal Care of the Injured Patient*, in publication.

IV. MODES OF TRANSPORTATION

Do no further harm is the most important principle when choosing the mode of patient transportation. Ground, water, and air transportation modalities can be safe and effective in fulfilling this principle.

Interhospital transfer of the critically injured is potentially hazardous unless patients are stabilized as optimally as possible before transport, transfer personnel are properly trained, and provision has been made for dealing with the unexpected crisis during transport. To ensure safe transfers, trauma surgeons must be involved in training, continuing education, and quality improvement programs designed for transfer personnel and procedures. Surgeons also should be actively involved in the development and maintenance of systems of trauma care.

V. TRANSFER PROTOCOLS

Where protocols for patient transfer do not exist, the following guidelines are suggested.

A. Referring Doctor

The local doctor wishing to transfer the patient should speak directly to the surgeon accepting the patient at the receiving hospital and provide this information:

1. Identification of the patient

2. A brief history of the incident, including pertinent prehospital data

3. Initial patient findings in the emergency department, and the patient's response to the therapy administered

B. Information to Transferring Personnel

Information regarding the patient's condition and needs during transfer should be communicated to the transporting personnel. This information should include, but not be limited to:

1. Airway maintenance

2. Fluid volume replacement

3. Special procedures that may be necessary

4. Revised Trauma Score, resuscitation procedures, and any changes that may occur en route. (See Table 2, page 288, Sample Transfer Form.)

C. Documentation

A written record of the problem, treatment given, and patient status at the time of transfer, as well as certain physical items, must accompany the patient. A facsimile transmission may be used to avoid delay in transfer. (See Table 2, page 288, Sample Transfer Form.)

D. Prior to Transfer

The patient should be resuscitated and attempts made to stabilize the patient's conditions as completely as possible based on this suggested outline.

1. Airway

a. Insert an airway or endotracheal tube, if needed.

b. Provide suction.

c. Insert a gastric tube to reduce the risk of aspiration.

2. Breathing

a. Determine rate and administer supplementary oxygen.

b. Provide mechanical ventilation when needed.

c. Insert a chest tube if needed.

3. Circulation

a. Control external bleeding.

b. Establish 2 large-caliber IVs and begin crystalloid solution infusion.

c. Restore blood volume losses with crystalloid or blood, and continue replacement during transfer.

d. Insert an indwelling catheter to monitor urinary output.

e. Monitor the patient's cardiac rhythm and rate.

4. Central nervous system

a. Assist ventilations for the unconscious patient.

b. Administer mannitol or diuretics, if needed.

c. Immobilize head, neck, thoracic, and/or lumbar spine injuries.

TRANSFER TO DEFINITIVE CARE

Table 2–Sample Transfer Form
(Suggested information to send with the patient)

Patient Information	Diagnostic Studies:
Name_____	• Lab data: Attach all results to form
Address_____	• Basic imaging studies: Send all films with patient
City_____State_____Zip_____	• ECG
Age_____Sex_____Weight_____	• Specimens: Send all appropriate specimens with patient, eg, DPL fluid
Next of kin_____	**Treatment Rendered:**
Address_____	• Medications given, amount and time
City_____State_____Zip_____	
Phone #_____/ _____-_____	• IV fluids, type and amount
Date and Time	• Other
Date_____/ _____/ _____	
Time of Injury_____ am/pm	**Status of Patient at Transfer:**
Time admitted to ED_____ am/pm	
Time admitted to OR_____ am/pm	
Time transferred_____ am/pm	
Ample History:	**Management during Transport:**
Condition on Admission	**Referral Information:**
HR_____Rhythm_____	Doctor_____
BP_____/ _____RR_____Temp_____	Hospital_____
	Phone # _____/ _____-_____
Probable Diagnoses:	**Receiving Information:**
	Doctor_____
	Hospital_____
	Phone # _____/ _____-_____

Adapted with permission, ACS Committee on Trauma: *Resources for Optimal Care of the Injured Patient.* In publication.

5. Diagnostic studies

When indicated, obtaining these studies should not delay transfer.

a. X-rays of cervical spine, chest, pelvis, and extremities

b. Sophisticated diagnostic studies, eg, CT and aortography, usually not indicated

c. Hemoglobin or hematocrit, type and cross-match, arterial blood gas determinations, and pregnancy test on all females of childbearing age

d. Determination of cardiac rhythm and hemoglobin saturation (ECG and pulse oximetry)

6. Wounds

Performing these procedures should not delay transfer.

a. Clean and dress after external hemorrhage control

b. Administer tetanus prophylaxis

c. Administer antibiotics, when indicated

7. Fractures: Appropriate splinting and traction

E. Management during Transport

The appropriate personnel should transfer the patient, based on the patient's condition and potential problems.

1. Monitoring vital signs and pulse oximetry

2. Continued support of cardiorespiratory system

3. Continued blood volume replacement

4. Use of appropriate medications as ordered by a doctor or as provided by written protocol

5. Maintenance of communication with a doctor or institution during transfer

6. Maintenance of accurate records during transfer

VI. TRANSFER DATA

The information accompanying the patient should include both demographic and historical information pertinent to the patient's injury. Uniform trans-

mission of information is enhanced by the use of an established transfer form. Examples of appropriate data to include on a transfer form are outlined in Table 2, page 288, Sample Transfer Form. Other data that should accompany the patient are outlined in Appendix 5, Trauma Scores—Revised and Pediatric. In addition to the information already outlined, space should be provided for recording data in an organized, sequential fashion—vital signs, CNS function, and urinary output—during the initial resuscitation and transport period. (See Appendix 6, Sample Trauma Flow Sheet.)

VII. PITFALLS

Moving a patient from one location to another, regardless of the distance involved, is hazardous. The process must be approached with the same attention to detail as the resuscitation of the patient's vital functions. Problems during transportation must be anticipated to minimize their impact, should they occur. Endotracheal tubes may become dislodged or malpositioned during transport. The necessary equipment for reintubation must accompany the patient and the attendants must be capable of performing the procedure. Anticipation of deterioration in the patient's neurologic condition or hemodynamic status allows for planning for such a contingency if it occurs before the patient arrives at the referral center. The prudent doctor must review the steps to take to ensure that the patient's transfer to another level of care is as safe as possible. **Remember,** the doctor who begins the care of the injured patient must be committed to ensuring that the level of care does not deteriorate. This includes the care delivered during patient transfer to definitive care.

The flurry of activity surrounding the initial evaluation, resuscitation, and preparations for transfer of trauma patients often takes precedence over other logistic details. This may result in the failure to include certain items in the information that is sent with the patient, eg, x-ray films, laboratory reports, or narrative descriptions of the evaluation process or treatments rendered at the local hospital. A list is helpful in this regard and can be printed or stamped on an x-ray jacket or patient chart folder to remind the referring doctor to include all pertinent information. The list should be kept in the resuscitation area.

Patients frequently spend more time than necessary at the initial hospital after the necessity for transfer is recognized, eg, additional diagnostic tests for "completeness." Once the decision to transfer the patient is made, little is gained by performing procedures other than those necessary to restore normal hemodynamic function. Delaying the transfer while waiting for test results is not appropriate. Delaying transfer of a patient with an obvious brain injury and focal neurologic findings to the care of a neurosurgeon while waiting to obtain a CT scan of the brain delays the patient's access to necessary specialty care. There are occasions when a patient cannot be hemodynamically normalized prior to transport. Direct consultation with the receiving doctor may be helpful in determining the most appropriate time to begin the transfer of a hemodynamically abnormal patient.

The process of transportation of patients to other medical facilities is not, in and of itself, a treatment or cure for any disease or injury. The very process of transporting patients has great potential for the level of care to deteriorate. The environment into which the patient is placed is often unpredictable and not well controlled. Careful planning can minimize the impact that these unintentional events may produce.

VIII. SUMMARY

A. The major principle of trauma management is to do no further harm.

B. Individual capabilities of the treating doctor, institutional capabilities, and indications for transfer should be known.

C. The referring doctor and receiving doctor should communicate directly.

D. Transfer personnel should be adequately skilled to administer the required patient care en route.

■ BIBLIOGRAPHY

1. American College of Surgeons Committee on Trauma: **Resources for Optimal Care of the Injured Patient.** Chicago. In publication.

2. Champion HR, Sacco WJ, Copes WS, et al: A revision of the trauma score. **Journal of Trauma** 1989; 29(5):623–629.

3. Mullins PJ, Veum-Stone J, Helfand M, et al: Outcome of hospitalized injured patients after institution of a trauma system in an urban area. **Journal of the American Medical Association** 1994; 271:1919–1924.

4. Phillips TF, Goldstein AS: Airway management. In: Mattox KL, Moore EE, Feliciano DD (eds): **Trauma, 2nd Edition**. East Norwalk, CT, Appleton & Lange, 1991.

5. Scarpio RJ, Wesson DE: Splenic trauma. In: Eichelberger MR: **Pediatric Trauma: Prevention, Acute Care, Rehabilitation.** St. Louis, Mosby Yearbook, 1993, pp 456–463.

6. Sharar SR, Luna GK, Rice CL, et al: Air transport following surgical stabilization: An extension of regionalized trauma care. **Journal of Trauma** 1988; 28:794–798.

Appendices

These appendices provide additional information to enhance the doctor's knowledge of trauma-related issues.

◼ TABLE OF CONTENTS

APPENDIX

Triage Scenarios

■ INTRODUCTION

This is a self-assessment exercise, to be completed **before** you arrive for the course. Please read through the introductory information on the following pages before reading the individual scenarios and answering the related questions. This skills station is conducted in a group discussion format in which your participation is expected. Upon completion of this session, you will receive a booklet of prepared responses for each scenario.

The **goal** of this station is to apply trauma triage principles in multiple patient scenarios.

Upon completion of this session, the participant will be able to:

A. Define triage.

B. Understand and describe the principles involved and the factors that must be considered in the triage process.

C. Apply the principles of triage with the use of actual scenarios.

TRIAGE SCENARIOS

I. DEFINITION OF TRIAGE

Triage is a process by which management of multiple patient casualties is prioritized.

II. PRINCIPLES OF TRIAGE

A. Degree of Life Threat Posed by the Injury (ABCDEs of Care)

The degree of life threat posed by each injury is determined by considering the order of priorities in the primary survey of an individual patient and applying these same principles to groups of patients. In this system the patient with an airway or breathing problem takes priority over a patient with a circulatory or neurologic disability.

B. Injury Severity

The overall severity of injury in a particular patient may be related not only to an individual injury, but also to the effects of different injuries and how the patient responds to all of these injuries in a global sense. For instance, an isolated fracture may be of low priority. However, when it is combined with another source of major hemorrhage, which increases the overall injury severity, the priority level in the triage process also may increase.

C. Salvageability

The patient with the most severe injury or the greatest threat to life is not necessarily the patient that receives top priority when dealing with multiple patient scenarios. Consideration must be given to the likelihood of survival of the patient. In this system the patient who is least likely to survive in spite of having the most severe injuries is often relegated to a lower priority and is managed after patients who are considered more salvageable.

D. Resources Including Capability of Personnel and Equipment

The patient whose needs exceed the resource capabilities is given a lower priority until the necessary resources are secured.

E. Time, Distance, Environment

An injury that can be managed very quickly, although of lower severity and lower life threat, may be treated as a higher priority because of the short length of time taken for correcting the identified problem. Distance for travel in transporting a patient to definitive care and other environmental factors also need to be considered in prioritizing management of multiple patient scenarios.

III. APPLICATION OF TRIAGE PRINCIPLES

Triage is often based on incomplete information because the detailed information on the status of a patient may not be immediately obvious. However, decisions have to be made on the best information available. Frequently it is not possible to obtain such parameters as vital signs on the victims in multiple casualties. Indeed, it is necessary in many instances to make decisions by surveying an entire situation at a distance and determining on that basis which of the patients is the most severely injured. Simple factors (eg, a patient shouting in agony as opposed to one lying still with noisy breathing that can be detected from a distance) could be cues that would allow a decision to approach one patient with a potential airway problem before approaching another patient who may have a fractured extremity causing intense pain but not necessarily producing a major threat to life.

An important concept is to avoid indecision and proceed quickly with incomplete information because time is of the essence in the entire triaging process. In some situations, it may be possible to obtain information such as vital signs, etc from prehospital personnel. Such information should be used in prioritizing the management of multiple victims.

As a general rule, the order of priorities in multiple victim scenarios is the same as in an individual patient where airway (A) takes priority over breathing (B) and circulation (C). Therefore, the patient with an airway problem is managed before a patient with a circulatory problem. However, in some instances it may be necessary to prioritize patients based on salvageability. For example, a patient who has the least chance of survival, although being the most severely injured, may not be managed before a patient who can be stabilized very quickly and who has a problem that can be easily and rapidly reversed.

Triage decisions involving salvageability, in most situations, are dependent on assessment of the need for definitive care and not emergency care. Available resources and time/distance factors must be considered when making these decisions. For example, 3 patients with intraabdominal injuries present with hypotension. They would be triaged differently if 1 had a fractured limb and the other 2 had severe head injuries. Additionally, the 2 with severe head injuries would be triaged differently if 1 also had a suspected aorta disruption.

The triage process also involves identification of the necessary resources for stabilizing patients. If these resources are not available, the patient may not be given the same priority in the triage process.

Part of the triage process also may involve a determination of the most appropriate mode of transfer as well as the most appropriate institution to which the patient should be transferred based on the nature of the injuries and the resources required for managing the patient definitively.

Triage Scenario I—Gas Explosion in the Gymnasium

Scenario: You are summoned to a triage area at a construction site where 5 workers are injured in a gas explosion during the renovation of a gymnasium ceiling. After you quickly survey the situation, the patient's conditions are as follows:

Patient A—A young man is screaming, "Please help me, my leg is killing me!"

Patient B—A young woman is cyanotic, tachypneic, and breathing very noisily

Patient C—A 50-year-old man is lying in a pool of blood with his left trouser leg soaked in blood

Patient D—A young man is lying face down on a stretcher and not moving

Patient E—A young man is swearing expletives and shouting that someone should help him or he will call his lawyer.

Questions for Response:

1. *Identify what you perceive to be the primary problem requiring treatment.*

   Patient A is a young man screaming "Please help me, my leg is killing me!"

   Possible Injury/Problem:_____

   Patient B appears cyanotic and tachypneic, and is breathing very noisily.

   Possible Injury/Problem:_____

   Patient C is a 50-year-old man lying in a pool of blood with his left trouser leg soaked in blood.

   Possible Injury/Problem:_____

   Patient D is lying face down on a stretcher and not moving.

   Possible Injury/Problem:_____

   Patient E is swearing expletives and shouting that someone should help him or he will call his lawyer.

   Possible Injury/Problem:_____

(Proceed to next page for continuation of Scenario I.)

TRIAGE SCENARIOS

Triage Scenario I—Gas Explosion in the Gymnasium continued

2. *Establish your patient priorities for further evaluation by placing a number #1 through #5 (with #1 being your highest priority and #5 being your lowest priority) in the space provided next to each patient letter.*

_____ Patient A

_____ Patient B

_____ Patient C

_____ Patient D

_____ Patient E

3. *Briefly outline your rationale for prioritizing these patients in the manner you did.*

Priority 1—Patient _____:
Rationale: _____

_____

_____

Priority 2—Patient _____:
Rationale: _____

_____

_____

_____

Priority 3—Patient _____:
Rationale: _____

_____

_____

_____

Priority 4—Patient _____:
Rationale: _____

_____

_____

_____

Priority 5—Patient _____:
Rationale: _____

_____

_____

_____

(Proceed to next page for continuation of Scenario I.)

Triage Scenario I—Gas Explosion in the Gymnasium continued

4. *Briefly, describe what basic life support maneuvers or additional assessment techniques you would employ to further evaluate the problem(s).*

Priority 1 – Patient _____ :
Basic life support maneuvers or additional assessment techniques:_____

_____

_____

_____

_____

Priority 2 – Patient _____ :
Basic life support maneuvers or additional assessment techniques:_____

_____

_____

_____

_____

Priority 3 – Patient _____ :
Basic life support maneuvers or additional assessment techniques:_____

_____

_____

_____

_____

Priority 4 – Patient _____ :
Basic life support maneuvers or additional assessment techniques:_____

_____

_____

_____

_____

Priority 5 – Patient _____ :
Basic life support maneuvers or additional assessment techniques:_____

_____

_____

_____

_____

(Proceed to Scenario II, which is a continuation of this scenario.)

TRIAGE SCENARIOS

Triage Scenario II—Gas Explosion in the Gymnasium continued

Continuation of Scenario I:

1. *Characterize the patients according to who receives basic or advanced life support care and describe what that care would be. List the patients in the priority order as you identified them in Scenario I, starting with your first priority. Insert a mark in the box under BLS and/or ALS according to your decision of what the patient needs.*

Patient	BLS	ALS	Description of Care
_____	☐	☐	_____
_____	☐	☐	_____
_____	☐	☐	_____
_____	☐	☐	_____
_____	☐	☐	_____

(Proceed to next page for continuation of Scenario II.)

American College of Surgeons

Triage Scenario II—Gas Explosion in the Gymnasium continued

2. *Prioritize patient transfers and identify destinations. Provide a brief rationale for your destination choice.*

Priority	Patient	Destination	
1	_____	❏ Trauma center	❏ Nearest hospital

_____
_____
_____

| 2 | _____ | ❏ Trauma center | ❏ Nearest hospital |

_____
_____
_____

| 3 | _____ | ❏ Trauma center | ❏ Nearest hospital |

_____
_____
_____

| 4 | _____ | ❏ Trauma center | ❏ Nearest hospital |

_____
_____
_____

| 5 | _____ | ❏ Trauma center | ❏ Nearest hospital |

_____
_____
_____

3. *In situations involving multiple patients, what criteria would you use to identify and prioritize the management of these patients?*

_____
_____
_____
_____

4. *What cues can you elicit that would be of assistance in triage?*

_____
_____
_____
_____

(Proceed to next page for continuation of Scenario II.)

TRIAGE SCENARIOS

Triage Scenario II—Gas Explosion in the Gymnasium continued

5. *Which patient injuries or complaints should receive treatment at the scene before prehospital personnel arrive?*

_____

_____

_____

_____

_____

6. *After prehospital personnel arrive, what techniques should be instituted and what principles govern the order of initiation of such techniques?* Attention should be directed at

_____

_____

_____

_____

_____

7. *In multiple patient situations, who should be transported? Who should be transported early?*

_____

_____

_____

_____

_____

8. *Who could have treatment delayed and be transported later?*

_____

_____

_____

_____

_____

(Proceed to next page for Scenario III.)

Triage Scenario III—Trailer-home Explosion and Fire

Scenario: An explosion and fire, due to a faulty gas line, has involved 1 trailer in a nearby trailer park. Because of the close proximity of the incident to the hospital, the prehospital personnel transport the patients directly to the hospital without prior notification. The 5 patients, all members of the same family, are immobilized on long spine boards when they arrive at your small hospital emergency department. The injured patients are:

Patient A—**A 45-year-old man** is coughing and expectorating carbonaceous material. Hairs on his face and head are singed. His voice is clear and he is complaining about pain in his hands, which have erythema and early blister formation.

> **VS: BP 120 mm Hg systolic, HR 100, and RR 30**

Patient B—**A 6-year-old girl** appears frightened and is crying. She complains of pain from burns (erythema/blisters) over her back, buttocks, and both legs posteriorly.

> **VS: BP 110/70 mm Hg, HR 100, and RR 25**

Patient C—**A 70-year-old man** is coughing, wheezing, and expectorating carbonaceous material. His voice is hoarse and he responds only to painful stimuli. There are erythema, blisters, and charred skin to the anterior chest and abdominal walls and circumferential burns of both thighs.

> **VS: BP 80/40 mm Hg, HR 140, and RR 35**

Patient D—**A 19-year-old woman** is obtunded but responds to pain when her right humerus and leg are moved. There is no obvious deformity of the arm, and the thigh is swollen while in a traction splint.

> **VS: BP 140/90 mm Hg, HR 110, and RR 32**

Patient E—**A 45-year-old man** is pale and spontaneously complaining of pain in his pelvis. There is clinical evidence of fracture with abdominal distention and tenderness to palpation. There is erythema and blister of the anterior chest and abdominal walls and thighs. He also has a laceration to the forehead.

> **VS: BP 130/90 mm Hg, HR 90, and RR 25**

Management priorities in this scenario can be based on information obtained by surveying the injured patients at a distance. Although there may be doubt as to which patient is more injured, based on the available information, a decision has to be made to proceed with the best information available at the time.

(Proceed to the next page for questions related to this scenario.)

TRIAGE SCENARIOS

Triage Scenario III—Trailer-home Explosion and Fire continued

1. *Identify which patient(s) has associated trauma and/or inhalation injury in addition to body surface burns, and place a check in the box next to the patient letter.*

   ❏ Patient A   ❏ Patient B   ❏ Patient C   ❏ Patient D   ❏ Patient E

2. *Using the table provided below,*

   a. *Establish priorities of care in your hospital emergency department by placing a number (#1 through #5, with #1 being your highest priority and #5 being your lowest priority) in the space provided for each patient letter in the column "Treatment Priority."*

   b. *Identify which patient has associated trauma and/or an airway injury and place a mark in the appropriate column under "Associated."*

   c. *Estimate the percent of body surface area (BSA) burn for each patient and enter the percent for each patient letter in the column "% BSA."*

   d. *Identify which patient is transferred to a burn center and/or to a trauma center and place a mark in the appropriate column under "Transfer."*

   e. *Establish your priorities for transfer and enter your priority number under "Transfer Priority."*

Patient	Associated		Treatment Priority	% BSA	Transfer		Transfer Priority
	Trauma	Airway Injury			Burn	Trauma	
A							
B							
C							
D							
E							

(Proceed to next page for Scenario IV.)

American College of Surgeons

Triage Scenario IV—Cold Injury

Scenario:
You are in your hospital when you receive a call that 5 members of a doctor's family were snowmobiling on a lake when the ice broke. Four family members fell into the lake water. The doctor was able to stop in time and left to seek help. The response time of basic and advanced life support assistance was 15 minutes. By the time basic and advanced life support units arrived, 1 individual crawled out of the lake and removed another victim from the water. Two individuals remained submerged, were found by rescue divers, and were removed from the lake. Rescuers from the scene provided the following information.

Patient A—The doctor's 10-year-old grandson was removed from the lake by rescuers. The ECG monitor shows asystole.

Patient B—The doctor's 65-year-old wife was removed from the lake by rescuers. The ECG monitor shows asystole.

Patient C—The doctor's 35-year-old daughter, who had been in the lake and was helped out of the water by her sister-in-law, has bruises to her anterior chest wall.
  VS: BP 90 mm Hg systolic

Patient D—The doctor's 35-year-old daughter-in-law, who had been submerged and crawled out of the lake, has no obvious signs of trauma.
  VS: BP 110 mm Hg systolic

Patient E—The 76-year-old retired doctor, who never went into the water, has no complaints except for cold hands and feet.

1. *Establish the priorities for transport from the scene to your emergency department and provide a brief rationale for your decisions.*

Rationale

Transport priority #1   Patient _____   _____
                                          _____

Transport priority #2   Patient _____   _____
                                          _____

Transport priority #3   Patient _____   _____
                                          _____

Transport priority #4   Patient _____   _____
                                          _____

Transport priority #5   Patient _____   _____
                                          _____

(Proceed to next page for continuation of Scenario IV.)

TRIAGE SCENARIOS

Triage Scenario IV—Cold Injury continued

2. Upon arrival in the emergency department, all patients should have their core temperature taken. *Briefly, outline your rationale for the remainder of the primary assessment, resuscitation, and secondary survey of each patient.*

Patient A: Priority #_____: _____

_____

_____

_____

Patient B: Priority #_____: _____

_____

_____

_____

Patient C: Priority #_____: _____

_____

_____

_____

Patient D: Priority #_____: _____

_____

_____

_____

Patient E: Priority #_____: _____

_____

_____

_____

(Proceed to next page for Scenario V.)

Triage Scenario V—Car Crash

Scenario: You are the only doctor available in a 100-bed community emergency department. One nurse and 1 nurse's aide are available to assist you. Ten minutes ago you were notified by radio that ambulances would be arriving with patients from a single motor vehicle crash. No further report is received. Two ambulances arrive with 5 patients who were occupants in an automobile traveling at 60 miles (96 km)/hour before it crashed. The injured patients are:

Patient A—A 45-year-old man was the driver of the car. He apparently was not wearing a seat belt. Upon impact, he was thrown against the windscreen. On admission, he is notably in severe respiratory distress. The prehospital personnel provide the following information to you after preliminary assessment. Injuries include (1) severe maxillofacial trauma with bleeding from the nose and mouth, (2) an angulated deformity of the left forearm, and (3) multiple abrasions over the anterior chest wall.

    VS: BP 150/80 mm Hg, HR 120, RR 40, GCS Score = 8

Patient B—A 38-year-old woman passenger was apparently thrown from the front seat and found 30 feet (9 meters) from the car. On admission she is awake, alert, and complains of abdominal and chest pain. The report you are given indicates that on palpating her hips, she complains bitterly of pain and fracture-related crepitus is felt.

    VS: BP 110/90 mm Hg, HR 140, RR 25

Patient C—A 48-year-old male passenger was found under the car. You are told that on admission he is confused and responds slowly to verbal stimuli. Injuries include multiple abrasions to his face, chest, and abdomen. Breath sounds are absent on the left, and his abdomen is tender to palpation.

    VS: BP 90/50 mm Hg, HR 140, RR 35, GCS Score = 10

Patient D—A 25-year-old hysterical woman was extricated from the back seat of the vehicle. She is 8 months pregnant and complains of abdominal pain. Injuries include multiple abrasions to her face and anterior abdominal wall. You are told that her abdomen is tender to palpation. She is in active labor.

    VS: BP 120/80 mm Hg, HR 100, RR 25

Patient E—A 6-year-old boy was extricated from the floor of the rear seat. At the scene, he was alert and talking. He now responds to painful stimuli by only crying out. Injuries include multiple abrasions and an angulated deformity of the right lower leg. There is dried blood around his nose and mouth. You are told that his vital signs are:

    VS: BP 110/70 mm Hg, HR 180, RR 35

(Proceed to next page for questions related to Scenario V.)

TRIAGE SCENARIOS

Triage Scenario V—Car Crash continued

1. Outline the steps you would take to triage these 5 patients.

_____
_____
_____
_____
_____
_____
_____

2/3. Establish your patient priorities by placing a number (#1 through #5, with #1 being your highest priority and #5 being your lowest priority) in the space provided next to each lettered patient. In the space provided here, also briefly outline your rationale for prioritizing these patients in the manner you did.

Priority #_____   **Patient A**
*Rationale:*_____
_____
_____

Priority #_____   **Patient B**
*Rationale:*_____
_____
_____

Priority #_____   **Patient C**
*Rationale:*_____
_____
_____

Priority #_____   **Patient D**
*Rationale:*_____
_____
_____

Priority #_____   **Patient E**
*Rationale:*_____
_____
_____

(Conclusion of Triage Scenarios)

APPENDIX

Injury Prevention

2

◼ INTRODUCTION

Injury should not be thought of as an "accident," a term that implies a random circumstance resulting in harm. In fact, injuries occur in patterns that are predictable and preventable. The expression "an accident looking for a place to happen" is both paradoxical and premonitory. There are high-risk individuals and high-risk environments. In combination, they provide a chain of events that result in trauma. With the changing perspective in today's health care from managing illness to promoting wellness, injury prevention takes on the added dimension of not only promoting good health but also of reducing health care costs.

Prevention is timely. Doctors who care for the injured have a unique opportunity to practice effective, preventive medicine. Although the true risk takers may be recalcitrant to any and all prevention messages, many persons injured through ignorance, carelessness, or temporary loss of self-control may be receptive to information likely to reduce their future vulnerability. Each doctor-patient encounter is an opportunity to reduce trauma recidivism. This is especially true for the surgeon who is involved daily during the acute postinjury period when there may be an opportunity to truly change behavior. The basic concepts of injury prevention are described and strategies for implementation through traditional public health methods are included in this appendix.

INJURY PREVENTION

I. CLASSIFICATION OF INJURY PREVENTION

Prevention may be considered as primary, secondary, or tertiary. Primary prevention refers to elimination of the trauma incident totally so that it does not happen. Examples of primary prevention measures include stoplights at intersections, window guards to prevent falls in toddlers, swimming pool fences to exclude nonswimmers from drowning, and medicine safety caps to prevent ingestions.

Secondary prevention accepts the fact that the injury may occur, but serves to reduce the severity of the injury sustained. Examples of secondary prevention include safety belts, motorcycle and bicycle helmets, and playground safety surfaces. Tertiary prevention means reducing the consequences of the injury after it has occurred. Trauma systems, including the coordination of emergency medical services, identification of trauma centers, and the integration of rehabilitation services to reduce impairment, constitute efforts as tertiary prevention.

II. HADDON MATRIX

In the early 1970s, Haddon described a useful approach to primary and secondary injury prevention that is now known as the Haddon Matrix. According to Haddon's conceptual framework, there are 3 principal factors in injury occurrence: (1) the injured person (host), (2) the injury mechanism (vehicle), and (3) the environment in which the injury occurs. There are 3 phases in which injury and its sever-

ity can be modified: (1) the preevent phase, (2) the event phase (injury), and (3) the postevent phase. Table 1, Haddon's Factor-phase Matrix for Motor Vehicle Crash Prevention, characterizes how the matrix serves to identify opportunities for injury prevention and can be extrapolated to address other injury causes. The adoption of this structured design by the National Highway Traffic Safety Administration (NHTSA) resulted in a sustained reduction in the fatality rate per vehicle mile driven over the past 2 decades.

III. THE FOUR Es OF INJURY PREVENTION

Injury prevention can be directed to human factors (behavioral issues), vectors of injury, and/or environmental factors and implemented according to the four Es of injury prevention.

1. Education
2. Enforcement
3. Engineering
4. Economics (incentives)

Education is the cornerstone of injury prevention. Educational efforts are relatively easy to implement, promote the development of constituencies, and also serve to bring the issue before the public. Without an informed and activist public, subsequent legislative efforts (enforcement) are likely to fail. Education is based on the premise that knowledge supports a change in behavior. While attrac-

Table 1—Haddon's Factor-phase Matrix for Motor Vehicle Crash Prevention

	PREEVENT	EVENT	POSTEVENT
Host	Avoid alcohol use	Use of safety belts	Bystander delivers care
Vehicle	Antilock brakes	Air bag deploys	
Environment	Speed limits	Impact-absorbing barriers	Access to trauma system

tive in theory, education has been disappointing in practice. Yet it provides the underpinning for implementation of subsequent strategy to reduce alcohol-related crash deaths. Mothers Against Drunk Driving (MADD) is an organization that exemplifies the effective use of a primary education strategy to reduce alcohol-related crash deaths. Through their efforts, an informed and aroused public facilitated the enactment of stricter drunk-driving laws, resulting in a decade of reduced alcohol-related vehicle fatalities. For education to work, it must be directed to the appropriate target group, it must be persistent, and it must be linked to other approaches.

Enforcement is a useful part of any effective injury prevention strategy because, regardless of the type of trauma, there always are those who resist changes needed to improve outcome, even if the improved outcome is their own. Where compliance with injury prevention efforts lags, legislation making certain behavior mandatory (or illegal) often results in dramatic differences. Safety belt laws resulted in measurable increases in usage where educational programs alone had minimal effect.

Engineering, often more expensive at first, clearly has the greatest long-term benefits. Despite proven effectiveness, engineering advances may require concomitant legislative and enforcement initiatives, enabling implementation on a larger scale. Adoption of air bags is a recent example of the application of advances in technology combined with features of enforcement. Other advances in highway design and safety have added tremendously to the margin of safety while driving.

Economic incentives, when used for the correct purpose, are quite effective. The linking of federal highway funds to the passage of motorcycle helmet laws motivated the states to pass such laws and enforce the wearing of helmets. This resulted in a 30% reduction in head injury fatalities. Although this economic incentive is no longer in effect and rates of head injury deaths have returned to their previous levels in states that have reversed their helmet statutes, the association between helmet laws and reduced fatalities confirmed the utility of economic incentives in injury prevention. Insurance companies have clear data on risk-taking behavior patterns, and the payments from insurance trusts, consequently, provide related discount premiums.

IV. DEVELOPING AN INJURY PREVENTION PROGRAM—THE PUBLIC APPROACH

There are 5 basic steps to developing an injury prevention program.

A. Define the Problem

The first step is a basic one—define the problem. This may appear to be self-evident, but both the magnitude and community impact of trauma may be elusive unless reliable data are available. Population-based data on injury incidence are essential to identify the problem and to provide a baseline for determining the impact of subsequent efforts at injury prevention. Information from death certificates, hospital and/or emergency department discharge statistics, and trauma registry printouts are, collectively, good places to start. While community sentinel events may identify an individual trauma problem and raise public concern, high-profile problems do not lend themselves to effective injury prevention unless they are part of a larger documented injury control issue.

B. Define Causes and Risk Factors

After a trauma problem is identified, causes and risk factors must be defined. The problem may need to be studied to determine what kind of injuries are involved and where, when, and why they are occurring. Injury prevention strategies may begin to emerge with this additional information. Some trauma problems may vary from community to community; however, there are certain risk factors that are likely to be constant across situations and across socioeconomic boundaries. Abuse of alcohol and other drugs is an example of a contributing factor that is likely to be pervasive regardless of whether the trauma is blunt or penetrating, the location is the inner city or the suburbs, fatalities alone or no injuries occur, and disabilities are included. Data are most meaningful when the injury problem is compared between populations with and without defined risk factors. In many instances, the injured persons may have multiple risk factors, and clearly defined populations may be difficult to sort out. In such cases, it is necessary to control for the confounding variables.

INJURY PREVENTION

C. Develop and Test Interventions

The next step is to develop and test interventions. This is the place for pilot programs to test intervention effectiveness. Rarely is an intervention likely to be picked up without some indication that it works. It is important to consider the views and values of the community if an injury prevention program is to be accepted. End points must be defined up front and outcomes reviewed without bias. It is sometimes not possible to determine the effectiveness of a test program, especially if it is a small-scale trial intervention. For example, a public information program on safety belt use conducted at a school can be assessed by monitoring the incoming and outgoing school traffic and showing a difference, whereas the usage rates in the community as a whole may not change. Nonetheless, the implication is clear—broad implementation of public education regarding safety belt use can have a beneficial effect within a controlled community population. Telephone surveys are not reliable measures to confirm behavioral change, but they can confirm that the intervention reached the target group.

D. Implement Injury Prevention Strategies

With confirmation that a given intervention may effect favorable change, the next step is implementation of injury prevention strategies. From this point, the possibilities are vast.

E. Evaluate Impact

With implementation comes the need to monitor the impact of the program or evaluation. An effective injury prevention program linked with an objective means to define its effectiveness can be a powerful message to the public, the press, and legislators, and ultimately may bring about a permanent change in behavior.

V. SUMMARY

If this seems like a large task, in many ways it is. Yet, it is important to remember that a pediatrician in Tennessee was able to validate the need for infant safety seats that led to the first infant safety seat law. Another example is that of a New York orthopaedic surgeon whose testimony played an important role in achieving the first safety belt law in the United States. Although not all doctors are destined to make as big an impact, all doctors can have an impact on their patients' behaviors. Injury prevention

measures do not have to be implemented on a grand scale to make a difference. Although doctors may not be able to prove a difference in their own patient population, if they all made injury prevention a part of their practice, the results could be significant. As preparations for hospital or emergency department discharge are being made, consideration should be given to patient education to prevent injury recurrence. Whether it is alcohol abuse, returning to an unchanged hostile home environment, riding without head protection on a motorcycle, or smoking while refueling the car, there are many opportunities for doctors to make a difference in their patients' future trauma vulnerability.

■ BIBLIOGRAPHY

1. ACS Committee on Trauma: Injury prevention and control. **Resources for Optimal Care of the Injured Patient.** Chicago, in publication.

2. Cooper A, Barlow B, Davidson L, et al: Epidemiology of pediatric trauma: Importance of population-based statistics. **Journal of Pediatric Surgery** 1992; 27:149–154.

3. Haddon W, Baker SP: Injury control. In: Clark DW, MacMahon B (eds): **Prevention and Community Medicine, 2nd Edition.** Boston, Little Brown Co, 1981, pp 109–140.

4. Laraque D, Barlow B: Prevention of pediatric injury. In: Ivatory R, Cayten G (eds): **The Textbook of Penetrating Trauma**, chapter 10. Baltimore, Williams & Wilkins, 1996.

5. National Committee for Injury Prevention and Control: **Injury Prevention: Meeting the Challenge.** New York, Education Development Center, 1989.

6. Rivera FP: Traumatic deaths of children in United States: Currently available prevention strategies. **Pediatrics** 1985; 85:456–462.

RESOURCES

1. British Columbia Injury Research and Prevention Unit, Centre for Community Health and Health Research, L408-4480 Oak Street, Vancouver, BC V6H 3V4, Canada; 604/875-3776, *www.injuryresearch.bc.ca*.

2. Harborview Injury Prevention and Research Center, University of Washington, Box 359960, 325 Ninth Avenue, Seattle, WA 98104-2499; 206/521-1520, *http://depts.washington.edu/hiprc/*.

3. Harvard Injury Control Research Center, Harvard School of Public Health, 677 Huntington Avenue, 2nd Floor, Boston, MA 02115; 617/432-3420; *www.hsph.harvard.edu/hicrc/.*

4. Injury Control Research Center, University of Alabama-Birmingham, CH19 UAB Station, Birmingham, AL 35294; 205/934-1643, *www.uab.edu/icrc/.*

5. Injury Prevention and Research Center, University of North Carolina, 137 East Franklin St., CB#7505 CTP, Chapel Hill, NC 27599-7505; 919/966-2251, *www.sph.unc.edu/iprc.*

6. Injury Free Coalition for Kids, Columbia University, Mailman School of Public Health, 722 West 168th Street, Rm 1711, New York, NY 10032; 212/342-0517; *www.injuryfree.org.*

7. Iowa Injury Prevention Research Center, University of Iowa, 158 IREH Oakdale Research Campus, Iowa City, IA 52242-5000; 319/335-4458, *www.pmeh.uiowa/iprc.*

8. Johns Hopkins Center for Injury Research and Policy, Hampton House, 624 N. Broadway, 5th Floor, Baltimore, MD 21205-1996; 410/614-4026, *www.jhsph.edu/Research/Centers/CIRP.*

9. National Center for Injury Prevention and Control, Centers for Disease Control, Program Development and Implementation, Mailstop K65, 4770 Buford Highway NE, Atlanta, GA 30341-3724; 770/488-1506, *www.cdc.gov/osp/data.htm.*

10. San Francisco Center for Injury Research and Prevention, San Francisco General Hospital, 1001 Potrero Avenue, Department of Surgery, Ward 3A, Box 0807, San Francisco, CA 94110; 415/206-4623, *www.surgery.ucsf.edu/sfic/.*

11. Slide Prevention Programs (Alcohol and Injury, Bicycle Helmet Safety), available from American College of Surgeons, Customer Service/Publications, 633 N. Saint Clair St., Chicago, IL 60611-3211; 312/202-5474; *https://secure.facs.org/commerce/2003/trauma.html.*

12. Southern California Injury Prevention and Research Center, UCLA School of Public Health, 10911 Weyburn Avenue, Suite 200, Los Angeles, CA, 90024-2884; 310/794-2706, *www.ph.ucla.edu/sciprc.*

13. State and Local Departments of Health, Injury Control Divisions.

14. The Children's Safety Network, National Injury and Violence Prevention Resource Center, Education Development Center, Inc., 55 Chapel Street, Newton, MA 02458-1060; 617/969-7100, *www.childrensafetynetwork.org.*

15. TIPP Sheets, available from American Academy of Pediatrics, 141 Northwest Point Boulevard, Elk Grove Village, IL 60007; 800/433-9016, *www.aap.org.*

APPENDIX 3

Biomechanics of Injury

■ INTRODUCTION

The details of the injury event can provide clues to the identification of 90% of a patient's injuries. Important information begins with details of events in the preinjury phase, eg, alcohol or other drug ingestion, seizure activity, chest pain, loss of consciousness before impact. History related to this phase should include:

1. The type of traumatic event, eg, vehicular collision, fall, penetrating injury
2. An estimation of the amount of energy exchange that occurred, eg, speed of the vehicle at impact, distance of the fall, and caliber and size of the weapon
3. The collision or impact of the patient with the object, eg, car, tree, knife, baseball bat, bullet

Mechanisms of injury may be classified as blunt, penetrating, thermal, and blast. In all cases, there is a transfer of energy to tissue, or in the case of freezing, a transfer of energy (heat) from tissue. Energy laws assist with an understanding of how tissues sustain injury. These include:

1. Energy is neither created nor destroyed; however, it can be changed in form.
2. A body in motion or a body at rest tends to remain in that state until acted on by an outside force.
3. Kinetic energy (KE) is equal to the mass (m) of the object in motion multiplied by the square of the velocity (v) and divided by two.

$$KE = \frac{(m)(v^2)}{2}$$

4. Force (F) is equal to the mass times deceleration (acceleration).
5. Injury is dependent upon the amount and speed of energy transmission, the surface area over which the energy is applied, and the elastic properties of the tissues to which the energy transfer is applied.

A definition of terms used in this section is necessary to avoid confusion.

Acceleration (a) is the change in velocity with respect to time. This is expressed as feet per second per second or meters per second per second. An object being pulled toward the earth would accelerate at 32.1 feet (9.81 meters) per second per second if there were no forces acting in the opposite direction.

Force (F) is the "push" or "pull" of one object on another, although the two do not necessarily have to be in contact. Force is the acceleration, or change in state of motion, that one object would impart to a given mass. (See the aforementioned energy law and formula #4.) Weight is an example of a specific force. A **load** refers to a force applied to a body or structure. The Newton (1 kg $\times$ m^{-1} $\times$ sec^{-2}) or dyne (1 g $\times$ cm^{-1} $\times$ sec^{-2}) are the common units used to describe force.

Mass (m) describes the inertial quality of matter, which is the inherent property of matter to resist a change in its state of motion. The greater the mass, the greater the inertia. Mass should not be confused with force or weight and only describes the amount of material.

Strain is defined as the internal deformation or change in dimension (relative to its original dimension) as the result of a force.

Stress can be considered the internal resistance (or opposite forces) that resists the deformation of a body. If the external forces exceed the internal forces that resist deformation, equilibrium is lost. Stress is expressed as force per unit area (Newton × m^2 or pounds × in^{-2}).

Weight describes the rate at which any given body is attracted toward the center of a gravitational body, such as the earth. Since a 70-kg person standing on the ground is not accelerating toward the center of the earth, an opposite force (the ground) holds the person up. This force in the opposite direction is denoted as weight.

Velocity (v) is the change in distance with respect to time, eg, miles or kilometers per hour, feet per second, etc.

I. ENERGY TRANSFER AND CAVITATION

Energy transfer can be considered as a shock wave (identical to a sound wave) that moves at various speeds through different media. Energy is carried at the front of the wave and is concentrated in a small space. In considering the propagation of these shock waves in an elastic medium such as human tissue, stress imparted to the tissue is dependent on (1) the velocity of the material particles initiating the shock wave, (2) the velocity of the waves in the material (tissue), and (3) the mass density of the material. This theory holds true for any wave, such as sound waves, arterial pressure waves, or the shock wave produced in liver or cortical bone on impact with an object that results in the transfer of energy. Because mass density and the velocity of sound in any given tissue are constant, the stress level in the tissue at impact is controlled by the velocity of the material particles of the tissue and is directly proportional to it. If the velocity exceeds the tolerance level of the tissue, tissue disruption occurs, thereby producing injury.

Considering the propagation of these shock waves through tissue, it is easy to see that injury is likely to be produced at boundaries where different tissues make contact or at tissue/air interfaces. Stress induced in these areas by compression and reexpansion may produce pressure differences across the boundaries. Shock waves release energy in their propagation from dense to less dense tissues. Consider a shock wave that travels at 500 m/sec. Sound travels at 3500 m/sec in bone and 30 m/sec in lung parenchyma. The shock wave is relatively slow with respect to the speed of sound in bone, but is more than 15 times faster than sound waves in lung parenchyma. Such stress is responsible for hemorrhage, edema, or parenchymal disruption in the lung when subjected to the shock wave, but produces little damage to cortical bone.

For a moving object to lose speed its energy of motion must be transmitted to another object or the energy changed to some other form. Direct energy transfer occurs when the human body tissue cells are placed in motion directly away from the site of impact. The rapid movement of tissue particles away from the point of impact produces damage by tissue compression, as well as at a distance from the point of initial impact as the shock wave progresses and the cavity expands. (See Figure 1, page 318, Cavitation.)

These same principles apply irrespective of whether the skin is penetrated. Assessing the extent of injury is more difficult when no skin penetration or disruption is apparent than when an open wound is present. A baseball bat swung with equal force into a metal or foam rubber barrel transmits the same amount of energy, yet the effect of the energy transfer is readily apparent to one barrel and not the other. A fist driven into the abdominal cavity of a victim may sink in deeply but leaves no visible depression after the assailant's fist is removed. Without evidence of fracture or tissue destruction, the extent of injury cannot be determined by simple inspection of the tissue. A history of the injury-producing event must be obtained. The visible cavity after impact is referred to as a permanent cavity, and the invisible cavity is referred to as a temporary cavity. The elastic properties of the tissues under consideration contribute to the size of each cavitation, just as in the example of the barrels, but the elastic properties of tissue have a more important role in the size of the permanent cavity produced than in the temporary cavity.

The size of the temporary cavitation also is determined by the magnitude of energy exchanged. Energy exchange is determined by the number of tissue particles impacted by the moving object and the kinetic energy of the moving object. The larger the surface area and the denser the tissue, the greater the number of particles affected. The reverse also is true. A narrow object, with a small surface area, passing through tissue that is not very dense, eg, small bowel or lung, does not create much of a cavity because only a relatively few tissue particles are affected. Bone is very dense, and when impacted by an object with a large cross-sectional area, it breaks and shatters, and fragments frequently travel some distance from the point of initial impact. These 2 scenarios represent the extremes. Most energy exchange lies somewhere in between.

Another factor to consider when determining injury mechanisms is the physical state of the tissue when the energy is applied. An example to consider is the effect of applying a needle to a surgical glove that is stretched longitudinally and one that is tensely inflated. One explodes the glove while the other produces only a small hole. This is due to the fact that the polymer strands of the inflated glove are under triaxial stress or loading. Polymer chains in every direction at the site of puncture are stretched and disrupt when punctured with a needle. The chains

BIOMECHANICS OF INJURY

FIGURE 1
Cavitation

in the glove stretched longitudinally are under uni-axial stress and only those chains are disrupted. Frequently, dull scissors have difficulty cutting suture unless the suture is placed under some tension. The force applied to the relaxed suture is only the shear force applied by the scissors, whereas the total force in the taut suture is the sum of initial stress plus the shear forces. Numerous clinical examples should come to mind. The suture is similar to blood vessels or ligaments. Many organs, such as the heart, liver, diaphragm, and urinary bladder, are subjected to multi-axial forces, accounting for the burst injuries commonly seen in clinical practice.

II. HISTORY

Information obtained from prehospital personnel related to a vehicle's interior and exterior damage frequently provides clues to injuries sustained by its occupants. Prehospital personnel are trained to make such observations, and this information facilitates the suspicion and subsequent identification of occult injuries. A bent steering wheel usually indicates chest impact. This should alert the

doctor to the possibility of injury to the anterior bony thorax and mediastinal organs, in addition to pulmonary parenchymal injury. Rapid deceleration from a high-speed vehicular crash, significant compression of the passenger compartment, a bent steering wheel, and an indistinct aortic arch shadow should lead to the aggressive exclusion of a thoracic aortic injury. A "bull's-eye" break of the windscreen usually indicated impact with the individual's head and the possibility of cervical spine injury. An indentation in the lower dashboard indicated a knee impact and the possibility of dislocation of the knee or hip or a femur fracture. Lateral intrusion into the passenger compartment suggests the potential for lateral injury to the patient's chest, abdomen, pelvis, or neck. Additionally, historical information about the injury-producing event can suggest the need for surgical intervention. Penetrating injury to the trunk from which the patient rapidly becomes hypotensive usually indicates major vascular injury and the need for prompt surgical intervention. Patients with head injuries as the result of causes **other than** vehicular crashes and who have focal abnormalities or asymmetry by neurologic examination have a high probability of requiring surgical exploration. Burns that occur from conflagration in a closed space are commonly associated with inhalation injuries and carbon monoxide poisoning. These examples indicate the value of historical details concerning the injury events.

III. BLUNT TRAUMA

The common injury patterns and types of injuries identified with blunt trauma include:

1. Vehicular impact in which the patient is inside the vehicle
2. Pedestrian impact
3. Motorcycle crashes
4. Assaults (intentional injury)
5. Falls
6. Blasts

A. Vehicular Impact

Vehicular collisions can be subdivided further into (1) collision between the patient and the vehicle, or between patient and some stationary object outside the vehicle if the patient is ejected (eg, tree, earth), and (2) the collision between the patient's organ(s) and the external framework of the body (organ compression).

The interactions between the patient and the vehicle depend on the type of crash. Five crashes depict the possible scenarios—frontal, lateral, rear, angular (front quarter or rear quarter), and rollover.

1. Occupant collision

a. Frontal impact

A frontal impact is defined as a collision with an object in front of the vehicle, which suddenly reduces its speed. Consider 2 identical vehicles traveling at the same speed. Each vehicle possesses the same kinetic energy [KE = $(m \times v2)/2$]. One vehicle strikes a concrete bridge abutment while the other brakes to a stop. The vehicle involved in the application of its brakes loses the same amount of energy as the crashing vehicle, but over a longer period. The first energy law states that energy cannot be created or destroyed. Therefore, this energy must be transferred to another form and is absorbed by the crashing vehicle and its oc-

cupants. The individual in the braking vehicle has the same **total** amount of energy applied, but the energy is distributed over a broad range of surfaces (eg, seat friction, foot to floorboard, tire braking, tire to road surface, hand to steering wheel) and over a longer time period.

The unrestrained occupant of the vehicle involved in the collision experiences an event much like the vehicle in which the occupant is riding. As the collision brings the vehicle to an abrupt stop, the passenger continues to move forward with the same initial velocity until something abruptly terminates the forward motion, eg, the steering wheel, dashboard, windscreen, or earth if the occupant is ejected. This kinetic energy is transformed into shock waves that the tissues must absorb and is equal to the product of the mass times the change in acceleration/deceleration with respect to the time interval [$F = (m \times \Delta v)/\Delta t$]. A quantitative example of the amount of energy that can be transferred is provided in the section on restraint injury.

On impact, the patient may follow a down-and-under pathway with the lower extremities being the initial point of impact and the knees or feet receiving the initial energy exchange. The forward motion of the torso onto the extremities may result in:

1) Fracture-dislocation of the ankle
2) Knee dislocation as the femur overrides the tibia and fibula
3) Femur fracture
4) Posterior dislocation of the femoral head from the acetabulum as the pelvis overrides the femur

The second component of this down-and-under motion is the forward motion of the torso into the steering column or dashboard. If the structure of the seat and the patient's position are such that the patient's head becomes the lead point, the skull impacts the windscreen or the framework around the windscreen. The cervical spine absorbs some of the initial energy while the chest and abdomen absorb the energy from the impact on the steering column or dashboard. (See Figure 2, page 320, Frontal Impact, Unrestrained Driver.) Depending on the position of the head at impact, the transfer

BIOMECHANICS OF INJURY

FIGURE 2
Frontal Impact, Unrestrained Driver

of energy may produce direct or shear forces to brain tissue, rotational, flexion, or extension forces to the cervical spine, as well as direct compressive forces to facial structures. Lacerations to soft tissues from broken components of the vehicle also can occur.

b. Lateral impact

Lateral impact is defined as a collision against the side of a vehicle that accelerates the occupant away from the point of impact (acceleration as opposed to deceleration). This type of impact is second only to frontal impact in terms of injury and fatality. As much as 31% of all automobile crash fatalities occur as the result of lateral impact. Interestingly, more than 75% of victims of side impacts are over the age of 50 years, whereas 25% of victims involved in frontal impacts are over 50 years. Many of the same types of injuries occur as with a frontal

impact. Additionally, compression injuries to the torso and pelvis may occur. Internal injuries are related to the side on which the force was applied, the position of the occupant (driver or passenger), and the force of impact and the time over which the force was applied (intrusion of the passenger cabin). The driver who is struck on the driver's side is at greater risk for left-sided injuries, including left rib fractures, left-sided pulmonary injury, splenic injury, and left-sided skeletal fractures, including pelvic compression fractures. A passenger struck on the passenger side of the vehicle may experience similar right-sided skeletal and thoracic injuries, with liver injuries being common.

In lateral impacts, the head acts as a large mass that rotates and laterally bends the neck as the torso is accelerated away from the side of the collision. Injury mechanisms, therefore, involve a variety of specific forces, which include shear, torque, and lateral compression and distraction. With sufficient rotation and torque, nerve root avulsion and brachial plexus injury can occur. The examining doctor also must consider acceleration as well as deceleration forces and lateral anatomic considerations when examining the patient.

c. Rear impact

Rear impact involves different biomechanical properties. More commonly, this type of impact occurs when a vehicle is at a complete stop and is struck from behind by another vehicle. The vehicle, including its occupant, is accelerated forward from the energy transfer from impact. Because of the apposition of the seat back and the torso, the torso is accelerated along with the car. The occupant's head often is not accelerated with the rest of the body due to the absence of a functional headrest. As a result, hyperextension of the neck occurs. This stretches the supporting structures of the neck and produces a "whiplash" injury. (See Figure 3, Rear Impact, Improper and Proper Headrest Use.) Fractures of the posterior elements of the cervical spine, eg, laminar fractures, pedicle fractures, spinous process fractures, may re-

sult and are equally distributed through the cervical vertebrae. Fractures at multiple levels are common and are usually due to direct bony contact. A frontal impact also may occur after the vehicle has been set in motion.

d. Quarter panel impact

A quarter panel impact, front or rear, produces a variation of lateral and frontal impact collision injury patterns or lateral and rear impact collision injury patterns.

e. Rollover

During a rollover, the unrestrained occupant can impact any part of the interior of the passenger compartment. Injuries may be predicted from the impact points on the patient's skin. As a general rule, this type of mechanism produces more severe injuries because of the violent, multiple motions that occur during the rollover. This is especially true for the unbelted occupant.

f. Ejection

The injuries sustained by the occupant during the process of ejection may be greater than

FIGURE 3
Rear Impact, Improper and Proper Headrest Use

Improper Headrest Use   Proper Headrest Use

BIOMECHANICS OF INJURY

when the individual impacts the ground. The likelihood of serious injury is increased by more than 300% if the patient is ejected from the vehicle. The doctor caring for the ejected patient must search carefully for occult injuries.

B. Organ Collision

1. Compression injury

Compression injuries occur when the anterior portion of the torso ceases to move forward and the posterior portion and internal organs continue their motion. The organs are eventually compressed from behind by the advancing posterior thoracoabdominal wall and the vertebral column, and in front by the impacted anterior structures. Blunt myocardial injury is a typical example of this type of injury mechanism. (See Figure 2, page 320, Frontal Impact, Unrestrained Driver.)

Similar injury can occur in lung parenchyma or abdominal organs. The lungs and abdominal viscera represent a particular variation of this mechanism of injury and accentuate the principle that the state of the tissue at the time of energy transfer influences the tissue damage. Holding a crumpled paper bag in 1 hand and crushing it with the opposite hand does not produce any additional damage to the bag. Blowing it up, holding the neck tight, and crushing the bag causes it to rupture, similar to the rubber glove example given earlier. In a collision, it is instinctive for the patient to take a deep breath and hold it, closing the glottis. Compression of the thorax produces alveolar rupture with a resultant pneumothorax and/or tension pneumothorax. (See Figure 2, page 320, Frontal Impact, Unrestrained Driver.) The increase in intraabdominal pressure may produce diaphragmatic rupture and translocation of abdominal organs into the thoracic cavity. Transient hepatic congestion with blood from this transient valsalva maneuver may cause the liver to burst when compressive forces are applied. In a similar fashion, small bowel rupture can occur if a closed loop is compressed between the vertebral column and an improperly worn seat belt.

Compression injuries to brain substance also can occur. Movement of the head associated with the application of a force through impact can be associated with rapid acceleration forces applied to the brain. This produces stress and deformation of the intracranial gray and white matter. Angular acceleration can also produce movement of the brain over the irregular surfaces of the internal bony calvarium, thereby producing injury. Accelerated brain in any axis can produce compressive injury to central nervous system tissue opposite the point of impact, the contra coup injury. Accelerated brain also produces stress and stretch forces at critical junctions, eg, the brain and brainstem or spinal cord, and at the junction of brain parenchyma and meningeal membranes. Compression injuries also can occur from depressed skull fractures.

2. Deceleration injury

Deceleration injuries occur as the stabilizing portion of an organ, eg, renal pedicle, ligamentum teres, or descending thoracic aorta, ceases forward motion with the torso while the movable body part, eg, spleen, kidney or heart and aortic arch, continues to move forward. Shear force is developed in the aorta by the continued forward motion of the aortic arch with respect to the stationary descending aorta. The distal aorta is anchored to the spine and decelerates more rapidly with the torso. The shear forces are greatest where the arch and stable, descending aorta join at the ligamentum arteriosum. This mechanism of injury also may be operative with the spleen and kidney at their pedicle junctions; with the liver as the right and left lobes decelerate around the ligamentum teres, producing a central hepatic laceration; and in the skull when the posterior part of the brain separates from the skull, tearing vessels and producing space-occupying lesions. The numerous attachments of the dura, arachnoid, and pia inside the cranial vault effectively separate the brain into multiple compartments. These compartments are subjected to shear stress by both acceleration and deceleration forces. Another example is the flexible cervical spine attached to the relatively immobile thoracic spine accounting for the frequent injury identified at the C7 to T1 junction.

3. Restraint injury

The value of passenger restraints in reducing injury has been so well established that it is no longer a debatable issue. The history of restraining devices has its origins in the World War I era. In 1903, a modification of the "luggage strap" was placed in army aircraft to keep pilots from falling

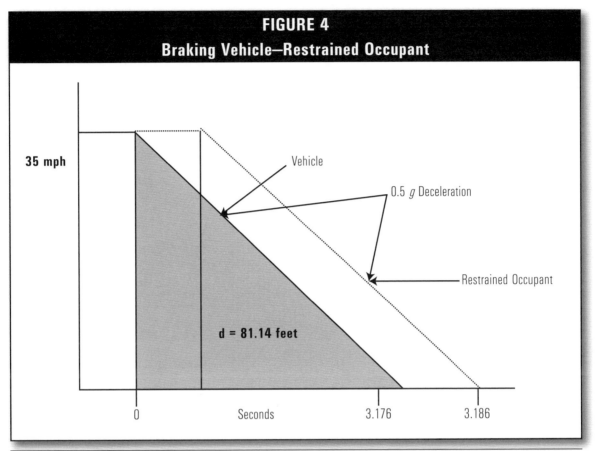

FIGURE 4
Braking Vehicle—Restrained Occupant

Modified with permission from Eppinger R, Occupant restraint systems. In: Nahum AM, Melvin JW (eds): *Accidental Injury: Biomechanics and Prevention.* New York, Springer-Verlag, 1993.

A restrained driver and the vehicle travel at the same speed and brake to a stop with a deceleration of 0.5 g (16 feet $\times$ sec^{-2} or 4.8 m $\times$ sec^{-2}). During the 0.01 second it takes for the inertial mechanism to lock the safety belt and couple the driver to the vehicle, the driver moves an additional 6.1 inches (15.25 cm) inside the passenger compartment.

out of the cockpit. Like today, the use of these safety devices did not gain unanimous popularity. In 1955, the United States Air Force recognized that more of their airmen were killed in automobile crashes than in aviation crashes and began aggressive automobile restraining system testing. The current 3-point restraints, when used properly, have been shown to reduce fatalities by 65% to 70% and produce a 10-fold reduction in serious injury. Presently, the greatest failure of the device is the occupant's refusal to use the system.

The value of occupant restraint devices, as well as a quantitative description of the energy transfers than can occur during a vehicular crash, are illustrated by a modification of an example published by Eppinger. (See Figure 4, Braking Vehicle—Restrained Occupant, and Figure 5, page 324, Colli-

sion—Unrestrained Occupant.) Consider a 70-kg person traveling in a vehicle at 35 mph (56 kph) that slows to a stop by braking. Further consider the difference in energy transferred to the restrained and unrestrained occupants if the vehicle were to crash into an immovable object at 35 mph (56 kph). The dynamics of the energy transfer are illustrated graphically in Figure 4, Braking Vehicle—Restrained Occupant. The speeds of the vehicle and its passenger are shown on the y-axis and time in seconds on the x-axis. The integral, or area under the curve, represents the distance traveled with respect to the ground, and the slope of the curve is the deceleration. The deceleration can be compared with the acceleration due to gravity, or the g forces, experienced by the vehicle and the occupant.

BIOMECHANICS OF INJURY

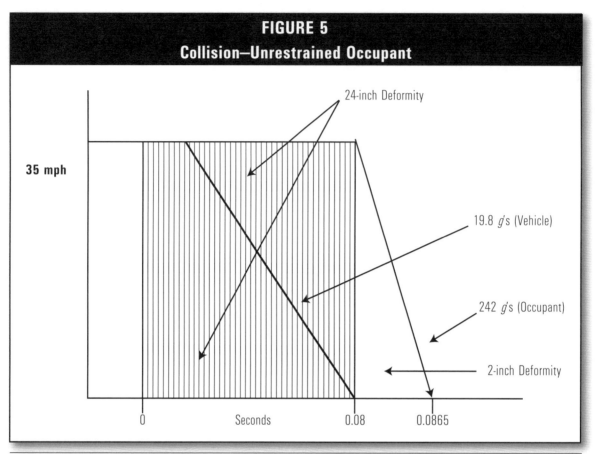

FIGURE 5
Collision—Unrestrained Occupant

35 mph

24-inch Deformity

19.8 *g*'s (Vehicle)

242 *g*'s (Occupant)

2-inch Deformity

0   Seconds   0.08   0.0865

Modified with permission from Eppinger R, Occupant restraint systems. In: Nahum AM, Melvin JW (eds): *Accidental Injury: Biomechanics and Prevention.* New York, Springer-Verlag, 1993.

Crashing into an immovable object from 35 mph (56 kph), the vehicle deforms by 24 inches (60 cm) and impacts the dashboard just as the vehicle comes to a stop. If the driver sustains only a 2-inch (5-cm) deformity, the driver decelerates at a velocity of 242 *g* over the 0.00653 second it takes to cease forward motion. The vehicle loses its kinetic energy over a longer period and sustains fewer *g* forces, although the initial velocity is identical.

In Figure 4, page 323, Braking Vehicle—Restrained Occupant, the brakes are applied to effect a 0.5 *g* deceleration (32.1739 feet × sec⁻² × 0.5 = 16.09 feet × sec⁻²) (or 9.7 m × sec⁻² × 0.5 = 4.8 m × sec⁻²). It takes just over 3 seconds for the vehicle to come to a complete stop and the distance traveled is 81 feet or 24.3 meters. Because the deceleration is relatively slow, the inertial lock of the restraint system does not engage. The forces acting on the occupant to slow the person's forward momentum (eg, seat friction) are of the same magnitude and timing as the vehicle. If for some reason there is a delay in the application of these forces to the occupant, the person continues to move forward inside the passenger compartment until the occupant is once again coupled to the

vehicle in some manner. For example, suppose the deceleration is of sufficient magnitude to lock the restraint system, but this requires 0.01 second after initiating the braking process. The occupant then moves another 6.1 inches (15.25 cm) inside the passenger compartment.

The unrestrained passenger of a car that crashes into a concrete wall is graphically illustrated in Figure 5, Collision—Unrestrained Occupant. If the vehicle deforms by 24 inches (60 cm) from the force of impact, forward motion ceases after 0.078 second and a force of 19.85 *g* is applied to the car. The unrestrained occupant continues to move forward after the impact. Assuming the first interior surface is 24 inches (60 cm) from

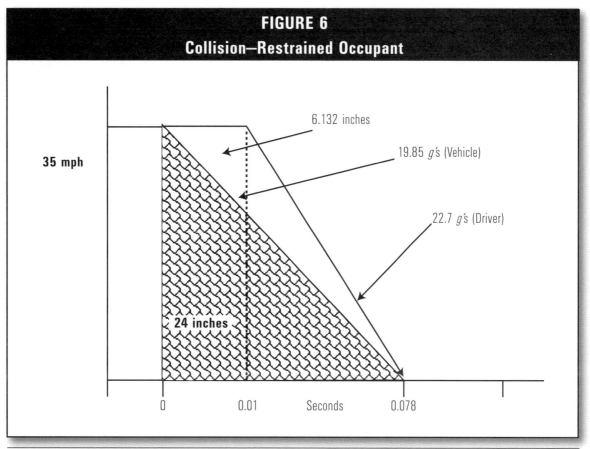

FIGURE 6
Collision—Restrained Occupant

35 mph

6.132 inches

19.85 *g*'s (Vehicle)

22.7 *g*'s (Driver)

24 inches

0   0.01   Seconds   0.078

Modified with permission from Eppinger R, Occupant restraint systems. In: Nahum AM, Melvin JW (eds): *Accidental Injury: Biomechanics and Prevention.* New York, Springer-Verlag, 1993.

Both driver and vehicle come to rest at the same time after impact. The inertial locking mechanism requires 0.01 seconds to engage, bringing the driver to a stop over 0.068 second. This accounts for the difference in *g* forces, but compared with the unrestrained driver, the force is significantly less forward motion. The vehicle loses its kinetic energy over a longer period and sustains fewer *g* forces, although the initial velocity is identical.

the force of impact, forward motion ceases (eg, dashboard, windscreen) at 2 feet (0.6 m) in front of the person, and the occupant impacts this surface just as the vehicle comes to rest. If the body of the passenger compresses by 2 inches (5 cm), the unrestrained passenger sustains a force of more than 242 *g* in 0.0065 second. By comparison, the restrained driver sustains only 22.7 *g* over 0.068 second. (See Figure 6, Collision—Restrained Occupant.) The 70-kg person who refuses to utilize the restraint system in the vehicle, thinking "I can brace myself," must be able to bench press 16,975 pounds (7639 kg), or more than 8.5 tons (7.65 tonnes), in a crash at just 35 mph (56 kph).

From the examples provided in Figures 4 through 6 one can see that the benefit of the restraint sys-

tem is to couple the occupant to the frame of the moving vehicle while the kinetic energy of the system is dissipated through maximum deformation of the vehicle over as great a time period as possible. This minimizes the transfer of energy to the occupant and is termed "ride down" in the biomechanics literature.

Increasing availability of the air bag in vehicles may significantly reduce injuries sustained in frontal impacts. However, air bags are beneficial only in approximately 70% of collisions. These devices are **not** replacements for the safety belt and must be considered **supplemental** protective devices. Occupants in head-on collisions may benefit from the air bag, but only on the first impact. If there is a second impact into another

BIOMECHANICS OF INJURY

object, the bag is already deployed and deflated, and is no longer available for protection. Air bags provide no protection in rollovers, second crashes, or lateral or rear impact. The 3-point restraint system must be used. Side air bag systems offer promise for safer passenger compartments. Currently, **maximum protection is provided only with the simultaneous use of both systems.**

When worn **correctly**, the safety belt can reduce injuries. With increasing use of the restraint system it is not surprising that the number of injuries related to safety belt use is increasing. However, it must not be forgotten that the seriousness of injuries sustained is dramatically reduced with restraint system use. If worn correctly, the device can reduce injuries. To function properly, the belt must be below the anterior/superior iliac spines and above the femur. It must be tight enough to remain in place during the motion of the crash and securely couple the occupant to the frame of the vehicle. If worn **incorrectly,** eg, above the anterior/superior iliac spines, the forward motion of the posterior abdominal wall and vertebral column traps the pancreas, liver, spleen, small bowel, duodenum, or kidney against the belt in front. Burst injuries and lacerations of these organs can occur. Hyperflexion over an incorrectly applied belt can produce anterior compression fractures of the lumbar spine (Chance fractures). (See Figure 7, page 327, Proper Versus Improper Lap Belt Application.) Energy exchange occurring in the chest during collision may be so great that injuries can result even with a properly worn safety belt. Clavicular fractures, blunt cardiac injury, and pneumothorax can result. In these instances, the patient would not have survived the crash without the protection of the restraint system.

Extensive investigation is under way to devise means to improve the efficiency of automotive safety systems. Utilizing the maxims for good restraint performance, a number of modifications of current belt and air bag systems are under study. An automatic belt retractor is activated by sensors detecting the onset of a crash. Retractors decrease delay between collision onset and seat-belt loading, thus lowering the acceleration curve. This maximizes time and distance over which the restraint forces are applied and dissipates these forces earlier in the collision event. Depowered air bags are now available in some countries. These deploy with less force, assuming the occupant is restrained, and minimize the potential

for air bag-related injury. Smart air bags take note of the weight and location of the seat belt and the use of restraints and vary air bag deployment speeds accordingly. Variable pedal adjustments allow the drivers to position themselves further from the steering column. Variable stiffness of seat cushions may prevent the down-and-under motion of the pelvis (described previously) and maintain correct belt application to the body. More extensive use of soft materials is being integrated into automobile interiors. Safety belts are being designed to stretch and absorb energy over a greater distance. A collapsible steering column that lengthens the interval from crash to occupant impact by increasing the distance between occupant and interior would provide additional protection. Currently, some automobiles have crash sensors that automatically notify an emergency services agency when a crash occurs. Finally, side impact protection is improving, with stiff door members to minimize intrusion and side air bag deployment.

C. Pedestrian Injury

More than 7000 pedestrians are killed in the United States each year after being struck by a motor vehicle. Another 110,000 suffer serious nonfatal injuries after a collision with a vehicle in motion. The problem is primarily urban in nature, with nearly 80% of such injuries occurring in cities or on residential roads. Evidence of braking is present in three-fourths of the incidents, reducing impact speeds to slightly over 10 mph (16 kph) on the average. It is estimated that nearly 90% of all pedestrian-auto interactions occur at speeds less than 30 mph (48 kph). Children constitute an exceptionally large percentage of those injured by collision with a vehicle. Thoracic, head, and lower extremity (in that order) account for the majority of injuries sustained by pedestrians.

There are 3 impact phases to the injuries sustained by a pedestrian. (See Figure 8, page 328, Adult Pedestrian Injury Triad.)

1. Vehicular bumper impact

Bumper height versus patient height is a critical factor in the specific injury produced. In the upright adult, the initial impact with the front bumper is usually against the legs and pelvis. Knee injuries are as common as are injuries to the pelvis. Children are more likely to receive chest and abdominal injuries from bumper im-

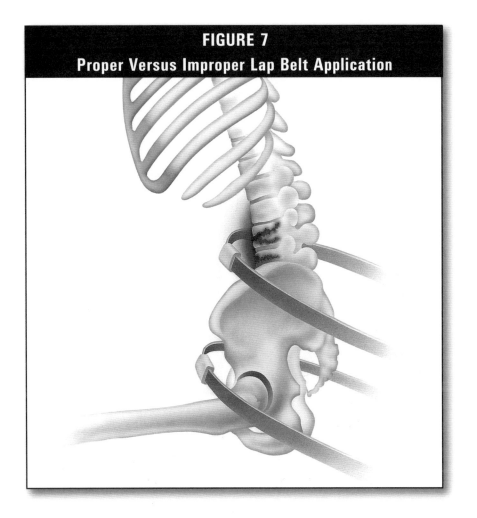

FIGURE 7
Proper Versus Improper Lap Belt Application

pact. As the design of vehicles change, so do the injury patterns seen when pedestrians are struck. Most recently manufactured passenger cars have lower front profiles and shorter hoods. This has shifted the injury patterns seen in both children and adults by altering the impact areas of the lower extremity. This trend may be offset to some degree by the increase in pickup trucks and recreational vehicles that are on the roadways.

2. Vehicular hood and windscreen impact

Torso and head injuries occur as the patient impacts with the hood and windscreen of the vehicle.

3. Ground impact

Head and spine injuries result as the patient falls off the vehicle to the ground or is accelerated into another object, resulting in an additional collision. Organ compression injuries also occur as described previously.

D. Injury to Cyclists

Two-wheeled and multiwheeled cycles are used extensively in the world for means of transportation, business, and recreation. More than 100 million bicycles are in use in the United States and many more than that number in other countries. Nearly half of all Americans ride bicycles. Bicycle-related injuries are the most common recreational injury in the United States, accounting for more than 600,000 emergency department visits per year. Each year, bicycle crashes account for more than 1200 deaths and motorcycle collisions for nearly 5000. Motorcycle crashes result in injuries that are severe enough to require hospital admission to more than 360,000 individuals each year. Interestingly, the bicycle is

BIOMECHANICS OF INJURY

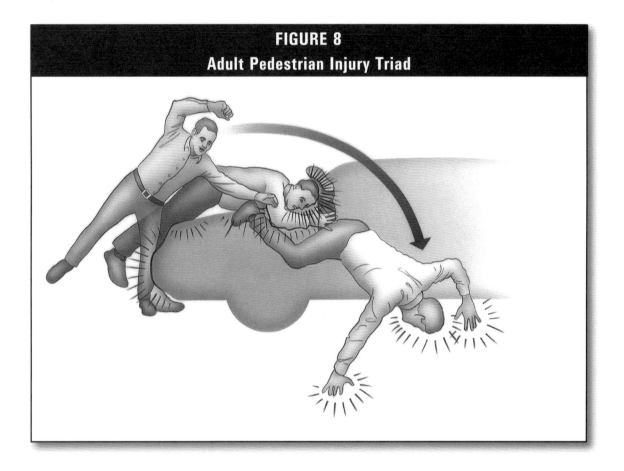

FIGURE 8
Adult Pedestrian Injury Triad

on the hazardous products list developed by the Consumer Product Safety Commission.

Cyclists and/or their passengers also may sustain compression, acceleration/deceleration, and shearing-type injuries. Cyclists are not protected by the vehicle's structure or restraining devices, as are the occupants of an automobile. Cyclists are protected only by clothing and safety devices worn on their bodies, eg, helmets, boots, or protective clothing. Only the helmet has the ability to redistribute the energy transmission and reduce its intensity, and even this capability is limited. Obviously, the less protection that is worn, the greater the risk for injury. The extent of protective equipment worn by the patient is important precrash information to obtain from the prehospital personnel.

Mechanisms of injury that may occur with cycle collisions include frontal impact, lateral impact, ejection, and "laying the bike down." Additionally, the rider may be injured from simply falling off the vehicle or becoming entangled with the cycle's mechanical components.

1. Frontal impact/ejection

The pivot point of the cycle is the front axle and the center of gravity is above this point near the seat. If the front wheel of the motorcycle collides with an object and stops, the motorcycle rotates forward on an arch with the moment arm directed toward the axle. Forward momentum is maintained until the cyclist and the rest of the cycle are acted on by forces to deplete the kinetic energy, such as secondary collision with the ground or stationary object. During this forward projection, the cyclist's head, chest, or abdomen may impact with the handlebars. If the cyclist is projected over the handlebars and ejected from the bike, the thighs may impact with the handlebars, resulting in bilateral femur fractures. The degree of injury sustained during the secondary collision is dependent upon the site of impact, the kinetic energy of the cyclist, and the time interval over which the energy is depleted.

2. Lateral impact/ejection

In a lateral impact, open or closed fractures of the lower extremity may occur. Crush injury to the extremities is frequently encountered. If the cyclist is struck by a moving vehicle, the rider is vulnerable to the same type of injuries sustained by an occupant in an automobile involved in a lateral collision. Unlike the occupant of an automobile, the cyclist does not have the passenger compartment structure to transfer the kinetic energy of impact into forces of deformation and reduce the energy transfer to the rider. The cyclist receives the full energy of the impact. As in the frontal impact, additional injury is sustained during the secondary impact with the ground or a stationary object.

3. "Laying the bike down"

To avoid entrapment between the motorcycle and a stationary object, the motorcyclist may turn the motorcycle sideways, dropping the bike and inside leg onto the pavement or ground. This strategy is intended to slow the speed of the rider and separate the cyclist from the bike. Significant soft-tissue injury can occur with this practice in addition to the spectrum of injuries described previously.

4. Helmet

Helmet use for **all** cyclists, whether motorized or not, has been shown repeatedly to reduce the incidence of severe head injury, be associated with improved chances for survival, shorten hospital stay, reduce hospital costs, and perhaps be associated with less "risk-taking" behavior. Head injury occurs in more than one-third of all bicycle-related injuries, is responsible for 66% of hospital admissions, and is directly related to 85% of all bicycle-related fatalities. The statistics are similar for motorcyclists. Although the helmet's ability to protect the head is somewhat limited, its utility should not be underestimated. The helmet is designed to reduce the force to the head by changing the kinetic energy of impact to the work of deformation of the padding and to distribute the force over as large an area as possible. This reduces the amount of energy that is delivered to the head. Helmets obviously are effective in reducing energy transfer by translation. It is generally accepted, however, that rotational or angular acceleration is most likely to produce brain injury. It can be deduced that helmets must offer some protection from rotational forces as well, considering the effectiveness of the devices. The concern that the use of bicycle or motorcycle helmets increases the risk of injury below the head, especially cervical spine injury, **has not been substantiated.**

E. Falls

Falls are the leading cause of nonfatal injury in the United States and the second leading cause of both spinal and brain injury. Similar to motor vehicle crashes, falls produce injury by a relatively abrupt change in velocity (deceleration). Whenever an external force is applied to the human body, the severity of injury is the result of the interaction between the physical factors of the force and the tissues of the body. The extent of injury to a falling body is related to the ability of the stationary surface to arrest the forward motion of the body. At impact, differential motion of tissues within the organism causes tissue disruption. Decreasing the rate of the deceleration and enlarging the surface area to which the energy is dissipated increase the tolerance to deceleration by promoting more uniform motion of the tissues. The characteristics of the contact surface that arrests the fall are important as well. Concrete, asphalt, or hard surfaces increase the rate of deceleration and are associated with more severe injuries.

Injury also is dependent upon the elasticity and viscosity of body tissues. The tendency for a tissue to resume its prestressed condition following impact is related to its elasticity. Viscosity implies resistance to change of shape with changes in motion. The tolerance of the organism to deceleration forces is a function of these combined properties. The point beyond which additional force overcomes this tissue cohesion determines the magnitude of injury. Therefore, the severity of injury is determined by the kinematics of vertical deceleration, the viscoelastic properties of the tissue, and the physical characteristics of the impact surface. One other component that should be considered in determining the extent of injury is the position of the body relative to the impact surface. Consider the following examples. A man falls 15 feet (4.5 m) from the roof of a house. In the first example he lands on his feet, the second on his back, and in the last situation he lands on the back of his head with his neck in 15° of flexion. In the first example the entire energy transfer occurs over a surface area equivalent to the area of the man's feet, is transferred via the bones of the lower extremity to

BIOMECHANICS OF INJURY

the pelvis, and then to the spine. The soft tissue and visceral organs decelerate at a slower rate than the skeleton. Additionally, the spine is more likely to flex than extend due to the ventral position of the abdominal viscera. Calcaneal fractures, femoral neck fractures, anterior vertebral compression fractures, and spinal ligamentous injury can be suspected. Avulsion of abdominal viscera from their peritoneal attachments or mesentery is common. In the second example, the force is distributed over a much larger surface area, and while tissue damage may indeed occur, it is usually less severe. In the final example, the entire energy transfer is directed over a small area and focused on a point in the cervical spine where the apex of the angle of flexion occurs. It is easy to see how the injuries differ in each of these examples, yet the mechanism and total energy is identical.

F. Blast Injury

Explosions result from extremely rapid chemical transformation of relatively small volumes of solid, semisolid, liquid, or gaseous materials into gaseous products that rapidly expand to occupy a greater volume than the undetonated explosive occupied. If unimpeded, these rapidly expanding gaseous products assume the shape of a sphere. Inside this sphere the pressure greatly exceeds atmospheric pressure. The outward expansion of this sphere produces a thin, sharply defined shell of compressed gas that acts as a pressure wave at the periphery of the sphere. The pressure decreases rapidly as this pressure wave travels away from the site of detonation in proportion to the third power of the distance. Energy transfer occurs as the pressure wave induces oscillation in the media through which it travels. The positive pressure phase of the oscillation may reach several atmospheres in magnitude, but it is of extremely short duration, whereas the negative phase that follows is of longer duration. This latter fact accounts for the phenomenon of buildings falling inward.

Blast injuries may be classified into primary, secondary, or tertiary. **Primary blast injuries** result from the direct effects of the pressure wave and are most injurious to gas-containing organs. The tympanic membrane is the most vulnerable to the effects of primary blast and may rupture if pressures exceed 2 atmospheres. Lung tissue may develop evidence of contusion, edema, and rupture resulting in pneumothorax as the result of primary blast injury. Rupture of the alveoli and pulmonary veins produces

the potential for air embolism and sudden death. Intraocular hemorrhage and retinal detachments are common ocular manifestations of primary blast injury. Intestinal rupture also may occur. **Secondary blast injuries** result from flying objects striking an individual. **Tertiary blast injury** occurs when an individual becomes a missile and is thrown against a solid object or the ground. Secondary and tertiary blast injuries may cause trauma typical of penetrating and blunt mechanisms, respectively.

IV. PENETRATING TRAUMA

Cavitation, described previously, is the result of energy exchange between the moving missile and body tissues. The amount of cavitation or energy exchange is proportional to the surface area of the point of impact, the density of the tissue, and the velocity of the projectile at the time of impact. (See Figure 9, page 331, Cavitation Results.)

The wound at the point of impact is determined by:

1. The shape of the missile ("mushroom")
2. The relation of the missile and its position relative to the impact site (tumble, yaw) (see Figure 10, page 332, Ballistics Tumble and Yaw)
3. Fragmentation (shotgun, bullet fragments, special bullets)

A. Bullets

Most bullets fired from low- to medium-velocity weapons are made from lead. Lead melts when propelled above a velocity of 2000 feet per second (600 m per second). These high-velocity bullets may be fully jacketed (encased or covered) with copper-nickel or steel to prevent meltdown. Some bullets are specifically designed to increase the amount of damage they cause. Recall that it is the transfer of energy to the tissue, the time over which the energy transfer occurs, and the surface area over which the energy exchange is distributed that determine the degree of tissue damage. Bullets with hollow noses or semijacketed coverings are designed to flatten on impact, thereby increasing their cross-sectional area and resulting in more rapid deceleration and consequentially a greater transfer of kinetic energy. Some bullets have been especially designed to fragment on impact or even explode, which extends tissue damage. Magnum rounds refer to cartridges with a greater amount of gunpowder than the normal round, which is designed to increase the muzzle velocity of the missile.

FIGURE 9
Cavitation Results

Sharp missiles with small, cross-sectional fronts slow with tissue impact, resulting in little injury or cavitation.

Missiles with large, cross-sectional fronts, eg, hollow-point bullets that spread or mushroom on impact, cause more injury or cavitation.

B. Velocity

The velocity of the missile is the most significant determinant of its wounding potential. The importance of velocity is demonstrated by the formula relating mass and velocity to kinetic energy. Examples of this relationship are listed in Table 1, page 333, Missile Kinetic Energy.

$$\text{Kinetic energy} = \frac{(\text{mass} \times \text{velocity}^2)}{2}$$

Weapons are usually classified based on the amount of energy produced by the projectiles they launch.

1. Low energy—Knife or hand-energized missiles
2. Medium energy—handguns
3. High energy—Military or hunting rifles

The wounding capability of a bullet increases markedly above the critical velocity of 2000 feet per second (600 m per second). At this speed the bullet creates a temporary cavity due to tissue being compressed at the periphery of impact by the shock wave initiated by impact of the missile with tissue. Depending on the velocity of the missile, this cavity can have a diameter of up to 30 times that of the diameter of the bullet. The maximum diameter of this temporary cavity occurs at the area of the greatest resistance to the bullet. This also is where the greatest degree of deceleration and energy transfer occurs. A bullet fired from a handgun with a standard round may produce a temporary cavity of 5 to 6 times the diameter of the bullet. Knife injuries result in little or no cavitation. Tissue damage as the result of a high-velocity missile can occur at some distance from the bullet tract itself.

Some other aspects of missile trajectory are important in determining the amount of energy dissipated and the injuries produced. **Yaw** (the orientation of the longitudinal axis of the missile to its trajectory) and **tumble** increase the surface area of the bullet with respect to the tissue it contacts and, therefore, increase the amount of energy transferred. (See Figure 10, page 332, Ballistics Tumble and Yaw.) In general, the later the bullet begins to yaw after tissue penetration, the deeper the maximum injury. Bullet deformation and fragmentation of semijacketed ammunition increase surface area relative to the tissue and the dissipation of kinetic energy.

Wounds inflicted by shotguns require special considerations. The muzzle velocity of most of these weapons is generally 1200 feet per second (360 m per second). After firing, the shot radiates in a conical distribution from the muzzle. With a choked or

BIOMECHANICS OF INJURY

FIGURE 10
Ballistics Tumble and Yaw

narrowed muzzle, 70% of the pellets are deposited in a 30-inch (75-cm) diameter circle at 40 yards (36 m). However, the "shot" is spherical and the coefficient of drag through air and tissue is quite high. As a result, the velocity of the spherical pellets declines rapidly after firing and further after impact. This weapon may be lethal at close range, but its destructive potential rapidly dissipates as distance increases. The area of maximal injury to tissue is relatively superficial unless the weapon is fired at close range. Shotgun blasts may carry clothing or deposit wadding (the paper or plastic that separates the powder and pellets in the shell) into the depths of the wound and become a source of infection if not removed.

C. Entrance Versus Exit Wounds

It may be important to speculate on whether the wound is an entrance or exit wound for clinical reasons. Two holes may indicate 2 separate gunshot wounds of the entrance and exit of 1 bullet, suggesting the path the missile may have taken through the body. Missiles usually follow the path of least resistance once tissue has been entered, and the clinician should not assume that the trajectory of the bullet followed a linear path between the entrance and exit wound. The identification of the anatomic structures that may be damaged and even the type of surgical procedure that needs to be done may be influenced by such information.

The type of projectile (eg, jacketed or unjacketed, hollow point or ball ammunition), velocity, yaw, and the type of underlying tissue all influence the appearance of the bullet wound. If there is only 1 wound, it logically must be the entrance wound. An entrance wound usually lies against the underlying tissue due to the direction of the shock wave at impact, whereas an exit wound is not supported by the subcutaneous tissue for the same reason. Weapons most commonly used in the civilian sector cause a round or oval entrance wound with a surrounding 1- to 2-mm blackened area of burn or abrasion at the periphery of the wound from the spinning bullet passing through the skin. The injection of gas into the subcutaneous tissue from close-range injuries may produce crepitus around the entrance wound. Powder burns or tattooing of the edges of the entrance wound also may be identified. Exit wounds are usually ragged at the result of tissue tearing or splitting, which produces an irregular, or stellate, appearance.

V. INTERESTING FACTS FOR MEDICAL PERSONNEL TO USE

Often medical personnel are requested to give presentations to local service organizations, civic clubs, schools, or church groups on the topic of injury or injury prevention. The following "facts" (US data) regarding injury are presented in such a fashion as to be easily understood by the public. The use of this information is encouraged.

BIOMECHANICS OF INJURY

Table 1—Missile Kinetic Energy

CARTRIDGE	BULLET WEIGHT (Grains)	MUZZLE VELOCITY (Feet/Second)	MUZZLE ENERGY (Feet/Pound)
PISTOL/REVOLVER			
.22 Long rifle	40 CBC	1255	140
.25 ACP	50 FMJ	810	73
.38 Special	158 JHP	755	200
9-mm	115 FMJ	1160	345
.45 ACP	230 FMJ	835	356
.357 Magnum	158 Lead	1235	535
.44 Magnum	240 Lead	1350	971
RIFLE			
30-30 Winchester	170 SP	2200	1827
.243 Winchester	105 SP	2290	1988
7.62 × 51 mm NATO	168 HP-BT	2680	2680
30-06 Springfield	180 SP	2700	2913
.375 H&H Magnum	270 SP	2690	4337
.458 Winchester Magnum	510 SP	2040	4712
7.62 × 39 AK 47	123 FMJ	2300	1445
M16 A2	55 FMJ	3240	1282

Abbreviations: ACP = automatic Colt pistol; CBC = conical bullet cap; FMJ = full metal jacket; HP-BT = hollow point boat tail; JHP = jacketed hollow point; SP = soft point.

Adapted with permission from Barnes FC: *Cartridges of the World,* 9th edition, Frank C. Barnes and DBI Books, Inc., Northbrook, IL, 2000.

A. Automobile and Sports-related Facts

1. Eighty percent (80%) of all crashes take place near the home or workplace at speeds less than 35 mph (56 kph), the speed at which seat belts offer the greatest protection.

2. Statistics indicate that wearing a seat belt offers a 75% efficiency rate in preventing fatal injury and a 30% chance of preventing injury altogether.

3. Nearly 50% of all serious head injuries could be avoided through the use of safety belts.

4. People who consistently wear seat belts are less likely to be involved in a crash.

5. An unbelted adult holding a child in his/her lap in a 30-mph (48-kph) crash is thrown forward with the force of 1.5 tons (1350 tonnes).

6. An unrestrained occupant of a 35-mph (56-kph) vehicular crash must be able to bench press approximately 17,000 pounds (7727 kg) to "brace oneself."

7. Child safety seats are currently saving at least 160 lives each year. As many as 52,600 pediatric injuries can be avoided with their proper use.

8. A vehicle occupant is 25 times more likely to be injured if thrown from a car rather than being belted in place.

9. In a 30-mph (48-kph) collision an unbelted driver or passenger slams into the windscreen or other interior surface of the vehicle with the same impact as a fall from a 3-story building.

10. The majority of fatal motor vehicle crashes contain 1 or more of the following contributing factors: speed, alcohol, and failure to use the restraint system.

11. The majority of fatal vehicle crashes occur on a **dry, straight, rural** road! Environmental and highway design factors are rarely the cause.

12. Sports and recreational activities and equipment were associated with more injuries requiring treatment in emergency departments than all other consumer products and at a cost of more than $13 billion (USD) in 1992.

B. Bicycle Facts

1. Three hundred (300) children die each year from bicycle-related injuries. Ninety percent (90%) of these deaths are the result of collisions with motor vehicles. Eighty percent (80%) of the deaths are related to **head injury.**

2. Bicycle-related deaths are highest in children 10 to 14 years of age.

3. Bicycles are associated with more childhood injury than any other consumer product directly operated by children.

4. Four hundred thousand (400,000) children are treated each year in emergency departments for bicycle-related injuries. One-third of these are **head injuries**.

5. Bicycle helmets reduce the risk of head injury by **85%**.

6. Universal use of bicycle helmets would save 1 life every day and prevent 1 head injury every 4 minutes.

7. Mandatory bicycle helmet laws have reduced mortality by 80% in areas where they have been passed and enforced.

8. Every dollar spent on bicycle helmets saves $2 (USD) in medical care costs.

9. Twenty-two hundred (2200) children injured in bicycle-related incidents sustain permanent disability. Bicycle helmets would prevent 1700 of these injuries. Lifetime medical savings would total **$142 million (USD)**.

10. Bicycle helmets purchased in bulk can cost as little as $11 to $14 (USD).

11. The estimated annual cost of bicycle-related injuries and deaths is **$8 billion (USD)**.

12. Nearly half of all fatalities occur between 4 and 8 in the evening on Friday through Sunday.

Note: Bicycle safety information is provided by the National Safe Kids Campaign, 1301 Pennsylvania Avenue, NW, Suite 1000, Washington, DC 20004; 202/662-0600; FAX 202/393-2072.

■ BIBLIOGRAPHY

1. Collicott PE: Concepts of trauma management-epidemiology, mechanisms and prevention. In: Skinner DV (ed): **Cambridge Textbook of Emergency Medicine.** England, Cambridge University Press, 1996.

2. Eppinger R: Occupant restraint systems. In: Nahum AM, Melvin JW (eds): **Accidental Injury: Biomechanics and Prevention.** New York, Springer-Verlag, 1993, pp 186–197.

3. Fackler ML: Physics of missile injuries. In: McSwain NE Jr, Kerstein MD (eds): **Evaluation and Management of Trauma.** East Norwalk, CT, Appleton-Century-Crofts, 1987, pp 25–53.

4. Feliciano DV, Wall MJ Jr: Patterns of injury. In: Moore EE, Mattox KL, Feliciano DV: **Trauma, Second Edition.** East Norwalk, CT, Appleton & Lange, 1991, pp 81–96.

5. Fung YC: The application of biomechanics to the understanding and analysis of trauma. In: Nahum AM, Melvin JW (eds): **The Biomechanics of Trauma.** Norwalk, CT, Appleton-Century-Crofts, 1985, pp 1-16.

6. Greensher J: Non-automotive vehicle injuries in the adolescent. **Pediatric Annals** 1988; 17(2):114, 117–121.

7. Kraus JF, Fife D, Conroy C: Incidence, severity and outcomes of brain injuries involving bicycles. **American Journal of Public Health** 1987; 77(1):76–78.

8. Leads from the MMWR. Bicycle-related injuries: Data from the National Electronic Injury Surveillance System. **Journal of the American Medical Association** 1987; 257(24):3334, 3337.

9. Mackay M: Kinetics of vehicle crashes. In: Maull KI, Cleveland HC, Strauch GO, et al (eds): **Advances in Trauma, Volume 2.** Chicago, Yearbook Medical Publishers, 1987, pp 21–24.

10. Maull KI, Whitley RE, Cardea JA: Vertical deceleration injuries. **Surgery, Gynecology and Obstetrics** 1981; 153(2):233–236.

11. MacLaughlin TF, Zuby DS, Elias JC, et al: Vehicle interactions with pedestrians. In: Nahum AM, Melvin JW (eds): **Accidental Injury: Biomechanics and Prevention.** New York, Springer-Verlag, 1993, pp 539-566.

12. McSwain NE Jr: Abdominal trauma. In: McSwain NE Jr, Kerstein MD (eds): **Evaluation and Management of Trauma.** East Norwalk, CT, Appleton-Century-Crofts, 1987, pp 129–166.

13. McSwain NE Jr: Mechanisms of injury in blunt trauma. In: McSwain NE Jr, Kerstein MD (eds): **Evaluation and Management of Trauma.** East Norwalk, CT, Appleton-Century-Crofts, 1987, pp 1–24.

14. National Highway Traffic Safety Administration: The effect of helmet law repeal on motorcycle fatalities. **DOT Publication HS-807.** Washington, DC, 1987, p 605.

15. Offner PJ, Rivara FP, Maier RV: The impact of motorcycle helmet use. **Journal of Trauma** 1992; 32(5):636–642.

16. Rozycki GS, Maull KI: Injuries sustained by falls. **Archives of Emergency Medicine** 1991; 8(4):245-252.

17. Wagle VG, Perkins C, Vallera A: Is helmet use beneficial to motorcyclists? **Journal of Trauma** 1993; 34(1):120–122.

18. Weigelt JA, McCormack A: Mechanism of injury. In: Cardona VD, Hurn PD, Mason PBJ, et al: **Trauma Nursing from Resuscitation Through Rehabilitation.** Philadelphia, WB Saunders Company, 1988, pp 105–126.

19. United States Consumer Protection Agency: **1992 Annual Report.** Washington, DC.

20. Zador PL, Ciccone MA: Automobile driver fatalities in frontal impacts: Air bags compared with manual belts. **American Journal of Public Health** 1993; 83(5):661–666.

APPENDIX 4

Tetanus Immunization

◼ INTRODUCTION

Attention must be directed to adequate tetanus prophylaxis in the multiply injured patient, particularly if open-extremity trauma is present. The average incubation period for tetanus is 10 days; most often it is 4 to 21 days. In severe trauma cases, tetanus can appear as early as 1 to 2 days. All of the medical profession must be cognizant of this important fact when providing care to the injured patient.

Tetanus immunization depends on the patient's previous immunization status and the tetanus-prone nature of the wound. The following guidelines are adapted from "Prophylaxis Against Tetanus in Wound Management," prepared by the ACS Committee on Trauma, and information available from the Centers for Disease Control and Prevention (CDC). Because this information is reviewed and updated as new data become available, the Committee on Trauma recommends contacting the CDC for the latest information and detailed guidelines related to tetanus prophylaxis and immunization for the injured patient.

TETANUS IMMUNIZATION

I. GENERAL PRINCIPLES

A. Incidence Reduction

Active immunization against tetanus with tetanus toxoid markedly reduces the incidence of this disease and resulting death.

B. Recommendations for Prophylaxis

Recommendations for tetanus prophylaxis are based on the condition of the wound, especially as it relates to tetanus susceptibility and the patient's immunization history. (See Table 1, Wound Classification, for clinical features of wounds that are prone to develop tetanus.) The attending doctor must determine the requirements for adequate prophylaxis against tetanus for each injured patient.

C. Surgical Wound Care

Regardless of the active immunization status of the patient, meticulous surgical care—including removal of all devitalized tissue and foreign bodies—should be provided immediately for all wounds. If doubt exists about the adequacy of the debridement of the wound or a puncture injury is present, the wound should be left open and not closed by sutures. Such care is essential as part of the prophylaxis against tetanus.

D. Passive Immunization

Passive immunization with 250 units of human tetanus immune globulin (TIG), administered intramuscularly, must be considered individually for each patient. TIG provides longer protection than antitoxin of animal origin and causes few adverse reactions. The characteristics of the wound, conditions under which it occurred, its age, TIG treatment, and the previous active immunization status of the patient must be considered. (See Table 2, page 339, Summary of Tetanus Prophylaxis for the Injured Patient.) When tetanus toxoid and TIG are given concurrently, separate syringes and separate sites should be used. If the patient has ever received a series of 3 injections of toxoid, TIG is not indicated, unless the wound is judged to be tetanus prone and is more than 24 hours old.

E. Documentation

Information about the mechanism of injury, wound characteristics, wound age, previous active immunization status, history of neurologic or severe hypersensitivity reaction following a previous

Table 1—Wound Classification

CLINICAL FEATURES	NON–TETANUS-PRONE WOUNDS	TETANUS-PRONE WOUNDS
Age of wound	≤ 6 hours	> 6 hours
Configuration	Linear wound, abrasion	Stellate wound, avulsion
Depth	≤ 1 cm	> 1 cm
Mechanism of injury	Sharp surface, eg, knife, glass	Missile, crush, burn, frostbite
Signs of infection	Absent	Present
Devitalized tissue	Absent	Present
Contaminants (dirt, feces, soil, saliva, etc)	Absent	Present
Denervated and/or ischemic tissue	Absent	Present

Information adapted with permission from the Centers for Disease Control and Prevention, Atlanta, GA, www.cdc.gov/epo/mmwr/preview/mmwrhtml/00041645.htm., last updated 1991.

Table 2—Summary of Tetanus Prophylaxis for the Injured Patient

HISTORY OF ADSORBED TETANUS TOXOID (doses)	NONTETANUS-PRONE WOUNDS		TETANUS-PRONE WOUNDS	
	Td[1]	TIG	Td[1]	TIG
Unknown or < 3	Yes	No	Yes	Yes
≥ 3[2]	No[3]	No	No[4]	No

Information adapted with permission from the Centers for Disease Control and Prevention, Atlanta, GA, www.cdc.gov/epo/mmwr/preview/mmwrhtml/00041645.htm., last updated 1991.

Key to Table 2

[1] For children younger than 7 years old: DTP (DT, if pertussis vaccine is contraindicated) is preferred to tetanus toxoid alone. For persons 7 years old and older: Td is preferred to tetanus toxoid alone.

[2] If only 3 doses of fluid toxoid have been received, a fourth dose of toxoid, preferably an adsorbed toxoid, should be given.

[3] Yes, if more than 10 years since last dose.

[4] Yes, if more than 5 years since last dose. (More frequent boosters are not needed and can accentuate side effects.)

Td = Tetanus and diphtheria toxoids adsorbed, for adult use.

TIG = Tetanus immune globulin, human.

immunization treatment, and plans for follow-up should be documented for every injured patient. Each patient must be given a written record describing treatment rendered and follow-up instructions that outline wound care, drug therapy, immunization status, and potential complications. The patient should be referred to a doctor for comprehensive follow-up care, including completion of active immunizations.

A wallet-sized card documenting the immunization administered and date of immunization should be given to every injured patient. The patient should be instructed to carry the written record at all times and complete the active immunization process as indicated. For precise tetanus prophylaxis, an accurate and immediately available history regarding previous active immunization against tetanus is required. Otherwise, rapid laboratory titration is necessary to determine the patient's serum antitoxin level.

F. Antibiotics

The effectiveness of antibiotics for prophylaxis of tetanus is uncertain. In patients who need TIG as part of the treatment to prevent tetanus and it is not available for any reason, antibiotics like penicillin delay the onset of tetanus. This allows a period of 2 days in which to obtain the TIG and institute proper passive immunization.

G. Contraindications

The only contraindication to tetanus and diphtheria toxoids for the wounded patient is a history of neurologic or severe hypersensitivity reaction to a previous dose. Local side effects alone do not preclude its continued use. If a previous systemic reaction to equine tetanus antitoxin is suspected to represent allergic hypersensitivity, immunization should be postponed until appropriate skin testing is performed. If a tetanus toxoid-containing preparation is contraindicated, passive immunization against tetanus should be considered for a tetanus-prone wound.

Contraindications to pertussis vaccination in infants and children younger than 7 years old include either a previous adverse reaction after diphtheria and tetanus toxoids and pertussis vaccine adsorbed (DTP) or single-antigen pertussis vaccination and/or the presence of a neurologic finding. If such a contraindication to using pertussis vaccine adsorbed (P) exists, diphtheria and tetanus toxoids adsorbed (for pediatric use) (DT) is recommended. A static neurologic condition, such as cerebral palsy or a family history of convulsions or other central nervous system disorders, is not a contraindication to giving vaccines containing the pertussis antigen.

TETANUS IMMUNIZATION

H. Active Immunization for Normal Infants and Children

For children younger than 7 years of age, immunization requires 4 injections of DTP. A booster (fifth dose) injection is administered at 4 to 6 years of age. Thereafter, a routine booster of tetanus and diphtheria toxoids adsorbed (Td) is indicated at 10-year intervals.

I. Active Immunization for Adults

Immunization for adults requires at least 3 injections of Td. An injection of Td should be repeated every 10 years throughout the individual's life, providing no significant reactions to Td have occurred.

J. Active Immunization for Pregnant Women

Neonatal tetanus is preventable by active immunization of the pregnant mother during the first 6 months of pregnancy, with 2 injections of Td given 2 months apart. After delivery and 6 months after the second dose, the mother should be given the third dose of Td to complete the active immunization.

An injection of Td should be repeated every 10 years throughout life, providing no significant reactions to Td have occurred. In the event that a neonate is born to a nonimmunized mother without obstetric care, the infant should receive 250 units of TIG. Active and passive immunization of the mother also should be initiated.

K. Previously Immunized Individuals

1. Fully immunized

When the doctor determines that the patient is previously and fully immunized, and the last dose of toxoid was given within 10 years:

a. Administer 0.5 mL of adsorbed toxoid for tetanus-prone wounds, if more than 5 years has elapsed since the last dose.

b. This booster may be omitted if excessive toxoid injections have been given before.

2. Partially immunized

When the patient has received 2 or more injections of toxoid, and the last dose was received more than 10 years ago, 0.5 mL adsorbed toxoid is administered for both tetanus-prone and non-

tetanus-prone wounds. Passive immunization is not necessary.

L. Individuals Not Adequately Immunized

When the patient has received only 1 or no prior injections of toxoid or the immunization history is unknown:

1. **Nontetanus-prone wounds:** Administer 0.5 mL of adsorbed toxoid for nontetanus-prone wounds.

2. **Tetanus-prone wounds**

   a. Administer 0.5 mL adsorbed toxoid.

   b. Administer 250 units TIG.

   c. Consider administering antibiotics, although their effectiveness for prophylaxis of tetanus remains unproved.

   d. Administer medication using different syringes and sites for injection.

   e. A complete series of 3 tetanus toxoid vaccinations should be recommended.

M. Immunization Schedule

1. **Adult**

   a. Three injections of toxoid

   b. Booster every 10 years

2. **Children**

   a. Four injections of DTP

   b. Fifth dose at 4 to 6 years of age

   c. Booster every 10 years

■ BIBLIOGRAPHY

1. American College of Surgeons Committee on Trauma: Prophylaxis against tetanus in wound management. Poster, 1995.

2. U.S. Department of Health and Human Services, Centers for Disease Control and Prevention: Diphtheria, tetanus, and pertussis: Recommendation for vaccine use and other preventive measures, recommendations of the Immunization Practices Advisory Committee (ACIP). **Morbidity and Mortality Weekly Report Recommendations and Reports** August 8, 1991; 40(RR10):1–28.

APPENDIX 5

Trauma Scores: Revised and Pediatric

▪ INTRODUCTION

Correct triage is essential to effective function of regional trauma systems. Overtriage inundates trauma centers with minimally injured patients who then impede care for severely injured patients. Undertriage can produce inadequate initial care and may cause preventable morbidity and mortality. Unfortunately, the perfect triage tool does not exist.

TRAUMA SCORES: REVISED AND PEDIATRIC

I. REVISED TRAUMA SCORE

Experience with adult trauma scoring systems illustrates this problem by the multiplicity of scoring systems that have been proposed over the last decade. None of these scoring protocols is universally accepted as a completely effective triage tool. At present, most of adult trauma surgeons utilize the Revised Trauma Score (RTS) as a triage tool and the weighted variation of this score as a predictor of potential mortality. This score is based totally on physiologic derangement on initial evaluation and entails a categorization of blood pressure, respiratory rate, and the Glasgow Coma Scale. (See Table 1, page 343, Revised Trauma Score.)

II. PEDIATRIC TRAUMA SCORE

Application of these 3 components to the pediatric population is difficult and inconsistent. Respiratory rate is often inaccurately measured in the field and does not necessarily reflect respiratory insufficiency in the injured child. The Glasgow Coma Scale is an extremely effective neurologic assessment tool; however, it requires some revision for application to the preverbal child. These problems, in association with the lack of any identification of anatomic injury or quantification of patient size, undermine the applicability of the RTS to effectively triage the injured child. For these reasons, the Pediatric Trauma Score (PTS) was developed. The PTS is the sum of the severity grade of each category and has been demonstrated to predict potential for death and severe disability reliably. (See Table 2, page 344, Pediatric Trauma Score.)

A. Size

Size is a major consideration for the infant-toddler group, in which mortality from injury is the highest. **Airway** is assessed not just as a function, but as a descriptor of what care is required to provide adequate management. **Systolic blood pressure** assessment primarily identifies those children in whom evolving preventable shock may occur (50 to 90 mm Hg systolic blood pressure [+l]). Regardless of size, a child whose systolic blood pressure is below 50 mm Hg (-l) is in obvious jeopardy. On the other hand, a child whose systolic pressure exceeds 90 mm Hg (+2) probably falls into a better outcome category than a child with even a slight degree of hypotension.

B. Level of Consciousness

Level of consciousness is the most important factor in initially assessing the central nervous system. Because children frequently lose consciousness transiently during injury, the "obtunded" (+l) grade is given to any child who loses consciousness, no matter how fleeting the loss. This grade identifies a patient who may have sustained a head injury with potentially fatal—but often treatable—intracranial sequelae.

C. Musculoskeletal Injury

Skeletal injury is a component of the PTS because of its high incidence in the pediatric population and its potential contribution to mortality. Finally, **cutaneous injury,** both as an adjunct to common pediatric injury patterns and as an injury category that includes penetrating wounds, is considered in the computed PTS.

The PTS serves as a simple checklist, ensuring that all components critical to initial assessment of the injured child have been considered. It is useful for paramedics in the field, as well as for doctors in facilities other than pediatric trauma units. As a predictor of injury, the PTS has a statistically significant inverse relationship with the Injury Severity Score (ISS) and mortality. Analysis of this relationship has identified a threshold PTS of 8, above which injured children should have a mortality rate of 0%. All injured children with a PTS of less than 8 should be triaged to an appropriate pediatric trauma center, because they have the highest potential for preventable mortality, morbidity, and disability. According to the National Pediatric Trauma Registry statistics, they represent approximately 25% of all pediatric trauma victims, clearly requiring the most aggressive monitoring and observation.

Recent studies comparing the PTS with the RTS have identified similar performances of both scores in predicting potential for mortality. Unfortunately, the RTS produces unacceptable levels of undertriage, which is an inadequate trade-off for its greater simplicity. Perhaps more importantly, however, the PTS's function as an initial assessment checklist requires that each of the factors that may contribute to death or disability is considered during initial evaluation and becomes a source of concern for those individuals responsible for the initial assessment and management of the injured child.

TRAUMA SCORES: REVISED AND PEDIATRIC

Table 1—Revised Trauma Score

	VARIABLES	SCORE	START OF TRANSPORT	END OF TRANSPORT
A. Respiratory Rate (breaths/minute)	10–29 > 29 6–9 1–5 0	4 3 2 1 0	 _____	 _____
B. Systolic BP (mm Hg)	> 89 76–89 50–75 1–49 0	4 3 2 1 0	 _____	 _____
C. GCS Score Conversion $C = D + E^1 + F$ (adult) $C = D + E^2 + F$ (pediatric)	13–15 9–12 6–8 4–5 < 4	4 3 2 1 0	 _____	 _____
D. Eye Opening	Spontaneous To voice To pain None	4 3 2 1	 _____	 _____
E.¹ Verbal Response, Adult	Oriented Confused Inappropriate words Incomprehensible words None	5 4 3 2 1	 _____	 _____
E.² Verbal Response, Pediatric	Appropriate Cries, consolable Persistently irritable Restless, agitated None	5 4 3 2 1	 _____	 _____
F. Motor Response	Obeys commands Localizes pain Withdraws (pain) Flexion (pain) Extension (pain) None	6 5 4 3 2 1	 _____	 _____
Glasgow Coma Scale Score (Total = $D + E^{1\,or\,2} + F$)			_____	_____
REVISED TRAUMA SCORE = A + B + C			_____	_____

Adapted with permission from Champion HR, Sacco WJ, Copes WS, et al: A revision of the Trauma Score. *Journal of Trauma* 1989; 29(5):624.

TRAUMA SCORES: REVISED AND PEDIATRIC

Table 2—Pediatric Trauma Score

ASSESSMENT COMPONENT	SCORE		
	+2	+1	−1
Weight	> 20 kg (> 44 lb)	10–20 kg (22–44 lb)	< 10 kg (< 22 lb)
Airway	Normal	Oral or nasal airway, oxygen	Intubated, cricothyroid-otomy, or tracheostomy
Systolic Blood Pressure	> 90 mm Hg; good peripheral pulses and perfusion	50–90 mm Hg; carotid/femoral pulses palpable	< 50 mm Hg; weak or no pulses
Level of Consciousness	Awake	Obtunded or any LOC[1]	Coma, unresponsive
Fracture	None seen or suspected	Single, closed	Open or multiple
Cutaneous	None visible	Contusion, abrasion, laceration < 7 cm not through fascia	Tissue loss, any GSW[2]/SW[3] through fascia
Totals:			

[1]LOC = loss of consciousness, [2]GSW = gunshot wound, [3]SW = stab wound

Adapted with permission from Tepas JJ, Mollitt DL, Talbert JL, et al: The pediatric trauma score as a predictor of injury severity in the injured child. *Journal of Pediatric Surgery* 1987; 22(1):l5.

APPENDIX

6

Sample Trauma Flow Sheet*

SAMPLE TRAUMA FLOW SHEET*

Name:	Chief Complaint:
Date:	
Arrival time:	

PREHOSPITAL TRANSPORT INFORMATION	**MECHANISM OF INJURY**

PREHOSPITAL TRANSPORT INFORMATION

❑ Scene ❑ Ambulance ❑ Helicopter

❑ Police ❑ Private vehicle ❑ Ambulatory

❑ Wheelchair ❑ Other _____

❑ Referring doctor _____

❑ Referring hospital _____

❑ Other information _____

_____

_____

MECHANISM OF INJURY

❑ MCV: ❑ Driver ❑ Passenger ❑ Front ❑ Back
❑ Seat belt on ❑ Air bag inflated

❑ MCC: ❑ Driver ❑ Passenger
❑ Helmet on ❑ Protective clothing worn

❑ Pedestrian vs vehicle ❑ Vehicle vs bicycle

❑ Vehicle speed _____ mph/kph

❑ Fall _____ feet/meters

❑ GSW ❑ Stab ❑ Crush ❑ Burn/Cold
❑ Assault ❑ Hypothermia ❑ Other

PROCEDURES BEFORE ARRIVAL

❑ Oral airway ❑ Nasal airway ❑ EOA/PTL

❑ ETT # _____ ❑ NTT # _____ ❑ RSI

❑ Cric # _____ ❑ O_2 @ _____ L/min via _____

Breath sounds: L _____ R _____

❑ IVs # _____ ❑ Peripheral ❑ Central ❑ Intraosseous

❑ IV fluids: 1 2 3 4 5 6 ❑ Blood: 1 2 3 4 5

❑ CPR ❑ PASG: ❑ Legs ❑ Abdomen

❑ Urinary cath ❑ Gastric tube

❑ Chest tube: ❑ R ❑ L ❑ Both

❑ C-spine/spine protection Time on: _____

❑ Splints: Type _____

❑ Medications: _____

❑ Other procedures: _____

_____

AMPLE HISTORY

Allergies: _____

_____

Medications: _____

_____

Past illnesses: _____

_____

Last meal: _____ Last tetanus: _____

Events: _____

_____

Pregnant? ❑ Yes ❑ No LMP _____

Spine protection device removed @ _____

Other: _____

_____

_____

OTHER SERVICES CONTACTED (Time called/arrived)				PERSONNEL RESPONSE (Time called/arrived)			
Service	**Name**	**Called**	**Arrived**	**Service**	**Name**	**Called**	**Arrived**
				ED doctor			
				Trauma surgeon			
				Neurosurgery			
				Orthopaedics			
				Anesthesia			
				Pediatrics			
				ENT/OMFS			
				Plastics/burns			
				Urology			
				Nurse			
				Nurse			
				Other			

SAMPLE TRAUMA FLOW SHEET*

INITIAL ASSESSMENT	IDENTIFY INJURY SITE BY NUMBER

INITIAL ASSESSMENT

AIRWAY/BREATHING

❑ Patent ❑ Obstructed ❑ Symmetrical

❑ Asymmetrical ❑ Unlabored ❑ Labored

❑ Trachea midline? ❑ Yes ❑ No

Breath Sounds:

Present: ❑ Right ❑ Left

Clear: ❑ Right ❑ Left

Decreased ❑ Right ❑ Left

Absent ❑ Right ❑ Left

Rales/rhonchi ❑ Right ❑ Left

Crepitus? ❑ Yes ❑ No

CIRCULATION

Skin/mucous: ❑ Pink ❑ Pale

Membrane color: ❑ Flushed ❑ Jaundiced

❑ Ashen ❑ Cyanotic

Pulses: ❑ Normal, Site _____

❑ Bounding, Site _____

❑ Weak, Site _____

❑ Absent, Site _____

Rate:_____/minute Rhythm _____

Skin temp: ❑ Warm ❑ Hot ❑ Cool/cold

Skin moisture: ❑ WNL ❑ Dry ❑ Moist

DISABILITY

GCS Score: Eye opening _____

Verbal _____

Best motor _____

TOTAL GCS SCORE _____

Revised Trauma Respiratory _____

Score (RTS) Systolic BP _____

GCS _____

TOTAL RTS _____

Pupil Reaction: OS Size OD Size

❑ Brisk _____mm _____mm

❑ Constricted _____mm _____mm

❑ Sluggish _____mm _____mm

❑ Dilated _____mm _____mm

❑ Nonreactive _____mm _____mm

IDENTIFY INJURY SITE BY NUMBER

1. Laceration 6. Open fracture 11. Edema
2. Abrasion 7. GSW 12. Amputation
3. Hematoma 8. Stab 13. Avulsion
4. Contusion 9. Burn 14. Pain
5. Deformity 10. Cold

Head: _____

Maxillofacial: _____

C-spine/neck: _____

Chest: _____

Abdomen: _____

Perineum: _____

Musculoskeletal: _____

SAMPLE TRAUMA FLOW SHEET*

TRAUMA RESUSCITATION ORDERS						
Time	Laboratory	Time	X-rays	Time	Procedures	
	Type/cross # units		Chest		O_2 @ L/min via	
	Type/hold		Pelvis		ETT # by:	
	CBC Screen		Lateral c-spine		NTT # by:	
	ETOH		Swimmers		Cric # by:	
	Drug screen		Thoracic spine		Needle thoracostomy by:	
	PT/PTT		Lumbar spine		Chest tube# by:	
	ABGs		Skull		R return: L return:	
	Urinalysis		Facial series		ED thoracotomy by:	
	DPL fluid		Mandible		Autotransfuser	
	Pregnancy test + −		Abdomen		R IV site: size:	
	HIV + −		Extremity: LUE/RUE		R IV site: size:	
			Extremity: LLE/RLE		L IV site: size:	
	Other:		IVP		L IV site: size:	
			Cystogram		C IV site: size:	
			Urethrogram		CVP site: size:	
			Arteriogram/Aorto		Pericardiocentesis by:	
			CT head		ECG	
			CT chest		Gastric tube# by:	
			CT abdomen		Return	
			CT pelvis		Color	
			Helical CT		Rectal tone:	
					Urinary cath# by:	
					Urine dip + −	
					Spontaneous void dip + −	
					DPL + −	
					FAST by:	
					Results	
					Suturing by:	
					Restraints: UE LE	

FLUID INTAKE/OUTPUT		ABGs				
Intake	**Ouput**	O_2 LPM	pH	P_{CO_2}	P_{O_2}	Time
Total fluids prehospital_____mL	Urine _____ mL					
ED Total fluids_____mL	Gastric_____ mL					
Total blood prehospital_____mL	Blood_____ mL					
ED Total PRBCs_____mL	TOTAL _____ mL					
FFP Total_____mL		**MEDICATIONS**				
Platelets_____mL		Med	Dose	By	Route/Site	Time
Other:		Tetanus				
TOTAL_____mL						

American College of Surgeons

SAMPLE TRAUMA FLOW SHEET*

TIME									
Cuff BP	/	/	/	/	/	/	/	/	/
Pulse									
Rhythm									
Respirations									
Temperature									
MAP line									
O₂/Hgb Sat									
Carboximetry									
CVP									
Urinary output									
Blood output									
GCS SCORE									
1. Eye opening									
2. Verbal									
3. Best motor									
TOTAL (1+2+3)									
R pupil size and reaction									
L pupil size and reaction									

TIME	NOTES

DISPOSITION: ❑ Alive: Time out: _____am/pm   To: _____   Service: _____

❑ Dead: Time out: _____am/pm   To: _____

❑ Operative permit signed   ❑ Family notified   ❑ Pastoral service notified   ❑ Social services notified

Valuables/clothing: _____

Forensic evidence: _____

Doctor's Signature: _____

NOTE: This flow sheet is only an example of information that may be required. All institutions that receive trauma patients should develop a form that meets the needs of the institution.

APPENDIX

Ocular Trauma
(Optional Lecture)

■ OBJECTIVES:

Upon completion of this topic, the participant will be able to assess and manage sight-threatening eye injuries. Specifically, the participant will be able to:

A. Obtain patient and event histories.

B. Perform a systematic examination of the orbit and its contents.

C. Identify and discuss those eyelid injuries that can be treated by the primary care doctor, as well as those that must be referred to an ophthalmologist for treatment.

D. Discuss how to examine the eye for a foreign body, and how to remove superficial foreign bodies to prevent further injury.

E. Identify a corneal abrasion, and discuss its management.

F. Identify a hyphema, and discuss the initial management and necessity for referral to an ophthalmologist.

G. Identify those eye injuries requiring referral to an ophthalmologist.

H. Identify a ruptured globe injury, and discuss the initial management required prior to referral to an ophthalmologist.

I. Evaluate and treat eye injuries resulting from chemicals.

J. Evaluate a patient with an orbital fracture, and discuss the initial management and necessity for referral.

K. Identify a retrobulbar hematoma, and discuss the necessity for immediate referral.

OCULAR TRAUMA

I. INTRODUCTION

The initial assessment of a patient with ocular injury requires a systematic approach. The physical examination should proceed in an organized, step-by-step manner, and does not require extensive, complicated instrumentation in the multiple-trauma setting. Simple therapeutic measures often can save the patient's vision and prevent severe sequelae before an ophthalmologist is available. This optional lecture provides the pertinent information regarding early identification and treatment of ocular injuries that enhances the doctor's basic knowledge and may save the patient's sight.

II. ASSESSMENT

A. History

Obtain a history of any preexisting ocular disease.

1. Does the patient wear corrective lenses?

2. Is there a history of glaucoma or previous eye surgery?

3. What medications does the patient use, eg, pilocarpine?

B. Injury Incident

Obtain a detailed description of the circumstances surrounding the injury. This information often raises the index of suspicion for certain potential injuries and their sequelae, eg, the higher risk of infection from certain foreign bodies—wood versus metallic.

1. Was there blunt trauma?

2. Was there penetrating injury? In motor vehicular crashes there is potential for glass or metallic foreign bodies.

3. Was there a missile injury?

4. Was there a possible thermal, chemical, or flash burn?

C. Initial Symptoms/Complaint

1. What were the patient's initial symptoms?

2. Did the patient complain of pain or photophobia?

3. Was there an immediate decrease in vision that has remained stable or is it progressive?

The physical examination must be systematic so that function as well as anatomic structures are evaluated. As with injuries to other organ systems, the pathology also may evolve with time, and the patient must be periodically reevaluated. A directed approach to the ocular examination, beginning with the most external structures in an "outside-to-inside" manner, ensures that injuries are not missed.

D. Visual Acuity

Visual acuity is evaluated first by any means possible and recorded, eg, patient counting fingers at 3 feet (0.9 meters).

E. Eyelids

The most external structures to be examined are the eyelids. The eyelids should be assessed for the following: (1) edema; (2) ecchymosis; (3) evidence of burns or chemical injury; (4) laceration(s)—medial, lateral, lid margin, canaliculi; (5) ptosis; (6) foreign bodies that contact the globe; and (7) avulsion of the canthal tendon.

F. Orbital Rim

Gently palpate the orbital rim for a step-off deformity and crepitus. Subcutaneous emphysema may result from a fracture of the medial orbit into the ethmoids or a fracture of the orbital floor into the maxillary antrum.

G. Globe

The eyelids should be retracted to examine the globe without applying pressure to the globe. Specially designed retractors are available for this purpose. Cotton-tipped applicators can also be used by placing them gently against the superior and inferior orbital rims and rolling the eyes open. The globe is then assessed anteriorly for displacement resulting from a retrobulbar hematoma and for posterior or inferior displacement due to a fracture of the orbit. The globes also are assessed for normal ocular movement, diplopia, and evidence of entrapment.

H. Pupil

The pupils are assessed for roundness with regular shape, equality, and reaction to light stimulus. It is important to test for an afferent pupil defect. Optic nerve trauma usually results in failure of both pupils to constrict when a light is directed at the affected eye.

I. Cornea

The cornea is assessed for opacity, ulceration, and foreign bodies. Fluorescein and a blue light facilitate this assessment.

J. Conjunctiva

The conjunctivae are assessed for chemosis, subconjunctival emphysema (indicating probable fracture of the orbit into the ethmoid or maxillary sinus), subconjunctival hemorrhage, and foreign bodies.

K. Anterior Chamber

Examine the anterior chamber for a hyphema (blood in the anterior chamber). The depth of the anterior chamber can be assessed by shining a light into the eye from the lateral aspect of the eye. If the light does not illuminate the entire surface of the iris, a shallow anterior chamber should be suspected. A shallow anterior chamber may result from an anterior penetrating wound. A deep anterior chamber may result from a posterior penetrating wound of the globe.

L. Iris

The iris should be reactive and regular in shape. Assess the iris for iridodialysis (a tear of the iris) or iridodonesis (a floppy or tremulous iris).

M. Lens

The lens should be transparent. Assess the lens for possible anterior displacement into the anterior chamber, partial dislocation with displacement into the posterior chamber, and dislocation into the vitreous.

N. Vitreous

The vitreous also should be transparent, allowing for easy visualization of the fundus. Visualization may be difficult if vitreous hemorrhage has occurred. In this situation, a black rather than red reflex is seen by ophthalmoscopy. A vitreous bleed usually indicates a significant underlying ocular injury. The vitreous also should be assessed for an intraocular foreign body.

O. Retina

The retina is examined for hemorrhage, possible tears, or detachment. A detached retina is opalescent, and the blood columns are darker.

III. SPECIFIC INJURIES

A. Lid

Lid injuries often result in marked ecchymosis, making examination of the globe and lid injury difficult. However, a more serious injury to the underlying structures must be excluded. Look beneath the lid as well to exclude damage to the globe. Lid retractors or cotton-tipped applicators should be used if necessary to forcibly open the eye to inspect the globe. Ptosis may be secondary to edema, damage to the levator palpebrae, or oculomotor nerve injury.

Lacerations of the upper or lower lid that are horizontal, superficial, and do not involve the levator in the upper lid may be closed by the examining doctor using interrupted 6-0 (silk, nylon) skin sutures. The doctor also should examine the eye beneath the lid to rule out damage to the globe.

Lid injuries to be treated by an ophthalmologist include (1) wounds involving the medial canthus that may have damaged the medial canaliculus; (2) injury to the lacrimal sac or nasal lacrimal duct, which can lead to obstruction if not properly repaired; (3) deep horizontal lacerations of the upper lid that may involve the levator and result in ptosis if not repaired correctly; and (4) lacerations of the lid margin that are difficult to close and may lead to notching, entropion, or ectropion. These wounds may be covered with a saline dressing pending emergency ophthalmologic consultation.

Foreign bodies of the lid result in profuse tearing, pain, and a foreign-body sensation that increases with lid movement. The conjunctiva should be inspected, and the upper and lower lids should be everted to examine the inner surface. Topical anesthetic drops may be used, but only for initial examination and removal of the foreign body.

Impaled, penetrating foreign bodies are not disturbed and are removed only in the operating room by an ophthalmologist or appropriate specialist. If the patient requires transport to another facility for treatment of this injury or others, consult an oph-

OCULAR TRAUMA

thalmologist regarding management of the eye during transport.

B. Cornea

Corneal abrasions result in pain, foreign body sensation, photophobia, decreased visual acuity, and chemosis. The injured epithelium stains with fluorescein.

Corneal foreign bodies sometimes can be removed with irrigation. However, if the foreign body is embedded, the patient should be referred to an ophthalmologist. Corneal abrasions are treated with antibiotic drops or ointment to prevent ulcers. Recent clinical studies have demonstrated no advantage to patching in terms of patient comfort or time required for the abrasion to heal. The patient should be instructed to instill the drops or ointment and should be seen in follow-up within 24 to 48 hours.

C. Anterior Chamber

Hyphema is blood in the anterior chamber, which may be difficult to see if there is only a small amount. In extreme cases, the entire anterior chamber is filled. The hyphema can often be seen with a penlight. Hyphema usually indicates severe intraocular trauma.

Glaucoma develops in 7% of patients with hyphema. Corneal staining also may occur. **Remember,** hyphema may be the result of serious underlying ocular injury. Even in the case of a small bleed, spontaneous rebleeding often occurs within the first 5 days, which may lead to total hyphema. Therefore, the patient must be referred. The affected eye is patched, and the patient usually is hospitalized, placed at bed rest, and reevaluated frequently. Pain after hyphema usually indicates rebleeding and/or acute glaucoma.

D. Iris

Contusion injuries of the iris may cause traumatic mydriasis or miosis. There may be disruption of the iris from the ciliary body, causing an irregular pupil and hyphema.

E. Lens

Contusion of the lens may lead to later opacification or cataract formation. Blunt trauma can cause a break of the zonular fibers that encircle the lens and anchor it to the ciliary body. This results in subluxation of the lens, possibly into the anterior chamber, causing a shallow chamber. In cases of posterior subluxation, the anterior chamber deepens. Patients with these injuries should be referred to an ophthalmologist.

F. Vitreous

Blunt trauma also can lead to vitreous hemorrhage. This usually is secondary to retinal vessel damage and bleeding into the vitreous, resulting in a sudden, profound visual loss. Funduscopic examination may be impossible and the red reflex, seen with an ophthalmoscope light, is lost. A patient with this injury should be placed at bed rest with the eye shielded and be referred to an ophthalmologist.

G. Retina

Blunt trauma also causes retinal hemorrhage. The patient may or may not have decreased visual acuity, depending on involvement of the macula. Superficial retinal hemorrhages appear cherry red in color; the deeper lesions appear gray.

Retinal edema and detachment can occur with head trauma. A white, cloudy discoloration is observed. Retinal detachments appear "curtainlike." If the macula is involved, visual acuity is affected. An acute retinal tear usually occurs in conjunction with blunt trauma to an eye with preexisting vitreoretinal pathology. Retinal detachment most often occurs as a late sequelae of blunt trauma. The patient describes light flashes and a curtainlike defect in peripheral vision.

A rupture of the choroid initially appears as a beige area at the posterior pole. Later it becomes a yellow-white scar. If it transects the macula, vision is seriously and permanently impaired.

H. Globe

A patient with a ruptured globe has marked visual impairment. The eye is soft due to a decreased intraocular pressure, and the anterior chamber may be flattened or shallow. If the rupture is anterior, ocular contents may be seen extruding from the eye.

The goal of initial management of the ruptured globe is to protect the eye from any additional damage. As soon as a ruptured globe is suspected, no further manipulation of the eye should be performed. A sterile dressing and eye shield should be applied carefully to prevent any pressure to the eye that may cause further extrusion of the ocular contents. The patient should be instructed not to squeeze the injured eye shut. If not contraindicated by other injuries, the patient may be sedated while awaiting transport or treatment. Do not remove foreign objects, tissue, or clots before dressing placement. No topical analgesics are used—only oral or parenteral, if not contraindicated by any other injuries.

An **intraocular foreign body** should be suspected if the patient complains of sudden sharp pain with a decrease in visual acuity, particularly if the eye may have been struck by a small fragment of metal, glass, or wood. Inspect the surface of the globe carefully for any small lacerations and possible sites of entry. These may be difficult to find. In the anterior chamber, tiny foreign bodies may be hidden by blood or in the crypt of the iris. A tiny iris perforation may be impossible to see directly, but with a pen light the red reflex may be detected through the defect (if the lens and vitreous are not opaque).

I. Chemical Injuries

Chemical injuries require immediate intervention if sight is to be preserved. Acid precipitates proteins in the tissue and sets up somewhat of a natural barrier against extensive tissue penetration. However, alkali combines with lipids in the cell membrane, leading to disruption of the cell membranes, rapid penetration of the caustic agent, and extensive tissue destruction. Chemical injury to the cornea causes disruption of stromal mucopolysaccharides, leading to opacification.

The treatment is **copious and continuous irrigation.** Attempts should not be made to neutralize the agent. Intravenous solutions (sterile saline or Ringer's lactate solution) and tubing can be used to improvise continuous irrigation. Blepharospasm is extensive, and the lids must be manually opened during irrigation. Analgesics and sedation should be used, if not contraindicated by coexisting injuries. Thermal injuries usually occur to the lids only and rarely involve the cornea. However, burns of the globe occasionally occur. A sterile dressing should be applied and the patient referred to an ophthalmologist. Exposure of the cornea **must** be prevented or it can perforate, and the eye can be lost.

J. Fracture

Blunt trauma to the orbit causes rapid compression of the tissues and increased pressure within the orbit. One of the weakest points is the orbital floor, which fractures, allowing orbital contents to herniate into the antrum—hence the term "blowout."

Clinically the patient presents with pain, swelling, and ecchymosis of the lids and periorbital tissues. There may be subconjunctival hemorrhage. Facial asymmetry and possibly enophthalmos might be evident or masked by surrounding edema. Limitation of ocular motion and diplopia secondary to edema or entrapment of the orbital contents may be noted. Palpation of the rims may reveal a fracture step-off deformity.

Subcutaneous and/or subconjunctival emphysema can occur when the fracture is into the ethmoid or maxillary sinuses. Hypoesthesia of the cheek occurs secondary to injury of the infraorbital nerve. The Waters view and Caldwell view (straight on) are very helpful for evaluating orbital fractures. Examine the orbital floor, and look for soft tissue density in the maxillary sinus or an air fluid level (blood). Computed tomographic scans also are helpful and may be considered mandatory.

Treatment of fractures may be delayed up to 2 weeks. Watchful waiting has avoided unnecessary surgery by allowing the edema to decrease. Indications for orbital blowout repair include persistent diplopia in a functional field of gaze, enophthalmos greater than 2 mm, and fracture involving more than 50% of the orbital floor.

K. Retrobulbar Hematoma

A retrobulbar hematoma requires immediate treatment by an ophthalmologist. The resulting increased pressure within the orbit compromises the blood supply to the retina and optic nerve, resulting in blindness if not treated. If possible, the head should be elevated and no direct pressure placed on the eye.

L. Fat Emboli

Patients with long-bone fractures are at risk for fat emboli. Remember, this is a possible cause of a sudden change in vision for a patient who has sustained multiple injuries.

OCULAR TRAUMA

IV. SUMMARY

Thorough, systematic evaluation of the injured eye results in few significant injuries being missed. Once the injuries have been identified, treat the eye injury using simple, systematic measures, prevent further damage, and help preserve sight until the patient is in the ophthalmologist's care.

■ BIBLIOGRAPHY

1. Arbour JD, Brunette I, Boisjoly HM, et al: Should we patch corneal erosions? **Archives of Ophthalomology** 1997; 115(3):313–317.

2. Campanile TM, St Clair DA, Benaim M: The evaluation of eye patching in the treatment of traumatic corneal epithelial defects. **Journal of Emergency Medicine** 1997; 15(6):769–774.

3. Flynn CA, D'Amico F, Smith G: Should we patch corneal abrasions? A meta-analysis. **Journal of Family Practice** 1998; 47(4):264–270.

4. Hart A, White S, Conboy P, et al: The management of corneal abrasions in accident and emergency. **Injury** 1997; 28(8):527–529.

5. Mead MD: Evaluation and initial management of patients with ocular and adnexal trauma. In: Albert DM, Jakobiec FA (eds): **Principles and Practice of Ophthalmology.** Philadelphia, WB Saunders, 1994.

6. Patterson J, Fetzer D, Krall J, et al: Eye patch treatment for the pain of corneal abrasion. **Southern Medical Journal** 1996; 89(2):227–229.

7. Poon A, McCluskey PJ, Hill DA: Eye injuries in patients with major trauma. **Journal of Trauma** 1999; 46:494–499.

8. Sastry SM, Paul BK, Bain L, Champion HR: Ocular trauma among major trauma victims in a regional trauma center. **Journal of Trauma** 1993; 34:223–226.

9. Sternberg P: Trauma: principles and techniques of treatment. In: Ryan SJ (ed): **Retina, 2nd edition.** St. Louis, Mosby, 1994.

10. Tasman WS: Posterior vitreous detachment and peripheral retinal breaks. **Transactions — American Academy of Ophthalmology and Otolaryngology** 1968; 72:217.

APPENDIX

Injury Care in Austere and Hostile Environments
(Optional Lecture)

■ **OBJECTIVES:**

Upon completion of this session, the participant will be able to:

A. Define the austere and hostile environments.

B. Adapt ATLS standards for use in the austere and hostile environments.

C. Identify available resources and treatment options.

D. Apply the ABCDEs.

INJURY CARE IN AUSTERE AND HOSTILE ENVIRONMENTS

I. INTRODUCTION

Even the largest hospital or medical center can become an austere environment after natural or man-made disasters. During a war or after terrorist attack with chemical, biologic, or nuclear weapons, the environment may be both austere and hostile. In a hostile environment, the safety of the patients, medical care providers, and even the medical facility is threatened, and provision must be made to protect them. How do doctors support the ABCDEs of Airway, Breathing, and Circulation in such situations? The goal of this chapter is to discuss how and when to depart from the use of standard equipment and supplies and apply the principles of ATLS in austere and hostile environments.

II. BACKGROUND

Many countries of the world are able to commit significant resources to health care, including the care of the injured patient. The ATLS Course is written with such well-equipped and staffed hospital facilities in mind. However, not all the equipment for diagnostic testing and supplies mentioned are available to all doctors. Some countries and regions have few resources to devote to health care. The doctors who practice in these countries include local nationals, missionaries, military personnel, and members of charitable and relief organizations, eg, the International Red Cross. Remote and wilderness areas in any country are austere and may have hostile climates.

Some areas are thrust into austerity or become hostile environments from the destruction of their infrastructures by disasters, either natural or man-made (eg, terrorist actions or war). These situations are particularly challenging due to their unpredictability. Citizens of large countries with strong militaries should not believe themselves immune and fail to prepare.

III. AUSTERE/HOSTILE ENVIRONMENTS: COMPARISON WITH THE STANDARD

The ATLS Course focuses on treatment priorities of trauma patient care in a hospital environment. The austere or hostile environment is different for several reasons. Frequently, there is limited availability of specialty care. Because of this, the care provider may not be able to request specialty consultation, such as surgery. The care provider may not be able

to arrange for transport of the patient in certain circumstances. Additionally, there is blurring of subspecialty boundaries; the surgeon (or rarely non-surgeon) may be called upon to perform procedures typically performed by other specialties.

Limitations on what should be performed medically are different in austere or hostile environments. For example, frostbite should not be treated if the individual cannot subsequently be kept warm, because the risk of refreezing can cause more injury than simply leaving the part frozen for a longer period. The availability of supplies relative to the number of casualties may make it inadvisable to start an IV in every injured patient.

The austere or hostile environment has limited equipment resources. Even community hospital emergency departments are very well-supplied when compared with most out-of-hospital settings. Doctors need to understand that equipment that is either outdated, suboptimal, or intended for other uses can be used to save lives.

Personnel limitations are a key factor in the austere or hostile environment. Specialty and surgical care may not be available. Available care providers may be poorly trained or may be inadequate in terms of numbers to meet the current demand.

Definitive care is not usually possible in the austere or hostile environment. Diagnostic challenges include management of possible fractures without radiology support and blood pressure determination in the absence of blood pressure cuffs. Operative considerations in the austere or hostile environment include deciding which operating room procedures can be performed outside of the operating room under less than ideal circumstances versus which operative procedures should never be performed outside the operating room. Pharmacologic support may be minimal or nonexistent. The clinician must know how to make optimal use of a limited number of medications.

Military environments are the most hostile and austere. Hospitals of various sizes at sequential echelons of care may all become austere environments, depending on the number of casualties received within a certain time period. Today, Forward Surgical Teams (FST) are increasingly being used to provide surgical skills closer to where casualties are generated. Special operations units are by their nature austere in regard to medical support and

INJURY CARE IN AUSTERE AND HOSTILE ENVIRONMENTS

supplies, and also may be in the most hostile areas. Covert operations requiring medical decision making are the most challenging of all.

Although the military environments may be the most challenging, civilian austere or hostile environments are more likely to be encountered by the majority of doctors. A hostile act, eg, chemical terrorist incident, may contaminate medical facilities and health care personnel and rapidly can make even the largest hospital an austere environment.

Remote areas have problems that are unique. Identification of the occurrence of injury is a significant problem in remote areas. For this reason, highway call boxes are in place in many states and proposals have been made to fit road vehicles with emergency locator transmitters similar to those in airplanes. Additionally, the burden of rural and remote areas includes the problems that time and distance generate.

Wilderness activities such as hiking/biking, spelunking, and water sports create a special challenge for the medical care provider as the bulk and weight of medical supplies becomes a tremendous issue. When supplies must be carried by backpack, thoughtful selection of medications and provisions is required. These also are the activities that may result in the most challenging evacuation because of the difficulty of contacting help.

Natural disasters (eg, hurricanes, tornadoes, and floods) and man-made disasters (eg, terrorism, war/armed conflicts, and industrial accidents/chemical spills) can rapidly turn a nonaustere environment into an austere environment. Even doctors working in tertiary care centers should have training and knowledge of trauma care under these circumstances.

IV. PREPARATION AND PLANNING

Successful trauma care in the austere and hostile environments comes from careful preparation and planning.

A. Travel to an Austere or Hostile Environment

Doctors traveling to such an austere or hostile environment must first prepare for self-protection and survival, or they may become a burden rather than a help in the situation. Good physical health and fitness is a prerequisite. Appropriate shelter, clothing,

food, and water must be planned for, and, in many cases, brought with the individual. It cannot be assumed that such supplies are available. Careful pre-travel communication with the local authorities and an advance party must be accomplished.

Communication between members of the party, local and international authorities, and with the home base must be planned. Planning for the care of loved ones and the medical practice left behind includes wills, powers of attorney, and access to funds to pay bills.

Administrative preparations include passports, visas, local currency, and transportation. It is important to have an invitation by local authorities to enter either the country or austere/hostile environment—unwanted and unprepared volunteers only place a burden on the local system.

Personal health protection includes vaccinations, appropriate personal prescriptions, and over-the-counter medications.

B. Preparation of a Hospital for Becoming an Austere or Hostile Environment

Preparation of a hospital for disaster requires a city- or region-wide plan that includes communications with fire and rescue personnel, police, and civil and military authorities. Such a plan includes how and when to involve each of these authorities, and clearly delineates a chain of command as well as who is in charge. These plans determine how patients are sorted and routed to the appropriate hospital to avoid overwhelming any one institution.

An assessment of the threats is important. Those in the tropics may need to consider typhoons and volcanoes, while those in other regions may need to prepare for earthquakes. Terrorist threats are not predictable. The hospital needs to have a plan to recall key personnel and a personnel rotation plan to allow them to get some rest if the situation is prolonged.

Spare equipment and supplies need to be stored in protected areas in the event regular equipment and supplies are destroyed or contaminated. Plans need to include options for loss of electric power, water, steam sterilization ventilators, intensive care unit(s), etc.

Terrorist activities, industrial accidents, and war may contaminate the patients and facilities with

INJURY CARE IN AUSTERE AND HOSTILE ENVIRONMENTS

toxic chemical or biologic agents. A detailed discussion of these agents and specific protections and treatments are outside the scope of this chapter. However, the doctor must become familiar with the symptoms, signs, and treatment of these conditions.

Plans must include decontamination of patients prior to their being brought into the health care facility so that the health care workers do not become secondary casualties, and thus unable to help. Protective clothing and respiratory protection must be available. Detection equipment for various threat agents must be available, and caregivers must be familiar with the use of these items. Finally, the plan must be exercised as a "full-dress" rehearsal on a regular basis.

V. MANAGEMENT OF AIRWAY AND BREATHING (See Chapter 2, Airway and Ventilatory Management)

The procedures needed to treat problems in "A" and "B" may vary substantially in an austere environment. The problems facing treatment in this type of environment center primarily on the environment itself, the limited equipment that is usually available, and the evacuation constraints. If the patient is threatened with further injury due to environmental concerns, eg, rough terrain, preventing further injury to the patient and to the health care provider takes priority. Once the site is secure or the patient is moved to a safe location, then the doctor can attempt to aid the victim.

A. Airway

Discerning the patient's true airway status may be difficult. The "look, listen, and feel" approach remains important. However, under conditions of low light, high noise levels, etc., airway problem recognition may not be easy. It requires close attention, patience, and ingenuity to fully evaluate the patient. Feeling chest or abdominal movements may become the primary means of assessing airway patency and breathing efforts.

1. Airway Maintenance Techniques

Management of the compromised airway is usually performed in a standard fashion in the austere environment. However, because of limited equipment or personnel, other issues or mechanisms may become important. Foremost is the

decision to initiate treatment. If the patient with a compromised airway can be treated rapidly, and maintaining that airway does not risk the safety of others in the group, then the standard techniques remain unchanged.

Associated with initial airway management is protection of the cervical spine. Cervical collars and other devices normally used to protect the c-spine during transport and evaluation are sometimes not available. Ingenuity again is essential to protecting the neck. Common examples of stabilizing the neck include the use of blankets, pillows, shoes, sandbags, malleable splints, padded hip belts, etc.

a. Chin lift/jaw thrust

Performance of these maneuvers remains unchanged in the austere environment. A temporary means of lifting the tongue off the posterior pharynx can be performed by attaching the anterior tongue to the lower lip or chin with safety pins or sutures. Alternatively, the pins can be held forward with string attached to the patient's clothing. Placing the pins transversely through the tongue will keep them from pulling through.

b. Oral/nasopharyngeal airway

The use of these devices remains important. If placement of one of these airways relieves the airway obstruction, then it must be well-secured prior to evacuation. If ventilation must be assisted with a face mask, then the patient ties up additional valuable personnel resources prior to and during evacuation. When equipment is not available, a nasal airway can be made with a urinary catheter, radiator hose, or other small tube.

c. Laryngeal mask airway (LMA)

The laryngeal mask is an airway designed to be placed blindly into the posterior pharynx with its final position resting over the epiglottis. It should be viewed as an interim airway between the oral/nasopharyngeal airways and the endotracheal tube (ETT). Additionally, the modified LMA can be used as a conduit through which an ETT can be placed.

The LMA is viewed as an alternative to the face mask to establish and maintain control of the patient's airway, but it is not a substitute for an ETT. It establishes an airway in unconscious patients without a gag reflex, but because it does not totally occlude the tracheal inlet, it cannot reliably prevent aspiration. It can be inserted from virtually any position using 1 hand. As it is inserted blindly, the patient's head and neck are maintained in a neutral position.

d. Multilumen esophageal airway devices

These tubes contain 2 cuffs and 2 airway ports. They differ from the esophageal obturator airway in that lung insufflation does not require the use of a face mask and all of its inherent problems and difficulties. Use of these tubes requires minimal skill and equipment. As with the LMA, they can be inserted rapidly and blindly with minimal cervical spine manipulation. Ventilation does not require a seal of the face mask. Their design allows adequate ventilation regardless of whether the distal tube and cuff are in the esophagus or the trachea.

2. Definitive Airway

The definition of a definitive airway remains unchanged in the austere environment—a cuffed tube in the trachea. Endotracheal intubation with an ET tube and laryngoscope remain the gold standard to which all other airways' effectiveness is compared. However, under austere conditions, the environment or lack of required equipment may prevent the performance of standard endotracheal intubation.

a. Tactile/digital orotracheal intubation

This technique is potentially useful in a difficult environment. The procedure requires minimal equipment, is not hindered by blood or secretions, is performed blindly, and does not require manipulation of the c-spine. Once learned, it can be performed rapidly to obtain a secure, definitive airway. However, it does not provide visualization of the laryngeal cords and exposes the doctor to body fluids. Additionally, precautions must be made to protect the operator's hand from the patient's teeth. To perform this procedure, the patient must be unconscious.

b. Surgical airway

Inability to obtain an airway using any of the previously mentioned techniques is the main indication for a surgical airway. The operator's training to perform the procedure and the availability of necessary equipment may preclude this technique from being performed rapidly and safely.

1) Jet insufflation of the airway

Entering the cricothyroid membrane with a large-caliber intravenous catheter and insufflating the lung with pressurized oxygen is quick and easy. However, it requires an oxygen source. If the equipment is available, this technique can provide up to 45 minutes of oxygenation until a more stable airway can be established.

2) Surgical cricothyroidotomy

The procedure and its advantages and disadvantages are outlined in Chapter 2, Airway and Ventilatory Management, Skills Station III, Cricothyroidotomy. In the absence of an ET tube, an airway can be made from a syringe barrel, flashlight or pen casings, or other small diameter tubes.

3) Percutaneous puncture/dilation techniques

This technique uses 1 of several products on the market to penetrate the cricothyroid membrane. The opening in the cricothyroid membrane is dilated in a manner similar to the Seldinger technique to allow placement of the ET tube. It is performed in a manner similar to needle cricothyroidotomy for jet insufflation, yet permits a standard cuffed tube to be placed in the trachea. It does require special equipment and more time to perform, and has all of the inherent complications of other surgical airways.

B. Ventilation and Oxygenation

After an airway is established, sufficient oxygenation and ventilation must be supported. The challenges in the austere environment focus on the equipment needed to support the failing respiratory system and the number of personnel required to assist the patient. Because supplemental oxygen usually is not available, the ability to support a patient

INJURY CARE IN AUSTERE AND HOSTILE ENVIRONMENTS

with oxygen remains very difficult in an austere environment.

When oxygen is only available in limited amounts, it should be reserved for those with evidence of hypoxia on physical exam, by pulse oximetry readings, or blood gas analysis. Patients most likely to require the additional oxygen acutely are those with chest injuries associated with lung contusion.

Initiating ventilation in the austere environment commits personnel and resources to the patient. Maintaining the airway in these environments and during transport requires close vigilance because of the risk of the airway device becoming dislodged. Monitoring includes ensuring a secure, patent airway and adequate ventilation. Ideally, monitoring includes pulse oximetry and end tidal CO_2, if available.

C. Chest Injuries

Chest injury in an austere environment should be handled as discussed in Chapter 4, Thoracic Trauma. However, not all materials necessary to manage a chest wound may be available. Open chest wounds must be covered, but in the absence of a chest tube, an occlusive dressing using plastic bags, IV fluid bags, etc, can be used. Such ancillary devices are taped on 3 sides to prevent a tension pneumothorax.

Needle decompression of a tension pneumothorax is performed as described previously. (See Chapter 4, Thoracic Trauma, Skills Station VII, Chest Trauma Management.) However, a tube other than a large-caliber IV catheter may have to be improvised. The decompression ideally is performed with an over-the-needle catheter with the catheter left in place to prevent recurrence. A Heimlich valve can be attached to the catheter. If a Heimlich valve is not available, one can be improvised with a finger from a glove attached to the tube with a hole at the fingertip. This simulates the flutter valve of a Heimlich valve.

If air evacuation is planned, the effects of altitude, temperature, and other factors associated with flight must be considered. For airway management, endotracheal cuff pressures increase. If a manometer is not available for the flight, then the cuffs are filled with a nonexpanding liquid (water or saline) rather than air. Similarly, a pneumothorax also expands at altitude with the potential for unexpected respira-

tory compromise. Ideally supplemental oxygen should be made available due to the decreased partial pressure of oxygen at altitude. Finally, gastric distention can easily occur, and gastric tube placement should be considered.

VI. MANAGEMENT OF CIRCULATION

The tools and supplies used to treat injured patients become less plentiful as the environment becomes more austere. Nowhere is this more obvious than in management of hypovolemic shock. Fluids (crystalloid, colloid, and blood) that are the mainstay of restoring circulating volume are very bulky and heavy. They are usually found in only minimal amounts in most field kits, and are quickly used up in disasters.

While the presence of shock in the injured patient demands the immediate involvement of a surgeon, one may not be available, or the surgeon's skills may be negated without appropriate surgical equipment, anesthesia, and support personnel. The goal under such circumstances is to maintain life until a higher level of care can be delivered.

Successful treatment of hypovolemic shock under these conditions requires a thorough understanding of the compensatory mechanisms of the body. While the goals of resuscitation are unchanged, emphasis may shift in the austere environment. Less than ideal organ perfusion may have to be accepted. "Life-over-limb" and triage decisions assume a central role in saving as many lives as possible.

A. Hemostasis

Control of bleeding is of utmost importance when there is minimal or no fluid with which to replace the lost blood. Direct pressure remains important and may be augmented with the compression of the artery above the bleeding site at a pressure point. These points are where arteries pass superficially and are felt as pulses. Compression of the artery for 20 minutes may stop or decrease the bleeding sufficiently to allow a dressing to be placed. These pressure points are the radial, brachial, and axillary arteries in the arm; and the femoral, popliteal, and ankle arteries in the leg.

Elevation of the bleeding area above the level of the heart reduces the pressure to the bleeding area and aids hemostasis for arterial bleeding. Elevation and a dressing may be all that are necessary for venous

INJURY CARE IN AUSTERE AND HOSTILE ENVIRONMENTS

bleeding. The patient or another individual may be enlisted to hold pressure, while the doctor treats someone else. In the worst cases, tourniquets are used. While there is a real risk of limb loss with a tourniquet, blood loss must be stopped to save the life of the patient. Any flexible material of enough length (rope, wire, cloth strips) can be used to encircle the limb and be tied in place. A rigid device (eg, rod or stick) is placed through the loop and twisted to tighten it until bleeding ceases. Arterial flow to, as well as venous flow from, the extremity must be stopped to prevent paradoxically increased bleeding from venous injuries. Time of tourniquet application should be recorded and accompany the patient.

A technique that stops vigorous scalp bleeding from a large flap is to fold the flap outward onto itself. This crimps the vessels and stops the bleeding. After 20 minutes the bleeding should be stopped or slowed enough to return the flap to its normal position and apply direct pressure and dressings. Prior to surgical management, endogenous hemostatic mechanisms must be relied on to control unseen bleeding.

With the possibility of ongoing or barely clotted bleeding sites, rapid restoration of normal blood pressure with a vigorous fluid bolus should be avoided. Smaller amounts of fluid given more slowly and turned off when the blood pressure rises to an acceptable, yet less than normal level, may allow the clot to be maintained and still provide adequate organ perfusion.

B. Resuscitation

1. Venous access

Central venous access kits, intravenous needles, and intraosseous needles may be unavailable in the austere/hostile environment. Performing venous cutdown assumes a larger role in the austere/hostile situation. Fluid administration tubing, with the connectors cut off, nasogastric tubes, and urinary catheters may be used for venous access with a cutdown.

2. Alternate fluid routes

Although oral fluids are avoided in the usual clinical arena because of the possibility of aspiration, fluids may be administered orally to the awake patient, or via a gastric tube in the unconscious patient. Absorption may be decreased after in-jury, but it does occur, nonetheless. Similarly, rectal clysis allows excellent fluid absorption, as demonstrated during World War I. Only about 250 mL/hour can be absorbed safely by either of these routes, so they are most useful for dehydrated patients, rather than massive resuscitation.

Patients that do not partially stabilize with their own mechanisms or who do not respond to some fluid using these alternate methods are unlikely to respond to large amounts of fluid. This might be used as a triage consideration, and such patients may become expectant.

3. Fluid choices

The fluids used are those that are available. Usually this is crystalloid or colloid fluid. Blood transfusion can be considered from noninjured members of the group. Typing can be by patient report of blood type. Quick "crossing" of drops of blood from the patient and the donor on a smooth white surface may reveal major incompatibilities. Careful consideration of the goals of fluid therapy is necessary in planning the use of a limited quantity of fluids. Patients that seem to be compensating their fluid losses and maintaining organ perfusion may require no fluids. Units of fluid (bags, bottles, etc) can be split between several patients, giving only that amount absolutely necessary to maintain life. Local fluids such as commercial beverages may be used as oral rehydration fluids. When balancing rebleeding with organ perfusion, careful reevaluation is key to whether further small amounts of fluid are given to maintain the low level of perfusion as necessary to maintain life until definitive care is possible.

VII. PAIN MANAGEMENT

Control of pain and alleviation of suffering is a primary goal of all doctors. This is important not only as a kindness, but also to minimize the adverse physiologic consequences of pain. These include increased levels of catecholamines and cortisol, increased metabolic rate, and increased total body oxygen consumption. Management of pain in hospitals is facilitated not only through availability of many different analgesic agents and cardiovascular monitoring, but also through availability of anesthesiologists who are knowledgeable and helpful regarding pain management. Austere circumstances require alternatives to hospital-based pain management protocols.

INJURY CARE IN AUSTERE AND HOSTILE ENVIRONMENTS

Pain management is a challenge in austere military circumstances. This is due to limitations in numbers and types of personnel, equipment/drugs, and the potential for even a few casualties to overwhelm existing resources. The doctors in these locations should be familiar with all uses of the agents they have available. Civilian remote and wilderness situations provide similar challenges to relieving the patient's pain. A wide spectrum of therapeutic agents is not always available to the doctor in these venues. Agents must be selected with care, not only for ability to relieve pain but also with consideration for safety.

Principles of pain management in the austere environment include (1) type of environment; (2) available options; (3) anatomic location and severity of injury; (4) possibility of complications; (5) allergies; (6) associated injuries; and (7) availability, timing, and plan for evacuation. The choice of a drug or multiple drugs depends on many factors. Many different agents are available to relieve pain or act as adjuncts.

Patients in a low-flow state secondary to hypovolemic shock should not be given intramuscular injections of narcotics. These drugs may remain in the muscle until flow is restored. With restoration of flow, a bolus of drug is released, putting the patient at risk for respiratory depression. However, in the austere environment, with inadequate supply of IV catheters, it may be necessary to consider intramuscular use of narcotics. Oral use is reasonable in the absence of abdominal and head injury.

Local anesthetics are considered for hematoma blocks associated with fractures or regional blocks if the doctor is knowledgeable of the sites of injection and allowable doses. Remember, local anesthetics can cause seizures if too high a dosage is utilized. Epinephrine can be added to slow absorption and thereby decrease the likelihood of toxicity. A caveat is to not add epinephrine if the injection is used in fingers, toes, penis, or nose because of ischemic risk in these areas with arteriolae. Another point to remember is that the nonsteroidal antiinflammatory medications all inhibit platelet function, so they must be avoided if there is hemorrhage or an injury with significant risk of severe hemorrhage.

Ketamine, a dissociative anesthetic, can be used safely either intramuscularly or intravenously. It has an effect similar to general anesthetics in that the patient is unaware of his/her surroundings. Attention must be directed to keeping the airway free of secretions. Although ketamine is useful for suture repair of lacerations and setting of fractures with angulation or arterial compromise, the individual will not be able to function without assistance for 1 to 2 hours, making it necessary to carry the patient if evacuation is imminent. Other agents allow the patient to assist in his/her own transportation, injuries allowing.

VIII. MANAGEMENT OF SPECIFIC INJURIES

A. Abdomen

The evaluation and management of abdominal injury in the austere setting is very different from what is practiced in the well-equipped modern hospital. The mortality of untreated intraabdominal injury is high: patients either die quickly from uncontrolled hemorrhage or they die later from intraabdominal sepsis. For this reason, a high index of suspicion must be maintained in these patients. Those with suspected injury must be referred early for surgical consultation or evacuation. Sophisticated diagnostic techniques such as ultrasound and computed tomography (CT) are not available in the austere setting. Diagnostic peritoneal lavage (DPL), while potentially available, has very different indications and implications in this setting.

The actual mechanism of injury becomes paramount in establishing priorities in the limited resources setting. Gunshot wounds to the abdomen, unless clearly tangential, are associated with visceral injury in 90% of patients. These patients all require rapid surgical referral and celiotomy. Civilian stab wounds to the abdomen are associated with visceral injury in only 30% to 40% of the patients. Unless clear evidence of intraabdominal injury (eg, evisceration, pneumoperitoneum, peritoneal findings, shock, or blood in the nasogastric tube or rectum) is present, these patients are treated based on symptoms and wound exploration. Stab wounds usually can be explored under local anesthesia without much difficulty to see if the abdominal wall fascia is penetrated. If there is no fascial penetration or abdominal symptoms, the wound can be managed primarily.

Blunt injury to the abdomen is associated with a variety of solid and hollow organ injuries and may be less dramatic in appearance than penetrating injury. Abdominal pain, tenderness, distension, shock, or blood in the nasogastric tube or urinary catheter are all suggestive of blunt intraabdominal injury. Although CT and ultrasound are not available in the austere setting, DPL can serve as a field-expedient substitute.

DPL is accomplished with a minimum of resources and time, and is a reliable means to determine if a significant hemoperitoneum exists. If gross blood is not encountered and newsprint-sized writing can be read through IV tubing containing the lavage fluid, the DPL is negative for significant intraperitoneal bleeding. DPL is limited in that it does not provide any information about extraperitoneal organs and structures. It is contraindicated in patients with obvious intraabdominal injury and is only indicated in patients with a high probability of intraabdominal injury. Many of these patients eventually require celiotomy because of continued bleeding or peritonitis. DPL might help to identify these patients earlier and assist in triage if evacuation is possible.

In situations where evacuation is impossible or is significantly delayed, DPL has no role. If a significant intraabdominal injury exists, it becomes quite apparent with time. In this setting, DPL adds nothing to physical examination or treatment.

Patients with a definite abdominal injury (evisceration, shock, peritoneal findings, and pneumoperitoneum) are expeditiously referred for surgical management. They should receive a broad spectrum antibiotic and sufficient intravenous fluids to maintain urinary output. Open wounds should be cleaned of gross contamination and dressed. Eviscerations should be covered with moist gauze or dressings and the patient kept warm. If wounds are massive, resources are minimal, and evacuation unlikely, these patients are given comfort measures only and treated expectantly.

Every patient with a significant history of injury should be considered to have an intraabdominal injury until it is proven otherwise by clinical exam, diagnostic test, or celiotomy.

B. Extremities

Extremity injury is common in patients suffering trauma. While these injuries are not usually immediately life threatening, they are often dramatic in appearance and may divert attention from other injuries. A brief history of the injury and pertinent

past history should be followed by a complete examination of the extremity.

The management of extremity injuries depends to a great extent upon the available resources and the length of time it takes to transfer the patient to a definitive care facility. Vascular injuries, if the patient does not exsanguinate, must be definitively repaired early, within 6 hours of injury, to preserve limb function. Likewise, because of the risk of arterial injury and osteonecrosis, major dislocations should be reduced early. Finally, traumatic amputations usually require early surgical debridement.

The immediate treatment of extremity injury should include, at a minimum, control of active bleeding by application of direct pressure, cleaning grossly contaminated wounds, and immobilizing the injured extremity until the patient is evacuated. Use tourniquets sparingly, if ever, since they place the entire limb at risk. Dislocations and major angulation deformities should be carefully reduced, while monitoring the limb's neurovascular status before and after reduction.

If definitive treatment is delayed, administer antibiotics to the patient, perform limited irrigation and debridement of open wounds, and keep the extremity immobilized with some type of splint or cast. Patients with femur fractures should be put into some sort of traction to minimize further blood loss into the thigh.

Splints and traction devices can be improvised from equipment and resources at the scene. Any rigid item, if properly padded, can be used as a splint. Likewise, a makeshift frame can be constructed to provide traction to femur fractures, sometimes using the patient's own boot or shoe as the ankle hitch. These patients also should receive analgesics and sufficient hydration to prevent shock, if available.

Compartment syndrome, a late complication of extremity injury, can present insidiously in the injured patient especially after crush injury, where no fracture is present. If compartment pressures cannot be measured, early fasciotomy may be indicated, especially in the presence of any vascular injury.

Other late complications of extremity injuries include fat embolus syndrome, deep venous thrombosis, and osteomyelitis. These complications must be considered if transfer to definitive care is markedly delayed.

INJURY CARE IN AUSTERE AND HOSTILE ENVIRONMENTS

The management of pelvic fractures in the austere setting deserves some comment. Since the force required to fracture the pelvic ring is so great, pelvic fractures usually occur in association with intraabdominal or other injuries. These patients may go into shock from bleeding from the pelvic fracture itself and from both arterial and venous vessels in the pelvis. Patients also may have significant neurologic injury, as well as genitourinary or rectal injury.

Very little can be done in the austere environment except immobilization of the lower extremities and pelvis. A pneumatic antishock garment, if available, can be placed and inflated. If this device is not available, the patient should be kept immobilized and the pelvis stabilized as well as possible with sheets, sandbags, etc. If available, external fixation can be performed to reduce open-book pelvic fractures and help minimize bleeding.

Patients with musculoskeletal injuries are classified according to the severity of their injury and the need for orthopaedic evaluation and treatment. Patients with vascular injury and dislocations require urgent referral or evacuation, as do patients with significant pelvic fractures or suspected cervical or thoracolumbar spinal injuries. Patients with stable open or closed fractures also require referral or evacuation, though less urgently. If referral or evacuation is delayed (>6 hours), these patients should receive antibiotics, analgesia, hydration, immobilization, and wound management as resources allow. Patients with sprains and minor injuries can either be treated primarily or referred to orthopaedics in a more routine fashion.

C. Burn Injury

The mortality of major burn injuries is significant, even with unlimited resources. Burn-injury patients often require airway support, mechanical ventilation, and massive fluid resuscitation, in addition to management of their burn wounds. The initial evaluation and management of these patients follows closely the ABCDE algorithm. Remember, these patients often have other injuries in addition to their burn injury (eg, blast injury, injury from jumping in an attempt to get away from the fire).

Inhalation injury, either from heat or breathing toxic gases emitted during combustion, essentially doubles the mortality of burn injury. Patients with significant facial burns and smoke or steam inhalation, as well as those with toxic gas inhalation from burning plastics, require a definitive airway (ie, endotracheal intubation or tracheostomy) and mechanical ventilation. Probably the most impressive facet of the care of burn patients is the massive fluid replacement these patients require. They require urgent evacuation to a burn center; otherwise, they can quickly overwhelm even a well-equipped hospital. Under austere conditions, patients with severe burns may need to be treated expectantly.

The initial treatment of patients with smaller burns can be initiated in the austere setting by preventing further injury, limited debridement to ruptured blisters only, initiating fluid resuscitation (orally if necessary), preventing hypothermia, and application of topical antibiotics and sterile dressings. If circumferential burns are present, distal circulation and the need for escharotomy should be assessed. If local resources are limited but evacuation is possible, even if delayed, the patient with a significant burn should be stabilized as much as possible prior to transport. The airway should be secure and fluid resuscitation begun, if possible. If resources are limited and evacuation is difficult or impossible, small (<5%) burns often heal with nonoperative care, though not always without significant scarring or loss of function, especially if over joints.

IX. PREPARATION FOR TRANSPORT

The purpose of this discussion is to highlight principles applicable to preparation of the injured for evacuation from isolated circumstances where resources are limited: military operations, wilderness environment, or during civil disasters with delayed rescue. It may be necessary to provide care for hours to days in proximity to dangers, eg, fire from hostile weapons, persistently threatening weather, and imminent flood.

Under these circumstances, the first priority is to protect the caregivers and the patient from further injury. Generally, a minimum of medical care is attempted while the injured patient(s) and caregiver are exposed to danger. Once the danger has been mitigated, care of the injured may commence to the fullest extent possible, given limitations inherent in the circumstances, while applying ATLS principles with some modifications. The skills required are similar to those used by a military medic or corpsman in the field once the caregiver and the patient are no longer under hostile fire.

INJURY CARE IN AUSTERE AND HOSTILE ENVIRONMENTS

The odds of successful rescue/evacuation, if needed, increase dramatically when plans are made in advance for such contingencies. Initiating rescue and communicating with rescuers is beyond the scope of this discussion. However, it is essential that provisions be considered for establishing communications with or signaling rescuers. This requires a plan for rescue, which requires notification of individuals not involved in the movement or plan of action. A flight, float, or expedition plan should be filed with individuals who can initiate rescue, automatically and autonomously under certain conditions. It is easy to understand why emergency extraction and rescue plans are an essential part of any military operation.

Flexibility and improvisation while waiting for evacuation from isolation are important to a successful outcome. Seeking appropriate shelter until evacuation is possible is an early priority. Shelters of opportunity should be sought as soon as the patient and caregiver are out of immediate danger. High ground is generally preferable if the patient can be moved. Simple shelters of various types can be constructed from available materials with a minimum number of simple tools.

Utilize these principles while waiting to transport the patient(s).

- Move the patient as little as possible after shelter is achieved.
- Initiate appropriate medical interventions as soon as feasible, based on the available resources and the patient's injuries.
- Arrange for a stretcher or litter for the severely injured or unconscious patient while providing extra padding to pressure points.
- Generally, place the patient in a supine position.
- Place the patient with a thoracic injury in a lateral decubitus position with the injured side down or in a semielevated position (head and chest elevated at approximately 45°).
- Splint the patient's fractures with available materials or with the other extremity.
- Keep the patient as dry as possible and prevent hypothermia.
- Shield the patient from prolonged exposure to intense, direct sunlight.
- Do not leave unattended patients close to campfires.

If helicopter evacuation is a possibility, scout a landing site to facilitate rescue. The landing site should ideally be on level, flat terrain clear of obstructions. It may be necessary to mark the site with smoke, reflectors, or other devices that can be seen from the air (branch or stone pointer). Helicopter extraction also is a possibility, but is much more difficult and riskier to the patient.

X. ENVIRONMENTAL EXTREMES OF HEAT AND COLD

Preventing heat and cold injuries is preferable to treating them. Understanding the effects of environmental extremes on the human body helps to avoid these injuries. Unfortunately, accidental heat and cold injuries still occur despite adequate precautions.

A. Cold Injury and Hypothermia

A high index of suspicion is essential to making the diagnosis of hypothermia. Patients suffering overwhelming environmental exposures (eg, cold water drowning and cold exposure) are readily identified.

- Clothing must provide adequate insulation.
- Adequate shelter must be sought for adequate protection from the environment.
- Food consumption must be adequate for the increased caloric energy requirements.
- Activity level must be at an adequate exercise level to produce the heat required to keep warm.

Preventing hypothermia involves 2 strategies: (1) reducing heat loss and (2) increasing heat production. Heat is lost from the skin in 4 ways: convection, conduction, evaporation, and radiation. In a normal environment, an individual loses 50% to 60% of body heat due to radiation. In contrast, convection is the major source of heat loss in a cold environment, particularly with strong winds. Conduction is a major route of heat loss during cold water immersion. Heat losses from convection and conduction can be effectively reduced with currently available clothing materials.

The amount of heat lost by convection is determined by the temperature difference between the air and the body surface with which it is in contact and by the speed with which the air is moving. A wind of 8 mph (12.8 kph) removes 4 times as much heat as a

INJURY CARE IN AUSTERE AND HOSTILE ENVIRONMENTS

wind of 4 mph (6.4 kph). Windchill charts detail the relationship between the ambient temperature and the effective temperature based upon the prevailing wind speed.

Many different materials are used for cold weather clothing. The oldest is wool and is still one of the best because it has innumerable small air pockets that provide excellent insulation. One of the greatest values of wool is its ability to provide insulation when wet. Its major disadvantage is its weight. Down provides excellent insulation when dry, but provides little protection when it is wet.

Heat production by the body can only be increased significantly by muscular exercise, either shivering or by voluntary work. Large muscles (legs) produce more heat than small muscles. Vigorous exercising can produce more heat than shivering. If a threatening situation cannot be avoided, deliberate exercise that utilizes large muscles, such as repeatedly stepping up onto and off rocks or logs, produces more heat than just standing and shivering. No drugs or other behavior can substitute for exercise as a means of generating body heat.

When cold injury does occur in the austere environment, an important principle is to avoid rewarming until a sustained warm environment can be assured. Clearly, as with systemic cold injury, the best management of local cold injury is prevention.

B. Heat-related Illness or Injury

Heat illness is due to exposure to increased ambient temperature under conditions in which the body is unable to maintain appropriate homeostasis. The milder syndromes are exertional; the most severe may occur without exercise. Three entities are described herein: (1) heat cramps, (2) heat exhaustion, and (3) heat stroke.

1. Heat cramps

Painful muscles after exertion in a hot environment are often attributed to a salt deficit. However, it is likely that many cases represent exertional rhabdomyolysis. Acute muscle injury due to severe exertional effort beyond the limits for which the individual is trained can result in myoglobin-uria. This rarely affects kidney function unless heat stroke is present. Treatment includes rest in a cool environment and salt replacement with a 650-mg sodium chloride tablet in 500 mL of water or a commercially available balanced electrolyte replacement solution.

2. Heat exhaustion

Fatigue, muscular weakness, tachycardia, postural syncope, nausea, vomiting, and an urge to defecate may result from dehydration and heat stress. This occurs in unacclimated individuals exercising in the heat and results from loss of both salt and water. Body temperature is normal. There may be a continuum from heat exhaustion to heat stroke. Treatment consists of rest in a cool environment, acceleration of heat loss by fan evaporation, and fluid repletion with salt-containing solutions. After the patient recovers, exercise in a hot environment should be avoided for 2 to 3 days to avoid recurrence.

3. Heat stroke

Core body temperature exceeds 40°C (104°F) with heat stroke and severe central nervous system dysfunction and anhydrosis occur. Two types of heat stroke are described herein.

a. Classic heat stroke

Classic heat stroke occurs after several days of extreme heat exposure in individuals not acclimated. Risk factors include chronic illness, old age, high humidity, obesity, chronic cardiovascular disease, poverty, alcohol abuse, dehydration, and use of sedatives. Sedentary heat stroke is a disease of the elderly or infirm whose cardiovascular systems are unable to adapt to the hot environmental stress.

b. Exertional heat stroke

Exertional heat stroke occurs rapidly in unacclimatized individuals exercising in conditions of high ambient temperature and humidity. Each year about 4000 persons die in the United States from heat stroke. Exercise-induced heat stroke most often affects young people (eg, athletes, military recruits, and laborers). Individuals with this type of heat stroke are more likely to have disseminated intravascular coagulopathy, lactic acidosis, and rhabdomyolysis.

Therapy for heat stroke is rapid cooling. The most efficient method is to induce evaporative heat loss

INJURY CARE IN AUSTERE AND HOSTILE ENVIRONMENTS

by misting and fan cooling. Immersion in an ice water bath or use of ice packs also is effective but can cause vasoconstriction and shivering which limits cooling and monitoring. Approximately 20 mL/kg of balanced salt solution resuscitation are often required within the first 4 hours. Vigorous cooling should be stopped when the patient's temperature reaches 38.9°C (102°F). If myoglobinuria is present, intravenous mannitol (12.5 g) should be given early.

Bad prognostic signs are body temperatures of 42.2°C (108°F) or more, coma lasting over 2 hours, shock, and hyperkalemia. Mortality rates are about 10%.

As with all thermal environmental injuries, the best treatment for heat stress is prevention. Acclimation to extreme heat requires about 3 to 5 days. Best strategies for activity involve alternating work and rest cycles and emphasis on fluid intake. Water requirements for work in a desert environment at 49°C (120°F) are 2 liters per hour. Availability of shelter with shading from the sun is important.

XI. COMMUNICATIONS AND SIGNALING

The principles of effective communications in the austere environment are:

1. Have a working plan in place beforehand.
2. Know what your communications system can and cannot do.
3. Have a backup communications plan.

Doctor-to-doctor contact with at least a minimum of patient information for referral is the safest way to coordinate patient transfers. Unfortunately, the austere environment may not afford either a doctor or a reliable means of communication. Effective communications rely on a preestablished and tested means of communication, with contingencies for a backup system when the primary means of communication fail. Available technologies include handheld radios, cellular phones, and newer technologies, such as telemedicine. Limitations of a phone system in a disaster setting include destruction of the phone lines, power loss, bad weather, and an increase in phone calls that frequently result in system saturation and overload. Cellular phones should ideally serve as a backup to a VHF radio communication system, which emits a directional signal that could

be pinpointed. In addition, Global Positioning Systems (GPS) are becoming relatively inexpensive and afford the medical care provider the opportunity to identify his/her location in the austere setting with extreme accuracy.

Oral reporting should be efficient and clear, particularly in disaster settings where radio traffic is high. Information relayed should include scene safety, number of patients, and the patients' conditions. Use of a standardized phonetic alphabet and phonetic numerals is preferred. When no direct contact is made with the receiving facility or medical care providers, every effort must be made to provide an accurate record that survives with at least a minimum amount of transfer data, including patient identification, medical problem, treatment provided, and patient status at transfer. Online medical care protocols for nondoctor providers are critically important when direct medical control is not available.

Communications at a disaster site are frequently and severely disrupted. Effective means of communication in this setting may include handheld radios, messengers, and megaphones. Disaster management is a multidisciplinary community activity and effective communication among the disaster responders is best addressed through the Incident Command System (ICS). Military organizations can bring to these sites well-developed communication systems with the ability to communicate worldwide through a secure network. Hospitals are expected to report to their local emergency communications center about their bed availability, number of casualties they have received and are prepared to accept, and items in short supply. Most patients are not likely to access the emergency medical services (EMS) system in a disaster prior to arrival at medical facilities. Communication backup systems may address unique situations such as communication by medical staff while operating in hazardous material suits or a chemical or biologic "protective posture."

In the austere environment, available communications equipment is frequently limited to that which is carried into the field by the participants. In the event the use of electronic equipment is unavailable, the best signaling devices are either audio or visual. A universally recognized distress signal is essentially considered 3 of anything, eg, 3 whistle blasts, 3 gun shots, 3 columns of smoke. An effective ground-to-air device is a mirror reflecting sunlight, which may be seen up to 10 miles (16 km) away.

INJURY CARE IN AUSTERE AND HOSTILE ENVIRONMENTS

Ground signals should be as large as possible and contain straight lines and square corners. An "X" on the ground is the symbol internationally recognized as needing medical assistance. Both day-and night-signaling devices are readily available and include mirrors, smoke, dyes, flashlights, flares, Search and Rescue Transponders (SART), and other pyrotechnic and nonpyrotechnic devices.

XII. TRIAGE

Mass casualty triage is the process of sorting or prioritizing patients into specific care categories depending on the number and severity of casualties and the resources available at that point in time. By definition, there are inadequate resources to care for this number of patients in the usual manner. Triage is the process of prioritizing injured patients to determine which need medical care immediately, which can wait for care, and which are so severely injured that attempts at care are futile given the existing circumstances. The correct concept is to do the greatest good for the greatest number. Triage in the austere environment may be required when there are as few as 2 injured patients, which may easily overwhelm the resources available to a single doctor. A decision must be made regarding which patient should first receive the benefit of the doctor's full attention and application of available resources.

Even large, well-organized medical teams, such as disaster-response teams or military hospitals, may face overwhelming casualties. Preplanning and practice must occur prior to team deployment. Typically, the most experienced surgeon acts as the triage officer. In the event the surgeons are all needed to perform operations, another experienced doctor can act as the triage officer. This individual should have prior training in triage.

In wilderness austere environments, the doctor may not have the benefits of preplanning and must rely on experience. In these circumstances, it is particularly important for care providers to be very familiar with their equipment and supplies in order to do the most good for the largest number of individual patients. Only through knowledge of available resources and understanding of the way to make best use of them can the doctor save the most lives.

It must be recognized that the entire concept of triage is predicated on the fact that not every patient gets immediate attention for his or her most significant injury. In order to do the most good for the largest number of patients, it is critically important to have a basic understanding of triage methods and categories. The first step in a mass casualty event is to "sift" the patients rapidly. This may consist of an order for all patients able to get up and gather at a single, clearly visible site in the immediate area, eg, "Everyone who can, please move to the base of the large tree." This enables the medical care providers to pay immediate attention to the remaining patients. Next, a careful "sieve" of the more severely injured patients occurs. Patients with life-threatening injuries are cared for first, using the ABCDEs. The next priority is patients with limb-threatening or other injuries that are not immediately life-threatening, eg, abdominal injuries without hypotension.

In the austere environment and to do the most good using existing supplies, it may be necessary to make some patients expectant (expected to die). This category of patients are given pain medication, if available, so they do not suffer. Supplies in limited quantity, such as intravenous fluids, should not be used in the care of expectant patients.

Many mass casualty triage classification schemes exist. A simple and useful method of triage involves 4 categories:

1. Immediate (needs treatment of life-threatening injuries)

2. Delayed (can wait 1 to 2 hours or more before treatment)

3. Minimal or ambulatory (can wait many hours for treatment)

4. Expectant or expected to die (given current patient load and resources)

The names and number of triage categories are not as important as the fact that all care providers have an understanding of the system being used. Color-coded triage tags are useful in identifying the category into which a patient is placed (eg, red for immediate, yellow for delayed, green for minimal, and gray for expectant). Patients who are dead need transport to the morgue or other designated area.

Triage of mass casualty victims is not a one-time exercise. Triage may occur at several levels and needs to be both accurate and repetitive. Disaster scene triage may be performed by experienced paramedics initially and then later by an onsite doctor if evacuation of victims is prolonged due to the sheer number of victims or difficulties in extrication or transport to definitive care. It is extremely important

INJURY CARE IN AUSTERE AND HOSTILE ENVIRONMENTS

to understand the need for retriage. Patients who are placed into the expectant category because of lack of resources in a mass casualty scenario may become immediate category patients once operating room resources become available and no further patients are expected to arrive. This is only 1 of many possible scenarios that serves to underscore the need for triage to be continuous rather than discrete.

XIII. SUMMARY

ATLS provides an organized approach to care of the injured patient in an emergency department setting. There are many circumstances which may result in the doctor needing to work outside the normal environment. These include both military and civilian austere and/or hostile environments. These may be either planned (wilderness or military) or unplanned (natural disaster or terrorist attack) austere and hostile environments. Preparation and familiarity with principles of care of the injured patient under austere and hostile circumstances optimize the care provided using limited resources.

■ BIBLIOGRAPHY

1. Adkisson GA, Butler FK, et al. In: **Manual for Pre-Hospital Trauma Life Support,** 2002.

2. Allen RC, McAtee JM (eds): **USAF Special Tactics Medication and Procedure Handbook,** 1997.

3. American College of Surgeons: **Advanced Trauma Life Support Program for Doctors.** Chicago, 1997 and 2002.

4. Bellamy RF: The causes of death in conventional land warfare: Implications for combat casualty care research. **Military Medicine** 1984; 149: 55–62.

5. Bickell WH, Wall MJ, Pepe PE, et al: Immediate versus delayed fluid resuscitation for hypotensive patients with penetrating torso injuries. **New England Journal of Medicine** 1994; 331(17):1105–1109.

6. Bledsoe BE, et al. In: **Paramedic Emergency Care, 2nd Edition.** Englewood Cliffs, NJ, Prentice-Hall, Inc., 1994.

7. Bowen TE, Bellamy RF (eds): **Emergency War Surgery: Second United States Revision of the Emergency War Surgery NATO Handbook.** Washington, DC, United States Government Printing Office, 1988.

8. Bowman WD: Basic patient assessment and life support techniques (Chapter 4), Oxygen and other types of respiratory system support (Chapter 5), and Environmental emergencies (Chapter 18). In: **Outdoor Emergency Care.** National Ski Patrol System, 1993.

9. Bowman WD: Wilderness survival. In: Auerbach P (ed): **Wilderness Medicine.** St. Louis, MO, Mosby-Yearbook, Inc., 1995, p 390.

10. Butler FK Jr, Hagmann J, Butler EG: Tactical combat casualty care in special operations. **Military Medicine** 1996; 161 Suppl:3–16.

11. Calkins MD, Robinson TD: Alternative airway use in the special operations environment: A comparison of laryngeal mask airway and esophageal tracheal combitube to endotracheal tube. **Journal of Trauma** 1999; 46(5):927–932.

12. Casualty Care Research Center, Uniformed Services University of the Health Sciences: Airway management. In: **Operational and Emergency Services Handbook,** 1998.

13. Casualty Care Research Center, Uniformed Services University of the Health Sciences: Care under fire, Part I. In: **Emergency Medical Technician—Tactical Handbook,** 1998, pp 95–120.

14. Cicala RS, Grande CM, Stene JK, et al: Emergency and elective airway management for trauma patients. In: Grande CM (ed): **Textbook of Trauma Anesthesia and Critical Care.** St. Louis, MO, Mosby-Yearbook, Inc., 1993, pp 344–380.

15. Dehart RL: **Fundamentals of Aerospace Medicine.** Philadelphia, Lea & Febiger, 1985.

16. Farmer CJ: Temperature-related injuries. In: Civetta JM, Taylor RW, Kirby RR (eds): **Critical Care, 2nd Edition.** Philadelphia, JB Lippincott, 1992, p 899.

17. Gentile DA, Morris JA, Schimelpfenig T, et al: Wilderness injuries and illnesses. **Annals of Emergency Medicine** 1992; 21(7):853–861.

18. Kaweski SM, Sise MJ, Virgilio RW: The effect of prehospital fluids on survival in trauma patients. **Journal of Trauma** 1990; 30:1215–1218.

19. Lumley JSP, Ryan JM, Baxter PJ, et al: **Handbook of the Medical Care of Catastrophes.** London, The Royal Society of Medicine Press, Ltd., 1996.

INJURY CARE IN AUSTERE AND HOSTILE ENVIRONMENTS

20. Marohn MR: Hypothermia in the intensive care unit. In: Marohn ML, Muldoon SM (eds): **Problems in Anesthesia.** Philadelphia, JB Lippincott, 1994, pp 23–43.

21. Martin RR, Bickell WH, Pepe PE, et al: Prospective evaluation of preoperative fluid resuscitation in hypotensive patients with penetrating truncal injury: A preliminary report. **Journal of Trauma** 1992; 33:354–361.

22. Moss JF, Haklin M, Southwick HW, et al: A model for treatment of accidental severe hypothermia. **Journal of Trauma** 1986; 26(1):68–74.

23. Rosemurgy AS, Norris PA, Olson SM, et al: Prehospital traumatic cardiac arrest: The cost of futility. **Journal of Trauma** 1993; 35(3):468–473, discussion 473–474.

24. Sharp TW, Yip R, Malone JD, et al: US military forces and emergency international humanitarian assistance: Observations and recommendations from three recent missions. **Journal of the American Medical Association** 1994; 272: 386–390.

25. Slater MS, Trunkey DD: Terrorism in America: An evolving threat. **Archives of Surgery** 1997; 132(10):1059–1066.

26. Weiss EA, Donner HJ: Wilderness improvisation. In: Auerbach P (ed): **Wilderness Medicine.** St. Louis, MO, Mosby-Yearbook, Inc., 1995, 446–449.

27. Wilkerson JA, Bangs CC, Hayward JS: Hypothermia, frostbite and other cold injuries. Seattle, The Mountaineers, 1986.

28. Wilmore DW: **The Metabolic Management of the Critically Ill.** New York, Plenum Publishing, 1977, p 52.

29. Woodhouse P, Keatinage WR, Coleshaw SR: Factors associated with hypothermia in patients admitted to a group of inner city hospitals. **Lancet** 1989; 2:1201.

30. Yeskey KS, Llewellyn CH, Vayer JS: Operational medicine in disasters, **Emergency Medicine Clinics of North America** 1996; 14(2):429–438.

ATLS®
Student Manual Index

A

ABC priorities, 13
ABCDE, 13, 28
 Airway maintenance/cervical
  spine protection, 15–16,
  18
  Pitfalls, 16
 Breathing and ventilation, 16, 18
 Circulation with hemorrhage
  control, 16–17, 18–19
  Bleeding, 17, 18
  Blood volume and cardiac
   output, 16–17
 Disability (neurologic
  evaluation), 17–18
 Exposure/environmental control, 18
 Triage, 294
Abdomen
 Anatomy, 132–133
 Assessment, 133–139
 Back, 132
 Celiotomy, 139, 143
 Diagnostic studies, 135, 136–139,
  149–150
 Examination, 25, 40, 133–135
  Pitfalls, 25
  Skills/procedures, 36, 147–150
 Flank, 132
 Intubation, 135
 Laboratory tests, 135
 Pelvic cavity, 132
 Pelvic fracture, 141–142, 143
 Peritoneal cavity, 132
 Retroperitoneum
  and Blood loss in elderly
   people, 269
  Hematoma, 76
  Space, 132–133
 Specific injuries, 139–142
 Trauma, 25, 131–145
  Assessment, 133–139

Abdomen *continued*
  Associated with major pelvic
   disruption, 218
  Associated with spine
   fracture, 218
  Austere and hostile
   environments, 364–365
  Mechanisms of injury, 133
   Blunt, 133
   Penetrating, 133
  Pediatric trauma, 254–256
   Nonoperative
    management, 255
  Skills/procedures, 147–150
  Transfer criteria, 286
  X-ray studies, 135–136, 137, 138,
   139, 143
Abruptio placentae, 279
Abuse
 Child, 259–260
 Elderly people, 272
**Acceleration, biomechanics of
  injury**, 315
Acetabulum (*See* Musculoskeletal
  system)
Acid-base balance, 78, 104
 in Child, 250
Acid-pepsin disorder, 266
ACS COT (*See* American College of
  Surgeons Committee on
  Trauma)
Adult (*See* Age factors)
Advance directives, 272
Afterload, 70
Age factors, 3, 113, 186, 320
 Adult, 13, 57, 58, 71, 73, 77, 78, 79,
  139, 155, 328, 340
 Child, 13, 14, 15, 17, 25, 49, 58, 71,
  73, 76, 77, 78, 79, 93–94,
  155, 167, 183, 234, 243–
  262, 340
  Equipment needs, 262
  Vital functions, by age group
   Blood pressure, 252

Age factors *continued*
  Heart rate, 252
  Respiratory rate, 252
  Urinary output, 252
  Weight, 252
 Elderly people, 14, 15, 17, 20, 25,
  43, 71, 81, 82, 263–274
Aging (*See* Age factors *and* Elderly
  people, trauma in)
Air bag, 325–326
 Associated injuries, 140
Airway
 Algorithm, 47, 49
 Bag-valve/bag-valve-mask
  ventilation, 50, 55–56
  in Child, 248, 250
  Pitfalls, 16
 Burn injury, 232, 233–234
 Chest decompression, 18, 24, 250
  Needle, in austere and hostile
   environments, 362
 Complications of placement in
  children, 247
 Definitive, 18, 45–49, 235
  in Austere and hostile
   environments, 361
  Criteria for use, 45
  Surgical, 48–49
 in Elderly people, 264, 265, 266
  268
 Endotracheal intubation, 18,
  45–47
 Equipment needs, children, 262
 Esophageal, 45
 Fetus, 279
 Head trauma, pediatric, 258
 Hemorrhagic shock, 76
 Jet insufflation, 48–49
  Limitations, 48
 Laryngeal mask airway
  (LMA), 45
  in Austere and hostile
   environments, 360–361
 Laryngeal trauma, 42–43, 46, 104

Disability statistics (*See* Injury, disability, mortality statistics)
Disaster situations (*See* Austere and hostile environments)
Discharge instructions, mild head injury, 161
Distance and time, triage, 284, 294
Diuretics, 81
   in Burn injury, 238
   in Elderly people, 268, 272
   in Head trauma, 165
Doll's eye testing, 163
Domestic violence, 281
   Partner violence screen, 281
Dopamine, 241
Doppler evaluation, 209, 211, 224, 237
DPL (*See* Diagnostic peritoneal lavage [DPL])
Drugs, and trauma in elderly people, 265, 271–272
DT (*See* Tetanus)
DTP (*See* Tetanus)
Duodenum
   Hematoma, pediatric abdominal trauma, 255–256
   Rupture, 139–140
Dura mater, 152–153
Dysphonia, 43

E

Echocardiography, transesophageal (TEE) (*See* X-rays radiologic studies)
Eclampsia, 278
Economic considerations, injury prevention, 311
Education, injury prevention, 310–311
   Facts for use by medical personnel, 332–334
Ejection from vehicle, 14, 321–322, 328, 329
Elbow (*See* Musculoskeletal system)
Elderly people, trauma in, 263–274
      (*See also* Age factors)
   Abuse, 272
   Airway/breathing/ventilation, 264, 265, 266–268
      Cervical arthritis, 266
      Dentition, 266
      Intubation, 264, 266, 267
      Microstomia, 266
      Nasopharyngeal fragility, 266
   Biomechanics of injury, 264
   Brain injury, 269–270
   Circulation, 268–269
      Pitfalls, 268

Elderly people, trauma in *continued*
   Comorbid conditions, 264, 265–266
   Effects of aging, 264, 266–267, 268, 269, 270
   End-of-life decisions, 272
   Head trauma, 269–270
   Hypothermia, 270
   Immune system and infections, 271
   Medications, 264, 268, 269, 270, 271–272
   Metabolism, 271
   Musculoskeletal system, 270–271
   Nutritional status, 271
   Primary survey, 264–270
   Spinal cord injury, 269–270
Electrical burn, 237–238
Electrocardiographic changes in pregnancy, 277
Electrocardiographic (ECG) monitoring (*See* Monitoring)
Electromechanical dissociation (*See* Pulseless electrical activity [PEA])
Embolization, transcatheter, 269
   in Pelvic fracture, 143
Emphysema
   Mediastinal, 112
   Subcutaneous, 112–113, 121
Empyema, 113, 114
End-of-life decisions, 272
Endocrine system in pregnancy, 278
Endoscope, fiberoptic, 47
End-tidal CO$_2$ detectors, 60
Energy laws, 315
Energy transfer, 317–318
   Direct, 317
Enforcement, injury prevention, 311
Engineering, injury prevention, 311
Entrance wounds, 332
Environment (*See* Austere and hostile environments *and* Exposure/environmental control)
Epidural hematoma (*See* Hematoma)
Epilepsy in elderly people, 265
Equipment
   Pediatric needs, 262
   and Supplies in austere and hostile environments, 358, 359
   Triage, 294
Escharotomy, 236, 237
   in Austere and hostile environments, 366
Esophagus, rupture, 113
   Causes (traumatic; iatrogenic), 113

Esophagus, rupture *continued*
   Diagnosis, 113
   Treatment, 113
Etomidate, 48
   for Child, 248
Examination, physical, 21, 76
   Abdominal trauma, 133–135
      Auscultation, 134
      Gluteal examination, 135
      Inspection, 133–134
      Palpation, 134
      Pelvic stability, 134
      Penetrating wounds, evaluation, 134
      Penile, perineal, rectal examination, 134–135
      Percussion, 134
      Serial vs computed tomography, flank or back injury, 139
      Vaginal examination, 135
   Burn injury, 236
   Hemorrhagic shock, 76–77
   Musculoskeletal trauma, 208–210, 223–225
   Pitfalls, 23, 24, 25, 26
   Secondary survey, 23–26, 28, 39–40, 171–172, 197–198, 208–209, 236–237, 280
   Skills/procedures, 33–40
Exit wounds, 332
Exploration, wound, 134, 138
Explosion, 207
   Triage scenarios, 297–304
Exposure/environmental control, 18, 207
   in Elderly people, 270
   Hemorrhagic shock, 76
   Skills/procedures, 34
   Triage, 294
Extremes of age (*See* Age factors; Elderly people, trauma in; *and* Pediatric trauma)
Extremities (*See* Burn injury; Fractures; *and* Musculoskeletal system)
Eyelid (*See* Lid injury)

F

Face, injuries associated with restraints, 140
Falls, 14, 207
   Biomechanics of injury, 329–330
      Deceleration, 329
   Pediatric abdominal trauma, 254
   Pediatric trauma, 245
Fasciotomy, 237

Spinal cord/spine *continued*
Management, 187–188, 199–203
Odontoid fracture, types I–III, 183
Paraplegia, 182, 186, 188, 199
Pediatric, 258–259
Penetrating injuries, 184–185
Quadriplegia, 182, 186, 198
Sacral sparing, 179, 182
Skills/procedures, 191–203
Spinal cord injury without radiographic abnormalities (SCIWORA), 182
T1-T10 fractures, 184
T11-L1 fractures, 184
Thoracic spine fractures, 184
Thoracolumbar junction fractures, 184
Transfer
Criteria, 286
Management, 287
Myotomes, 179–180
Neurogenic shock, 73
vs Spinal shock, 181
Physiology, 178–179
Primary survey, 197
Secondary survey, 197–198
Sensory examination, 179, 198, 199
Dermatomes, 179, 199
Specific injuries, 183–185
Syndromes
Anterior cord, 182
Brown-Séquard's, 182
Central cord, 182
Spinal cord injury without radiographic abnormalities (SCIWORA), 182
Pediatric spinal cord injury, 258
Spinal shock (*See* Shock)
Spleen injury, 141
Pediatric abdominal trauma, 256
Splint
in Austere and hostile environments, 365
for Extremity injuries, 216–217, 225–227
Long-spine device, 142, 143, 211
for Rib fracture (contraindicated), 113
Traction, 226–227
Sporting activities, spinal cord injury, 258–259
Starling's law, 70
Statistics (*See* Injury, disability, mortality statistics)
Sternum, fracture, 113, 121
Steroids, 165, 188, 199

Stocking-glove distribution (sensory loss, musculoskeletal trauma), 209
Strain, biomechanics of injury, 316
Stress, 317
Definition and formula, biomechanics of injury, 316
Uniaxial, 317–318
Stridor, 43, 46, 104
Stroke, 265
Stroke volume, 82
Definition, 70
Subclavian venipuncture (*See* Vascular access)
Subdural hematoma (*See* Hematoma)
Subtalar joint (*See* Musculoskeletal system)
Succinylcholine, 48, 163
for Child, 248
Contraindications, 48
Sucking chest wound, 105–106
Suction tube sizes, children, 262
Superficial peroneal nerve injury (*See* Musculoskeletal system)
Syndromes, spinal cord (*See* Spinal cord/spine *or the specific syndrome*)

T

T1-T10 fractures, 184
T11-L1 fractures, 184
Tachycardia, 71
Tachypnea, 42, 46
Tamponade, cardiac (*See* Cardiac tamponade)
Taping for rib fracture (contraindicated), 113
Td (*See* Tetanus)
TEE (*See* X-rays/radiologic studies)
Tension pneumothorax (*See* Pneumothorax)
Tentorium, 153
Terrorist attack (*See* Austere and hostile environments)
Tertiary blast effect, 207
Tertiary injury prevention, 310
Tetanus, 337–340
Antibiotics, 339
Immunization, 337–340
Active
Adults, 340
Infants and children, 340
Pregnant women, 340
Contraindications, 339
Documentation, 338–339
Passive, 338

Tetanus *continued*
Previously immunized people, 340
Schedule, 340
Incubation period, 337
Non–tetanus-prone wounds, 338, 340
Prophylaxis/risk assessment
Burn injury, 237
Cold injury, 239
in Elderly people, 270, 272
Musculoskeletal trauma, 225, 227
Contusions and lacerations, 215
Open fractures and joint injuries, 212
Recommendations, 338, 339
Surgical wound care, 338
Tetanus-prone wounds, 338, 340
Wound classification, 338
Thermoregulation in child, 254
Thoracentesis, needle, 127
Complications, 127
Thoracic spine
Fractures, 184
Screening guidelines, 188
X-ray evaluation, 185–187, 194
Thoracic trauma (*See also* Chest; Hemothorax; Pneumothorax; *and specific sites*), 103–115
Aortic disruption, 110–111
Associated with displaced thoracic spine fracture, 218
Associated with clavicular, scapular, or shoulder injury, 218
Associated with major pelvic disruption, 218
in Austere and hostile environments, 362
Altitude, air evacuation, 362
Cardiac injury, 110
Cardiac tamponade, 107–108
Causes, 104
Contusion, pulmonary, 106, 110
Crushing injury (traumatic asphyxia), 113
Diaphragm, 111–112, 120
in Elderly people, 268
Emphysema, subcutaneous, 112–113
Esophagus, 113
Fractures, 113, 120–121
Initial assessment and management, 104
Life-threatening injuries, 104–115
Mediastinum, 112, 114
Pathophysiology, 104